Cardiac Arrest

Guest Editors

WILLIAM J. BRADY, MD
NATHAN P. CHARLTON, MD
BENJAMIN J. LAWNER, DO, EMT-P
SARA F. SUTHERLAND, MD

EMERGENCY MEDICINE CLINICS OF NORTH AMERICA

www.emed.theclinics.com

Consulting Editor
AMAL MATTU, MD

February 2012 • Volume 30 • Number 1

SAUNDERS an imprint of ELSEVIER, Inc.

W.B. SAUNDERS COMPANY

A Division of Elsevier Inc.

1600 John F. Kennedy Boulevard • Suite 1800 • Philadelphia, Pennsylvania 19103-2899

http://www.theclinics.com

EMERGENCY MEDICINE CLINICS OF NORTH AMERICA Volume 30, Number 1
February 2012 ISSN 0733-8627, ISBN-13: 978-1-4557-3854-0

Editor: Patrick Manley
Developmental Editor: Donald Mumford

Emergency Medicine Clinics of North America (ISSN 0733-8627) is published quarterly by Elsevier Inc., 360 Park Avenue South, New York, NY, 10010-1710. Months of issue are February, May, August, and November. Business and Editorial Offices: 1600 John F. Kennedy Boulevard, Suite 1800, Philadelphia, PA 19103-2899. Customer Service Office: 6277 Sea Harbor Drive, Orlando, FL 32887-4800. Periodicals postage paid at New York, NY, and additional mailing offices. Subscription prices are $142.00 per year (US students), $281.00 per year (US individuals), $478.00 per year (US institutions), $201.00 per year (international students), $404.00 per year (international individuals), $576.00 per year (international institutions), $201.00 per year (Canadian students), $347.00 per year (Canadian individuals), and $576.00 per year (Canadian institutions). International air speed delivery is included in all *Clinics'* subscription prices. All prices are subject to change without notice. **POSTMASTER:** Send address changes to *Emergency Medicine Clinics of North America*, Elsevier Periodicals Customer Service, 11830 Westline Industrial Drive, St. Louis, MO 63146. Customer Service (orders, claims, online, change of address): Elsevier Periodicals Customer Service, 11830 Westline Industrial Drive, St. Louis, MO 63146. Tel: 1-800-654-2452 (U.S. and Canada); 314-453-7041 (outside U.S. and Canada). Fax: 314-453-5170. E-mail: journalscustomerservice-usa@elsevier.com (for print support); journalsonline support-usa@elsevier.com (for online support).

Reprints. For copies of 100 or more of articles in this publication, please contact the Commercial Reprints Department, Elsevier Inc., 360 Park Avenue South, New York, NY 10010-1710. Tel.: 212-633-3812; Fax: 212-462-1935; E-mail: reprints@elsevier.com.

Emergency Medicine Clinics of North America is covered in *MEDLINE/PubMed (Index Medicus), Current Contents/Clinical Medicine, EMBASE/Excerpta Medica, BIOSIS, SciSearch, CINAHL, ISI/BIOMED,* and *Research Alert.*

Printed and bound by CPI Group (UK) Ltd, Croydon, CR0 4YY

Transferred to Digital Print 2012

Contributors

CONSULTING EDITOR

AMAL MATTU, MD, FAAEM, FACEP
Program Director, Emergency Medicine Residency; Professor, Department of Emergency Medicine, University of Maryland School of Medicine, Baltimore, Maryland

GUEST EDITORS

WILLIAM J. BRADY, MD, FACEP, FAAEM
Professor of Emergency Medicine and Medicine, Departments of Emergency Medicine and Medicine, University of Virginia School of Medicine; Chair, Resuscitation Committee and Medical Director, Center for Emergency Preparedness and Response, University of Virginia Health System; Operational Medical Director, Charlottesville-Albemarle Rescue Squad and Albemarle County Fire Rescue, Special Event Medical Management, Charlottesville, Virginia; Operational Medical Director, Madison County EMS, Madison, Virginia; Medical Director, Mondial Assistance, USA and Canada

NATHAN P. CHARLTON, MD, FACEP
Assistant Professor of Emergency Medicine, Department of Emergency Medicine; Consulting Physician, Division of Medical Toxicology, University of Virginia School of Medicine; Associate Medical Director, Blueridge Poison Control Center, University of Virginia Health System, Charlottesville, Virginia

BENJAMIN J. LAWNER, DO, EMT-P
Assistant Professor of Emergency Medicine, Department of Emergency Medicine, University of Maryland School of Medicine; Deputy EMS Medical Director, Baltimore City Fire Department, Baltimore, Maryland

SARA F. SUTHERLAND, MD, FACEP
Assistant Professor of Emergency Medicine, Department of Emergency Medicine, University of Virginia School of Medicine, Charlottesville, Virginia; Chief Medical Officer, Mondial Assistance, USA and Canada

AUTHORS

BENJAMIN S. ABELLA, MD, MPhil
Department of Emergency Medicine, Center for Resuscitation Science, University of Pennsylvania, Philadelphia, Pennsylvania

KOSTAS ALIBERTIS, BA, CCEMT-P
Lead Instructor, Center for Emergency Preparedness and Response, University of Virginia, Charlottesville, Virginia; Chief, Western Albemarle Rescue Squad, Crozet, Virginia; National Faculty, American Heart Association, Committee for Emergency for Cardiovascular Care, Dallas, Texas

SETH O. ALTHOFF, MD
Attending Physician, Department of Emergency Medicine, Bridgeport Hospital, Bridgeport, Connecticut

AMY BAERNSTEIN, MD
Associate Professor, Department of Medicine, University of Washington, Seattle, Washington

MICHAEL C. BOND, MD, FACEP, FAAEM
Assistant Professor of Emergency Medicine, Department of Emergency Medicine, University of Maryland School of Medicine, Baltimore, Maryland

HEATHER A. BOREK, MD
Medical Toxicology Fellow, Department of Emergency Medicine, University of Virginia, Charlottesville, Virginia

DANIEL BOUTSIKARIS, MD
Resident, Combined Emergency Medicine/Internal Medicine/Critical Care Program, University of Maryland Medical Center, Baltimore, Maryland

TANNER S. BOYD, MD
Emergency Medicine Residency, Department of Emergency Medicine, University of Virginia School of Medicine, University of Virginia, Charlottesville, Virginia

WILLIAM BRADY, MD, FACEP, FAAEM
Professor of Emergency Medicine and Medicine, Departments of Emergency Medicine and Medicine, University of Virginia School of Medicine; Chair, Resuscitation Committee and Medical Director, Center for Emergency Preparedness and Response, University of Virginia Health System; Operational Medical Director, Charlottesville-Albemarle Rescue Squad and Albemarle County Fire Rescue, Special Event Medical Management, Charlottesville, Virginia; Operational Medical Director, Madison County EMS, Madison, Virginia; Medical Director, Mondial Assistance, USA and Canada

MEGHAN BREED, BA, EMT-I
Department of Emergency Medicine, University of Virginia; Charlottesville-Albemarle Rescue Squad, Charlottesville, Virginia

STEVEN C. BROOKS, MD, MHSc, FRCPC
Assistant Professor, Division of Emergency Medicine, Department of Medicine, University of Toronto; Clinician-Scientist, Rescu, Li Ka Shing Knowledge Institute, St Michael's Hospital; Clinician-Scientist and Emergency Physician, Program for Trauma, Emergency and Critical Care, Sunnybrook Health Sciences Centre, Toronto, Canada

JOCELYN DE GUZMAN, MD
Clinical Assistant Professor, Department of Emergency Medicine, Brody School of Medicine, East Carolina University; Medical Director, Disaster Services, Pitt County Memorial Hospital, Greenville, North Carolina

JEFFREY D. FERGUSON, MD, NREMT-P
Assistant Professor, Department of Emergency Medicine, Brody School of Medicine, East Carolina University; Medical Director, EastCare Critical Care Transport, Pitt County Memorial Hospital, Greenville, North Carolina

JONATHAN HSU, BHSc
Undergraduate Medical Education Program, Faculty of Medicine, University of Toronto, Toronto, Canada

BENJAMIN J. LAWNER, DO, EMT-P
Assistant Professor of Emergency Medicine, Department of Emergency Medicine, University of Maryland School of Medicine; Deputy EMS Medical Director, Baltimore City Fire Department, Baltimore, Maryland

CHRISTINE M. LIN, MD
Chief Resident and Clinical Instructor, Department of Medicine, University of Virginia, Charlottesville, Virginia

JOSEPH P. MARTINEZ, MD
Assistant Professor of Emergency Medicine, Assistant Dean for Student Affairs, Department of Emergency Medicine, University of Maryland School of Medicine, Baltimore, Maryland

MICHAEL T. MCCURDY, MD
Assistant Professor, Division of Pulmonary & Critical Care Medicine, Department of Medicine; Assistant Professor, Department of Emergency Medicine, University of Maryland School of Medicine, Baltimore, Maryland

PETER P. MONTELEONE, MD
Chief Resident and Clinical Instructor, Department of Medicine, University of Virginia, Charlottesville, Virginia

JOSE V. NABLE, MD, NREMT-P
Resident Physician, Department of Emergency Medicine, University of Maryland Medical Center, Baltimore, Maryland

VINAY NADKARNI, MD, MS
Department of Anesthesiology and Critical Care Medicine, University of Pennsylvania and the Children's Hospital of Philadelphia, Philadelphia, Pennsylvania

GRAHAM NICHOL, MD, MPH
Professor of Medicine, Department of Medicine, University of Washington-Harborview Center for Prehospital Emergency Care, University of Washington, Seattle, Washington

ROBERT E. O'CONNOR, MD, MPH
Professor and Chair of Emergency Medicine, University of Virginia Health System, Charlottesville, Virginia

DEBRA G. PERINA, MD
Associate Professor of Emergency Medicine, Director, Division of Prehospital Care, Department of Emergency Medicine, University of Virginia School of Medicine, University of Virginia, Charlottesville, Virginia

JOSHUA C. REYNOLDS, MD
Senior Resident in Emergency Medicine, Department of Emergency Medicine, University of Maryland Medical Center, Baltimore, Maryland

SANOBER SHAIKH, MD
Senior Resident in Emergency Medicine, Department of Emergency Medicine, University of Maryland Medical Center, Baltimore, Maryland

CHRISTOPHER T. STEPHENS, MD, EMT-P
Director of Education, Division of Trauma Anesthesiology, Department of Anesthesiology, R Adams Cowley Shock Trauma Center, University of Maryland School of Medicine, Baltimore, Maryland

ROBERT M. SUTTON, MD, MSCE
Department of Anesthesiology and Critical Care Medicine, University of Pennsylvania and the Children's Hospital of Philadelphia, Philadelphia, Pennsylvania

DAWN TANIGUCHI, MD
Resident, Department of Internal Medicine Resident, University of Washington, Seattle, Washington

ALINA TOMA, MD, FRCPC
Critical Care Fellow, Department of Internal Medicine, Sunnybrook Health Sciences Centre, University of Toronto; Emergency Physician, St Michael's Hospital, Toronto, Canada

KELLY WILLIAMSON, MD
Chief Resident, Department of Emergency Medicine, Northwestern University, Chicago, Illinois

MICHAEL E. WINTERS, MD, FACEP, FAAEM
Associate Professor of Emergency Medicine and Medicine, Co-Director, Combined Emergency Medicine/Internal Medicine/Critical Care Program, University of Maryland School of Medicine, Baltimore, Maryland

SAMANTHA L. WOOD, MD
Fellow, Combined Emergency Medicine/Internal Medicine/Critical Care Program, University of Maryland Medical Center, Baltimore, Maryland

WILLIAM A. WOODS, MD
Associate Professor of Emergency Medicine, Pediatrics and Mechanical and Aerospace Engineering, Department of Emergency Medicine, University of Virginia, Charlottesville, Virginia

Contents

> This article reviews out-of-hospital cardiac arrest from a public health per-
> spective. Case definitions are discussed. Incidence, outcome, and fixed
> and modifiable risk factors for cardiac arrest are described. There is a large
> variation in survival between communities that is not explained by patient
> or community factors. Study of variation in outcome in other related con-
> ditions suggest that this is due to differences in organizational culture
> rather than processes of care. A public health approach to improving out-
> comes is recommended that includes ongoing monitoring and improve-
> ment of processes and outcome of care.

> Myocardial disease and death from cardiac arrest remain significant public
> health problems. Sudden death events and out-of-hospital cardiac arrests
> (OHCA) are encountered frequently by emergency medical services. De-
> spite more than 30 years of research, survival rates remain extremely
> low. This article reviews access and presentations, demographics,
> OHCA outcomes, and response systems and processes in treatment of
> patients with arrest in this setting.

> In-hospital sudden cardiac arrest and resuscitation is distinct from out-of-
> hospital sudden cardiac arrest (OOHSCA) and warrants specific attention.
> Sudden cardiac arrest (SCA) is a manifestation of an underlying process
> rather than a disease itself. The complex, multiorgan system dysfunction
> common among the inpatient population can precipitate SCA by both sim-
> ilar and very different mechanisms than OOHSCA. The diagnostic and
> treatment algorithms of SCA remain largely the same between the inpa-
> tient and outpatient arenas. The application of complex diagnostic and
> therapeutic interventions is permissible, but such tools must not interrupt
> or delay the important basics of cardiac arrest management in the inpa-
> tient setting, including adequate chest compressions and timely defibrilla-
> tion when appropriate.

strategies to increase the chance of survival to discharge. These strategies focus on suggestions for organizing a system prepared to care for critically ill children, incorporating the 2010 American Heart Association resuscitation guidelines into clinical practice, and encouraging physicians to become advocates of decreasing the occurrence of pediatric cardiac arrest. Providing the best-prepared system available to care for critically ill children will, it is hoped, decrease the number of preventable deaths in children.

In certain cardiac arrest situations, modifications to current cardiac resuscitation algorithms may improve patient outcome. These situations are often rare, but when they occur they house the potential for severe time and resource use, and in some cases specialized skill sets. The decision to apply these modifications to standard care for the cardiac arrest patient may be obvious in some cases or may be applied due to suspicion from the presenting medical history, history of present illness, or physical examination. However, with rare exception, general care of any cardiac arrest patient should include continuous high-quality chest compressions and appropriate airway and ventillatory management.

Even the best conventional manual cardiopulmonary resuscitation (CPR) is highly inefficient, producing only a fraction of normal cardiac output. Over the past several decades, many therapeutic devices have been designed to improve on conventional CPR during cardiac arrest and increase the probability of survival. This article reviews several adjuncts and mechanical alternatives to conventional CPR for use during cardiac arrest. Recent clinical studies comparing conventional resuscitation techniques with the use of devices during cardiac arrest are reviewed, with a focus on clinical implications and directions for future research.

GOAL STATEMENT

The goal of *Emergency Medicine Clinics of North America* is to keep practicing physicians up to date with current clinical practice in emergency medicine by providing timely articles reviewing the state of the art in patient care.

ACCREDITATION

The *Emergency Medical Clinics of North America* is planned and implemented in accordance with the Essential Areas and Policies of the Accreditation Council for Continuing Medical Education (ACCME) through the joint sponsorship of the University of Virginia School of Medicine and Elsevier. The University of Virginia School of Medicine is accredited by the ACCME to provide continuing medical education for physicians.

The University of Virginia School of Medicine designates this enduring material activity for a maximum of 15 *AMA PRA Category 1 Credit*(s)™ for each issue, 60 credits per year. Physicians should claim only the credit commensurate with the extent of their participation in the activity.

The American Medical Association has determined that physicians not licensed in the US who participate in this CME enduring material activity are eligible for a maximum of 15 *AMA PRA Category 1 Credit*(s)™ for each issue, 60 credits per year.

The Emergency Medicine Clinics of North America CME program is approved by the American College of Emergency Physicians for 60 hours of ACEP Category I Credit per year.

Credit can be earned by reading the text material, taking the CME examination online at http://www.theclinics.com/home/cme, and completing the evaluation. After taking the test, you will be required to review any and all incorrect answers. Following completion of the test and evaluation, your credit will be awarded and you may print your certificate.

FACULTY DISCLOSURE/CONFLICT OF INTEREST

The University of Virginia School of Medicine, as an ACCME accredited provider, endorses and strives to comply with the Accreditation Council for Continuing Medical Education (ACCME) Standards of Commercial Support, Commonwealth of Virginia statutes, University of Virginia policies and procedures, and associated federal and private regulations and guidelines on the need for disclosure and monitoring of proprietary and financial interests that may affect the scientific integrity and balance of content delivered in continuing medical education activities under our auspices.

The University of Virginia School of Medicine requires that all CME activities accredited through this institution be developed independently and be scientifically rigorous, balanced and objective in the presentation/discussion of its content, theories and practices.

All authors/editors participating in an accredited CME activity are expected to disclose to the readers relevant financial relationships with commercial entities occurring within the past 12 months (such as grants or research support, employee, consultant, stock holder, member of speakers bureau, etc.). The University of Virginia School of Medicine will employ appropriate mechanisms to resolve potential conflicts of interest to maintain the standards of fair and balanced education to the reader. Questions about specific strategies can be directed to the Office of Continuing Medical Education, University of Virginia School of Medicine, Charlottesville, Virginia.

The faculty and staff of the University of Virginia Office of Continuing Medical Education have no financial affiliations to disclose.

The authors/editors listed below have identified no professional or financial affiliations for themselves or their spouse/partner:
Seth O. Althoff, MD; Amy Baernstein, MD; Michael C. Bond, MD; Heather A. Borek, MD; Daniel Boutsikaris, MD; Tanner S. Boyd, MD; William J. Brady, MD (Guest Editor); Meghan Breed, BA, EMT-1; Steven C. Brooks, MD, MHSc, FRCPC; Nathan P. Charlton, MD (Guest Editor); Jocelyn De Guzman, MD; Jeffrey D. Ferguson, MD, NREMT-P; Jonathan Hsu, BHSc; Benjamin J. Lawner, DO, EMT-P (Guest Editor); Christine M. Lin, MD; Patrick Manley, (Acquisitions Editor); Joseph P. Martinez, MD; Amal Mattu, MD (Consulting Editor); Michael T. McCurdy, MD; Peter P. Monteleone, MD; Jose V. Nable, MD, NREMT-P; Vinay Nadkarni, MD, MS; Graham Nichol, MD, MPH; Robert E. O'Connor, MD, MPH; Debra G. Perina, MD; Joshua C. Reynolds, MD; Sanober Shaikh, MD; Christopher T. Stephens, MD, EMT-P; Sara F. Sutherland, MD (Guest Editor); Dawn Taniguchi, MD; Kelly Williamson, MD; Michael E. Winters, MD; Samantha L. Wood, MD; and William A. Woods, MD (Test Author).

The authors/editors listed below identified the following professional or financial affiliations for themselves or their spouse/partner:
Benjamin S. Abella, MD, MPhil receives research funding from NIH NHLBI, the Doris Duke Foundation, Philips Healthcare, Medtronic Foundation, and the American Heart Association; and receives honoraria from Medivance Corp. and Philips Healthcare.
Kostas Alibertis, BA, CCEMT-P is on the Advisory Board of the American Heart Association.
Robert M. Sutton, MD, MSCE receives research funding support from the Laerdal Foundation.
Alina Toma, MD, FRCPC 's partner is employed by Amgen Canada Inc.

Disclosure of Discussion of Non-FDA Approved Uses for Pharmaceutical Products and/or Medical Devices
The University of Virginia School of Medicine, as an ACCME provider, requires that all faculty presenters identify and disclose any off-label uses for pharmaceutical and medical device products. The University of Virginia School of Medicine recommends that each physician fully review all the available data on new products or procedures prior to clinical use.

TO ENROLL

To enroll in the Emergency Medicine Clinics of North America Continuing Medical Education program, call customer service at 1-800-654-2452 or visit us online at www.theclinics.com/home/cme. The CME program is available to subscribers for an additional fee of $190.00.

Foreword
Cardiac Arrest

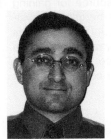

Amal Mattu, MD
Consulting Editor

"Cardiac arrest!" These two simple words conjure up images in our minds of sirens and flashing lights, doctors and nurses running, intubation, defibrillations, and an assortment of other similarly dramatic activities. It's unlikely that there's any other condition in medicine that has been the source of more research, teaching, discussion, and infatuation. The treatment of cardiac arrest, after all, is essentially to bring a dead patient back to life. It is in some respects man's attempt to play God...to bring back the dead is certainly the greatest achievement in the practice of medicine!

Despite decades of research and apparent advances in the management of cardiac arrest, however, we have been continually reminded that we are but mere mortals. The marvels of modern medicine are still little match for a lifeless heart or brain. Nevertheless, our continued efforts at advancing the cause *have* produced some tangible improvements in the rescue of these patients.

Cardiac arrest is a condition that affects all health care providers and practitioners in every specialty. This is exemplified by the fact that nearly all medical trainees, prehospital personnel, and in-hospital nurses are required to take courses in basic and sometimes advanced life support. But it's important for us to remember that out of all health care providers, *emergency physicians* must be the experts in cardiac arrest care. Frankly, there is no other specialty in the House of Medicine that receives such intense training in the combination of cardiac care, airway management, shock, and critical care pharmacology. Consequently, every emergency physician must commit himself or herself to attaining expertise in managing victims of cardiac arrest.

In this issue of *Emergency Medicine Clinics of North America*, Guest Editors William Brady, Nathan Charlton, Benjamin Lawner, and Sara Sutherland have presented us with the current state of practice with regards to management of cardiac arrest. The guest editors and their authors have summarized past attempts at advancing the practice that have failed, and they also discuss in detail the handful of management techniques that have actually been shown to work. Various articles address devices and pharmacological advances, as well as the basic techniques that have reemerged as

Emerg Med Clin N Am 30 (2012) xiii–xiv
doi:10.1016/j.emc.2011.10.001
0733-8627/12/$ – see front matter © 2012 Elsevier Inc. All rights reserved.

the key to success. Prehospital, in-hospital, and public health issues are addressed nicely. Special populations, such as pediatric, geriatric, and pregnant patients, are discussed. A thorough discussion of postresuscitation care is also provided, as this is now gaining attention as a critically important link in the "chain of survival."

This issue of *Emergency Medicine Clinics* is a tremendous resource for gaining expertise. This issue should be considered a must-read for emergency physicians...period. Other health care providers that work in high-acuity environments will also benefit tremendously by the wisdom in the pages that follow. Kudos to the guest editors and authors for providing this outstanding resource for emergency physicians and other health care providers and helping us all in our continuing quest to "bring back" a few more lives.

Amal Mattu, MD
Department of Emergency Medicine
University of Maryland School of Medicine
110 S. Paca Street, 6th Floor, Suite 200
Baltimore, MD 21201, USA

E-mail address:
amattu@smail.umaryland.edu

Preface

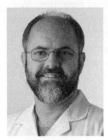 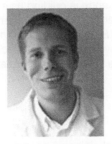 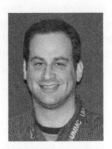 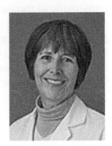

William J. Brady,   Nathan P. Charlton,   Benjamin J. Lawner,   Sara F. Sutherland,
MD   MD   DO, EMT-P   MD

Guest Editors

Medical resuscitation has been around for many thousands of years. The physician has performed resuscitation on a multitude of patients, using many methods, in a range of settings. Over these many millennia, the science of resuscitation has guided the clinician in the art of medical care. We have progressed from early methods, such as hanging an inverted patient from a tree limb and using a bellows inserted into the rectum, to more refined (and effective) contemporary interventions and strategies. Undoubtedly, clinicians of the future will look back at us with similar disbelief—*"can you believe it...they were actually pushing on the patient's chest...and shocking the heart!"* Nonetheless, the science of resuscitation has progressed to the point that we are now beginning to apply therapies, provide interventions, and offer management strategies in an evidence-based method—starting on the street and continuing in the hospital. Over the past 3 decades, resuscitation science and the resultant recommendations have changed markedly, from the early use of cardioactive medications and invasive airways to continuous chest compressions and early defibrillation.

Contemporary evidence suggests that the basic interventions—including appropriate cardiopulmonary resuscitation with activation of the emergency response system, adequate chest compressions, and early electrical defibrillation—that are provided early, correctly, and consistently, likely impact the cardiac arrest patient most favorably...as compared to the more advanced therapies. In fact, of the "five goals" noted in the American Heart Association's Guidelines 2010, three focus on such basic interventions[1]:

- Immediate recognition and activation of the emergency response team;
- Early CPR with emphasis on chest compressions;
- Rapid defibrillation;
- Effective advanced life support; and
- Integrated post–cardiac arrest care.

Interestingly, only one of these goals is listed as "effective advanced life support." And the "new actor" on the "resuscitation stage" is focused post–arrest care, ranging from the basics of optimization of oxygen, ventilation, and systemic perfusion to the more complex therapeutic hypothermia and emergent coronary reperfusion.

Emerg Med Clin N Am 30 (2012) xv–xvii
doi:10.1016/j.emc.2011.09.019   emed.theclinics.com

We are all involved in cardiac arrest resuscitation at a truly exciting time. We must focus on the basics of resuscitation. These interventions are likely the most beneficial, particularly at the early stage of arrest. The science is guiding us in that direction. We must strive to bring this science consistently and reliably to the patient's side in each and every resuscitation. This edition of the *Emergency Medicine Clinics of North America* is intended to provide a concise review of sudden cardiac arrest in all its facets of presentation and management. We hope that you, the clinician, will use it to care for our mutual patients.

DEDICATIONS

William J. Brady: This text is written for the clinicians who stand ready 24/7/365 to manage patients in extremis; these clinicians include law enforcement officers, fire rescue personnel, nurses, therapists, and physicians, among many others, who rush to the aid of others on a daily basis, often with no advanced warning and with minimal patient information. I am honored to work with such clinicians at the University of Virginia Medical Center and in the Thomas Jefferson EMS Region of Central Virginia—my thanks to all of you for your hard work, selfless efforts, and dedication to the patient, oftentimes in the most extreme circumstances. I must also give thanks to my wonderful, patient, and understanding wife, King, and my awesome children, Lauren, Anne, Chip, and Katherine—you guys are my love and inspiration, forever and always......the best thing that has ever happened to me.

Nathan Charlton: To Jennifer, Will, and Ben, whose patience and understanding are truly amazing. To the residents who make work worthwhile and to my colleagues who allow me to grow every day.

Benjamin Lawner: I would like to thank my colleagues at the University of Maryland Department of Emergency Medicine for their guidance and support, in particular, Dr Amal Mattu. Also, any expression of gratitude would be incomplete without mentioning my family—special thanks to April, Evan, and Eliot for their unconditional patience and support.

Sara Sutherland: I would like to dedicate my work on this book to all the bystanders and volunteer and professional EMTs who get to these patients in the first seconds or minutes of cardiac arrest and, by doing so, allow the advanced management of these patients to result in successful outcomes. Thank You.

William J. Brady, MD
Departments of Emergency Medicine and Medicine
University of Virginia School of Medicine
Charlottesville, VA 22908, USA

Nathan P. Charlton, MD
Department of Emergency Medicine
University of Virginia School of Medicine
Charlottesville, VA 22908, USA

Benjamin J. Lawner, DO, EMT-P
Department of Emergency Medicine
University of Maryland School of Medicine
110 South Paca Street, 6th Floor, Suite 200
Baltimore, MD 21201, USA

Sara F. Sutherland, MD
Department of Emergency Medicine
University of Virginia School of Medicine
Charlottesville, VA 22908, USA

E-mail addresses:
WB4Z@hscmail.mcc.virginia.edu (W.J. Brady)
NPC8A@hscmail.mcc.virginia.edu (N.P. Charlton)
blawn001@umaryland.edu (B.J. Lawner)
SAO4R@hscmail.mcc.virginia.edu (S.F. Sutherland)

REFERENCE

1. Field JM, Hazinski MF, Sayre MR, et al. 2010 American Heart Association Guidelines for cardiopulmonary resuscitation and emergency cardiovascular care science. Circulation 2010;122:S640–6.

Introduction

In April 2011, a 51-year-old man boards a plane with his wife for a well-deserved vacation. One hour into the flight, the man's wife is yelling for a doctor. The man is slumped over in his seat, unresponsive. Miraculously, another passenger comes to the rescue, performs CPR, and uses the plane's defibrillator to resuscitate the man to the cheers of passengers. Approximately 22 minutes later, the flight crew safely lands the plane, and the patient is able to thank his rescuer as he is taken to the hospital, where he fully recovers.

Someone suffers sudden cardiac arrest in the United States, on average, once every 90 seconds. This story is important because it shows what is possible if someone stops to help. It so happens that the rescuer works as an RN, but it could have been anyone.

This edition of *Emergency Medicine Clinics of North America* is devoted to CPR and other adjuncts used to link the Chain of Survival® and enhance survival. Readers who have saved a life using CPR know the profound sense of awe when the power of resuscitation is witnessed and a victim survives. It is miraculous that a person, who was as good as dead when they collapsed, rises to resume their life and experience the second chance shared by all survivors of sudden cardiac arrest. Celebration of survival is often fleeting, as the majority of victims of sudden cardiac arrest do not survive, even though recent advances in the science of resuscitation have led to bold innovation that has dramatically improved survival. Training programs in CPR were first developed in 1960 by the American Heart Association. While the "50th Anniversary" of CPR was officially recognized in 2010, its origins can be traced to early recorded history.

An early recorded reference to artificial breathing appears in the book of *Kings* in the *Old Testament*, where the prophet Elisha restored the life of a boy through a technique that included placing his mouth on the mouth of the child, and is the earliest account of mouth-to-mouth ventilation.[1]

"And when Elisha was come into the house, behold, the child was dead, and laid upon his bed. He went in therefore, and shut the door upon them twain, and prayed unto the LORD. And he went up, and lay upon the child, and put his mouth upon his mouth, and his eyes upon his eyes, and his hands upon his hands: and he stretched himself upon the child; and the flesh of the child waxed warm. Then he returned, and walked in the house to and fro; and went up, and stretched himself upon him: and the child sneezed seven times, and the child opened his eyes."

Despite this early "case report," mouth-to-mouth breathing was not officially recognized until 1740, when the Paris Academy of Sciences boldly recommended mouth-to-mouth resuscitation for drowning victims, followed in 1767 when the Society for the Recovery of Drowned Persons formed and became the first organized effort to deal with sudden and unexpected death. In 1768, the Dutch Humane Society was founded, in which physicians and laypersons collaborated to aid victims of drowning in the waterways. Mouth-to-mouth ventilation was systematically studied in the late 1950s and published in several leading medical journals, leading to its widespread acceptance and a means of ventilation support.[2–6] In 1957, the United States military adopted the mouth-to-mouth resuscitation method to revive unresponsive victims.

Emerg Med Clin N Am 30 (2012) xix–xxii
doi:10.1016/j.emc.2011.09.018
0733-8627/12/$ – see front matter © 2012 Elsevier Inc. All rights reserved.

Devices for ventilation were developed in the early 20th century and led to the development of negative pressure ventilators ("iron lung") housed in areas of the hospital that eventually became intensive care units. In 1952, an epidemic of poliomyelitis struck Copenhagen, which overwhelmed the supply of negative pressure ventilators. Positive pressure ventilation was developed as a substitute, and hundreds of volunteers were able to perform manual ventilation using an airway tube with an air reservoir. Endotracheal positive pressure ventilation eventually supplanted negative pressure ventilation and became the standard during the 1960s.

Palpation of pulses and heartbeat as a means to assess cardiovascular status has been used by health care providers for over 3000 years; however, descriptions of (open chest) cardiac massage did not appear until the 19th century. In 1891, Dr Friedrich Maass described the performance of chest compressions in humans; in 1903, Dr George Crile reported the first successful use of external chest compressions in human resuscitation, and in 1904, the first American case of closed-chest cardiac massage was performed by Dr George Crile. Several decades went by and in the late 1950s, Knickerbocker, Jude, and Kouwenhoven described external cardiac massage, or chest compressions, as a useful resuscitation technique that, in contrast to open cardiac massage, required little technical expertise.[7]

In 1955, Zoll described the first successful closed-chest human defibrillation. In 1979, the first portable automatic external defibrillator (AED) was developed, followed by the implantable defibrillator in 1981.[8] The combination of airway, breathing, circulation, and defibrillation (and the telephone) led to the American Heart Association description of the "chain of survival" with the four links of early access, early CPR, early defibrillation, and early advanced cardiac life support (ACLS).

How were each of these concepts integrated into a cogent set of resuscitation guidelines and then disseminated? By 1960, the key elements for modern day CPR were in place, namely airway, breathing, and circulation. Lay rescuers were first trained in 1961 in Cleveland. The first CPR guidelines were published in 1966, followed by large-scale training sessions in Seattle in the 1970s where upwards of 100,000 people were taught to perform CPR during a single session.[9] These efforts have paid off and Seattle has enjoyed the highest survival rates following out-of-hospital cardiac arrest in the nation.[10]

In 2000, the Cardiac Arrest Survival Act was passed, requiring AED programs to be instituted in all federal buildings. In addition, the use of AEDs was added to the list of protections under "Good Samaritan" laws, which were previously enacted in all 50 states to protect the lay public from liability if first aid or CPR was performed in an emergency. Getting back to our story, the FAA required that AEDs must be carried on commercial flights as minimum equipment, and that all members of the flight crew be trained in their use.

Chest compression rate and depth with minimal pauses in compressions are key determinants of return of spontaneous circulation and survival. In 2005, the benefits of bystander CPR with minimal interruptions to chest compressions were recognized and translated into modifications to the AHA emergency cardiovascular care (ECC) CPR Guidelines, which has resulted in widespread improvements in survival. The modern day success rates for survival from out-of-hospital cardiac arrest with intact neurologic function remains highly variable with ranges from 3% to 16.3% at sites participating in the Resuscitation Outcomes Consortium.[10] The great difference in survival rates are due to differences in incidence and risk, as well as how the community and health care system respond to cardiac arrest.

The 2010 AHA Guidelines for CPR and ECC recommend a change in the basic life support (BLS) sequence of steps from A-B-C (Airway, Breathing, Chest compressions) to C-A-B (Chest compressions, Airway, Breathing) for adults, children, and infants (excluding the newly born; see Neonatal Resuscitation section). This revolutionary change is intended to promote bystander CPR, even by untrained lay rescuers, and emphasizes that high-quality chest compressions alone, without intubation or supplemental ventilations, is the preferred approach to cardiac arrest resuscitation, even by trained rescuers.

There is increasing recognition that systematic post–cardiac arrest care after return of spontaneous circulation can improve the likelihood of patient survival with good quality of life. This recognition led to a fundamental change to the 2010 guidelines with the addition of a fifth link to the chain of survival—comprehensive and integrated postarrest care. Post–cardiac arrest care has significant potential to reduce early mortality caused by hemodynamic instability and later morbidity and mortality from multiorgan failure and brain injury.

Sudden cardiac arrest continues to be a leading cause of death in the United States, claiming the lives of more than 300,000 people each year, with half of those cases occurring out of hospital. While you were reading this, several people suffered sudden cardiac arrest in the United States. In this issue of *Emergency Medicine Clinics of North America*, leading experts in the field of resuscitation science share their knowledge with the readers to improve the care provided to victims of cardiac arrest. This comprehensive overview should prove of enormous benefit to clinicians who care for these patients by expanding our clinical armamentarium to combat the loss of life due to sudden cardiac arrest. It is incumbent on each of us to provide the level of community leadership that allows for prompt action to assist those who have suffered cardiac arrest. At least one airline passenger and his family are thankful for bystander assistance today.

Robert E. O'Connor, MD, MPH
Department of Emergency Medicine
University of Virginia School of Medicine
PO Box 800699
Charlottesville, VA 22908, USA

E-mail address:
REO4X@hscmail.mcc.virginia.edu

REFERENCES

1. Scherman N, editor. 2 Kings 4:32-35. Brooklyn, NY: Mesorah Publications Ltd; 2001. p. 886–7.
2. Safar P, McMahon M. Mouth-to-airway emergency artificial respiration. JAMA 1958;166:1459–60.
3. Safar P, Escarraga LA, Elam JO. A comparison of the mouth-to-mouth and mouth-to-airway methods of artificial respiration with the chest-pressure arm-lift methods. N Engl J Med 1958;258:671–7.
4. Gordon AS, Frye CW, Gittelson L, et al. Mouth-to-mouth versus manual artificial respiration for children and adults. JAMA 1958;167:320–8.
5. Elam JO, Greene DG, Brown ES, et al. Oxygen and carbon dioxide exchange and energy cost of expired air resuscitation. JAMA 1958;167:328–34.
6. Safar P. Ventilatory efficacy of mouth-to-mouth artificial respiration. JAMA 1958;167:335–41.
7. Kouwenhoven WB, Jude JR, Knickerbocker GG. Closed-chest cardiac massage. JAMA 1960;173:1064–7.

8. Zoll PM, Linenthal AJ, Gibson W, et al. Termination of ventricular fibrillation in man by externally applied electric countershock. N Engl J Med 1956;254:727.
9. Cobb LA, Alvarez H, Kopass MK. A rapid response system for out-of-hospital cardiac emergencies. Med Clin North Am 1976;60:283–90.
10. Nichol G, Thomas E, Callaway CW, et al. Resuscitation Outcomes Consortium Investigators. Regional variation in out-of-hospital cardiac arrest incidence and outcome. JAMA 2008;300(12):1423–31.

FURTHER READINGS

Safar P. History of cardiopulmonary cerebral resuscitation. In: Kaye W, Bircher N, editors. Cardiopulmonary resuscitation. New York: Churchill Livingstone; 1989. p. 1–53.
West JB. The physiological challenges of the 1952 Copenhagen poliomyelitis epidemic and a renaissance in clinical respiratory physiology. J Appl Physiol 2005;99:424–32.

Cardiac Arrest: A Public Health Perspective

Dawn Taniguchi, MD[a], Amy Baernstein, MD[b],
Graham Nichol, MD, MPH[c],*

KEYWORDS

- Cardiac arrest • Emergency medical services • Resuscitation

Cardiac arrest describes the loss of mechanical activity of the heart as confirmed by the absence of signs of circulation.[1] Sudden cardiac death is further described as a death from a cardiac cause within 1 hour from the onset of symptoms in a person without any prior condition that would appear fatal.[2] The World Health Organization proposed an alternate definition based on the recognition that many cardiac arrests are not witnessed: an unexpected, unexplained death within 1 hour of symptom onset for witnessed events, or within 24 hours of last observed alive and symptom-free, for unwitnessed events.[3] Sudden cardiac arrest is a term commonly applied to such an event when the patient survives.[4]

Episodes of cardiac arrest have multiple causes. In addition to primary cardiac events, respiratory arrest, pulmonary embolism, trauma, cerebral events, and many other conditions can lead to sudden unexpected death. For the purposes of surveillance, research, and treatment, it would be ideal to reserve sudden cardiac arrest for only primary cardiac events. However, this goal is elusive. Even with a full narrative of the death, experts often disagree on appropriate classification.[5] In survivors of out-of-hospital cardiac arrest, 12-lead electrocardiogram and history are poor predictors of which patients have "significant" cardiac lesions at the time of emergency catheterization.[6] Among victims of cardiac arrest who had high-grade coronary stenosis at autopsy, only a small minority were previously known to have coronary heart disease.[7] Classification of causes of arrest based on information acquired in-hospital is conditioned on survival to hospital, making it susceptible to selection bias. There is significant and important variation in the proportion of patients with cardiac arrest who are treated or transported by emergency medical services (EMS) providers,[8] so relying on data from this source does not distinguish reliably among causes of cardiac arrest.

[a] Department of Internal Medicine, University of Washington, 1959 NE Pacific Street, Box 356421, Seattle, WA 98195, USA
[b] Department of Medicine, University of Washington, 325 Ninth Avenue, Seattle, WA 98104, USA
[c] Department of Medicine, University of Washington-Harborview Center for Prehospital Emergency Care, University of Washington, Box 359727, 325 Ninth Avenue, Seattle, WA 98104, USA
* Corresponding author. Box 359727, 325 Ninth Avenue, Seattle, WA 98104.
E-mail address: nichol@uw.edu

Emerg Med Clin N Am 30 (2012) 1–12
doi:10.1016/j.emc.2011.09.003
0733-8627/12/$ – see front matter © 2012 Elsevier Inc. All rights reserved.

These observations suggest that the cause of arrest can accurately be determined only by conducting a postmortem examination.

Because it would be impractical to perform an autopsy on every fatal arrest, classification must rely on information available to paramedics in the out-of-hospital setting. For the purpose of evaluation of prehospital emergency care of cardiac arrest, a pragmatic alternative definition of sudden cardiac arrest[9,10] includes patients with nontraumatic, out-of-hospital cardiac arrest, who are assessed by EMS personnel and (1) receive attempts at external defibrillation (by lay responders or emergency personnel), or receive chest compressions by organized EMS personnel; or (2) are pulseless but do not receive attempts to defibrillate or CPR by EMS personnel. The latter includes patients with (1) a do not attempt resuscitation directive signed and dated by a physician, (2) extensive history of terminal illness or intractable disease, or (3) request from the patient's family.

Each of these definitions has inherent limitations. The suddenness (ie, time course) and cause are difficult to assess because only about two-thirds of cases are witnessed and, in most cases, an autopsy is not performed. Consequently, information from other sources is used to assess timeline and cause, including death certificates, EMS reports, medical records, and medical examiner reports. These sources are used independently or in combinations with each other. Information from death certificates tends to exclude patients who are successfully resuscitated and have been found to overestimate death by cardiac cause.[11] Studies limited to patients with cardiac arrest who are treated by EMS take into account patients who are assessed but not treated because of futility (ie, those with late recognition of death), resulting in an underestimation of incidence and overestimation of survival relative to those that include all patients with cardiac arrest who are assessed or treated by EMS. Surveillance using multiple sources is needed to capture all appropriate cases of cardiac arrest.[12]

INCIDENCE

Incidence of disease is defined as the occurrence rate per year for the condition within a population at risk. It is calculated by taking a ratio of the number of persons developing a disease each year divided by the population at risk. Given some of the complications with data collection described above, it is difficult to establish an accurate incidence. The incidence of cardiac arrest treated by EMS is greater than 55 per 100,000 person-years in the United States.[11] Combining information from death certificates, EMS reports and hospital record review suggests that the incidence of cardiac arrest is 95 per 100,000 person years,[10] or 8.04 per 100,000 person-years among children and 126.52 per 100,000 person-years among persons older than 20.[13] Another factor that affects incidence rates is that the number of individuals within a given area may fluctuate by time of day and day of week. Large cities that have more people during the working week may seem, falsely, to have a higher rate of cardiac arrest than would be expected based on the corresponding census population.

There is virtually no data available on incidence of cardiac arrest in the developing world.[4]

The incidence of cardiac arrest has markedly declined during the last 30 years (**Fig. 1**).[14–16] This decline is correlated with a decrease in overall cardiovascular mortality.[17] The reasons for this decline are likely multifactorial, but are mostly attributed to improvements in primary and secondary prevention of coronary heart disease.

SURVIVAL

Survival is defined as the number of survivors divided by the number of individuals who experienced the event of interest. Survival after cardiac arrest depends, in part, on the

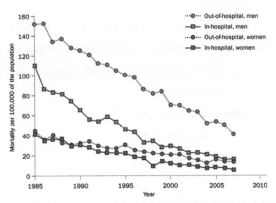

Fig. 1. Incidence of cardiac arrest over time. (*From* Adabag AS, Luepker RV, Roger VL, et al. Sudden cardiac death: epidemiology and risk factors. Nat Rev Cardiol 2010;7(4):216–25; with permission.)

population considered.[18] Among 39 sites worldwide that published their outcomes over time, median survival for all rhythm groups to hospital discharge was 6.4% (interquartile range [IQR], 3.7%–10.3%).[19] Among 10 sites in North American that collated data describing patients with cardiac arrest using similar definitions contemporaneously with each other, survival for all rhythm groups to hospital discharge was median of 8.4% (IQR, 5.4%–10.4%).[10] Experts have attempted to standardize reporting and comparison of outcomes by disseminating the Utstein template for cardiac arrest.[1] Despite this standardization, there is a greater than fivefold regional variation in survival among patients with any initial rhythm, as well as among patients with ventricular fibrillation.[10] This large variation reemphasizes that cardiac arrest is a treatable condition. However, regional variation in outcome after cardiac arrest is not fully explained by the Utstein factors, which include patient factors, such as age, gender, and initial rhythm; and EMS factors, such as time to arrival and time to first defibrillation.[20] Moreover, despite the marked decline in coronary artery disease mortality during the last 30 years,[21] few communities have been able to achieve sustained improvements in survival after cardiac arrest.[17,22–24]

NET BURDEN

Out-of-hospital cardiac arrest affects approximately 490,000 individuals in Europe each year[25] and approximately 350,000 individuals in the United States.[10] It is the third leading cause of death in the United States (**Fig. 2**; extrapolated from[10] and http://www.cdc.gov/nchs/fastats/deaths.htm, accessed March 11, 2011). The related condition of in-hospital cardiac arrest affects approximately 200,000 individuals in the United States (R Merchant, personal communication, March 10, 2011). Thus, reduction of the burden of illness associated with cardiac arrest is a critical public health issue.

NEED FOR PUBLIC HEALTH SURVEILLANCE OF CARDIAC ARREST

The true incidence of out-of-hospital cardiac arrest and survival from cardiac arrest are unknown. Current health surveillance systems cannot accurately determine the burden of out-of-hospital cardiac arrest, nor measure progress toward reducing this

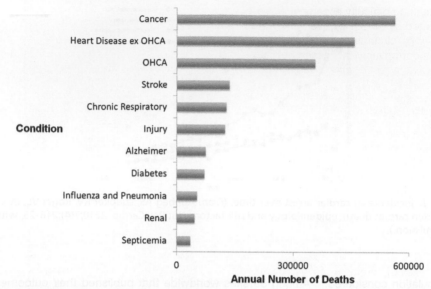

Fig. 2. Leading causes of death in United States.

burden. The Cardiac Arrest Registry to Enhance Survival (CARES) collates cases of out-of-hospital cardiac arrest from participating agencies in the United States, but includes only cases of presumed cardiac origin.[26] The National EMS Information System (NEMSIS) is an ongoing effort to create a national EMS database.[27] Because NEMSIS relies on self-report, events submitted by states do not necessarily represent all EMS events occurring within a state and states vary in criteria used to determine the types of EMS events submitted to the NEMSIS dataset.[28] Moreover, NEMESIS has a high rate of missing the vital data on functional status at discharge, limiting its ability to assess the comparative effectiveness of resuscitation interventions. The International Resuscitation Network demonstrated that data related to out-of-hospital cardiac arrest can be collated from five different countries, but does not collect data on an ongoing basis.[29] Other registries have focused on assessment of specific resuscitation interventions (eg, European Resuscitation Council Hypothermia Network).[30] Get With the Guidelines-Resuscitation (formerly known as American Heart Association National Registry for Cardiopulmonary Resuscitation) collates cases of in-hospital cardiac or respiratory arrest from institutions that are primarily in the United States,[31–34] but excludes cases of out-of-hospital cardiac arrest. Thus, although there are several prior and existing multicenter electronic clinical databases, none comprehensively assesses the benefits and harms of emergency cardiovascular care interventions in real-world settings on an ongoing basis through the continuum of care from EMS to hospital discharge by using a scalable, sustainable method.

Clinicians and policy makers need improved estimates of incidence to determine the absolute clinical and public health burden of cardiac arrest. Preventive and treatment measures aimed at reducing mortality from cardiac arrest can only derive from a reliable and valid estimate of its incidence and outcome. However, several barriers to effective surveillance of cardiac arrest exist. A common obstacle is that EMS and hospital systems may be reluctant to share outcome data because of concerns about how the data will be used and potential violation of regulations that protect personal health information. Even before the advent of the Health Insurance Portability and Accountability Act (HIPAA), EMS providers, quality assurance staff, and researchers often had difficulty ascertaining the functional status at hospital discharge of patients treated by EMS. However, under HIPAA, disclosure of information is permitted under specific circumstances, including public health disease reporting (http://www.hhs.gov/ocr/privacy/, accessed February 24, 2011). This is a strong argument for making cardiac arrest a reportable event.

PATIENT-LEVEL RISK FACTORS

Our understanding of why some individuals experience sudden cardiac arrest while other clinically comparable persons do not is incomplete and contributes to the ongoing public health challenge posed by cardiac arrest. Patient-level risk factors include fixed and modifiable factors. Overall, about 80% of people who suffer cardiac arrest have coronary artery disease (often undiagnosed), 10% to 15% have cardiomyopathy, and 5% to 10% have another problem, such as congenital heart disease or primary arrhythmogenic problem (eg, long QT syndrome or Brugada syndrome).[35]

Fixed

The risk of cardiac arrest increases with age, peaking in people aged 75 to 84 years. Females have a lower incidence of cardiac arrest than males.[11] Genetic risk factors for cardiac arrest include polygenetic factors that contribute to atherosclerosis, in addition to relatively rare genetic syndromes that directly cause arrhythmia such as congenital long QT syndrome and Brugada syndrome. However, the marked reduction in the incidence of ventricular fibrillation over the last few decades[15] suggests that genetics have a relatively small contribution to population-attributable risk. It remains unclear how to incorporate increased understanding of genetic risk into mass screening of individuals to cardiac arrest.

Modifiable

Health behaviors affect cardiac arrest risk. Given that 80% of sudden cardiac arrest is attributable to coronary disease, modification of risk factors, such as hypertension, diabetes, hyperlipidemia, and smoking, logically reduces both sudden and non-sudden cardiac deaths.[17] Regular exercise lowers cardiac arrest risk and can decrease mortality in people with established cardiac disease; however, risk is acutely increased during the period of exertion.[36] This relationship may reflect the balance between sympathetic and parasympathetic tone.

Cigarette smoking is thought to be the single most important cause of preventable death in the United States. An estimated 443,000 persons in the United States die prematurely each year due to exposure to tobacco smoke.[37] The deleterious effects of smoking may be mediated through increased plasma catecholamines, heart rate, and arterial blood pressure, resulting in coronary spasm and increases in myocardial work and oxygen supply. Collectively these effects lower ventricular fibrillation (VF) thresholds. In patients who successfully quit smoking, rates of cardiac arrest return to near normal over time. Of great concern is the effect of "passive smoking," which has been associated with an increase in smoking-related disease, primarily heart disease.

People who consume a moderate amount of alcohol (2–6 drinks per week) have a lower risk of sudden cardiac arrest when compared with nondrinkers. However, heavy consumption has been associated with increased risk. The interplay between alcohol and cardiac arrest is unclear but its protective effects are thought to be mediated via increased levels of high-density lipoprotein.[38,39]

A diet that includes fatty fish is rich in n-3 polyunsaturated fatty acids and has been associated with a lower risk of VF.[40] Research suggests that the acids stabilize action potentials by altering sodium and calcium ion channels in cardiac myocytes.

Diabetes may be a risk factor for cardiac arrest, independent of its contribution to coronary artery disease.[41,42] A proposed mechanism is abnormal prolongation of the QT interval due to diabetic autonomic dysfunction, although this has not been proved.[43] Moderate or vigorous, but not lesser, physical exertion is associated with increased risk of cardiac arrest.[44] Acute[45] and chronic[46] mental health conditions are associated with increased risk of cardiac arrest. However, it is difficult to objectively measure characteristics such as anger, anxiety, hostility, and aggressiveness because there are many confounding issues.

Structural

Dilated or hypertrophic cardiomyopathy accounts for about 10% to 15% of cases of cardiac arrest.[35] Decreased left ventricular function, regardless of ischemic or nonischemic cause, is a strong predictor of cardiac arrest.[47] Despite that severe left ventricular dysfunction is the best available risk predictor for sudden cardiac arrest, it was observed in less than a third of all cases in one community.[48] Other structural abnormalities, such as congenital malformations, scar from prior myocardial infarction, infiltrative diseases, and myocarditis, also predispose to cardiac arrest.[49]

Coronary Ischemia

Up to 71% of patients with cardiac arrest have coronary atherosclerosis and nearly half have an acute coronary occlusion.[6,50,51] Moreover, there is a high incidence (97%) of coronary artery disease in patients resuscitated from out-of-hospital cardiac arrest who undergo immediate angiography.[6] Among these, 50% have acute coronary occlusion. However, the absence of ST elevation on a surface 12-lead ECG after resuscitation from cardiac arrest is not strongly predictive of the absence of coronary occlusion on acute angiography. A case series of patients with unsuccessful field resuscitation suggested that in such patients VF is more likely to be associated with coronary atherosclerosis than was asystole or pulseless electric activity.[52] An autopsy study compared case subjects who died within 6 hours of symptom onset due to ischemic heart disease and who were not seen by a physician within 3 weeks with control subjects who died within 6 hours of symptom onset due to natural or unnatural noncardiac causes. Control subjects were matched to case subjects by age, gender, and socioeconomic status.[53] Intraluminal thrombosis was observed in 93% of case subjects versus 4% of control subjects. Collectively, these studies suggest that patients who are resuscitated from out-of-hospital VF have a high likelihood of having an acute coronary occlusion.

Medications

Medications that reduce coronary disease would logically reduce the rate of cardiac arrest. Indeed, statins decrease mortality due to cardiac arrest,[54,55] most likely acting via anti-ischemic rather than antiarrhythmic mechanisms.[56] Beta-blockers, aldosterone antagonists, angiotensin-converting enzyme inhibitors, angiotensin receptor-blockers, and omega-3 fatty acids may also contribute to reduced risk of cardiac arrest.[57]

Medications also have the potential to promote cardiac arrest. Medications that prolong the QT interval, including antiarrhythmics, antipsychotics, and many other classes of medications, may cause ventricular arrhythmias and, therefore, cardiac arrest. Hypokalemia and hypomagnesemia may have the same effect. However, it is unknown how much medication-induced or electrolyte-induced arrhythmias contribute to the overall incidence of cardiac arrest.[58]

Initial Rhythm

The exact mechanism of collapse in an individual patient is often difficult to establish because more than 40% of all cases present without prior warning[59] and are not readily under close observation. Therefore, much of what we understand is hypothesized from information obtained or observed after the event has begun. In the vast majority of cases, individuals who suffer cardiac arrest have evidence of structural heart disease. In general, approximately 80% have coronary atherosclerosis, another 10% to 15% have nonischemic cardiomyopathy, and the remaining 5% to 10% have a congenital disorder or no evidence of structural disease.[51] Usually this underlying structural abnormality predisposes an individual to a fatal or near fatal arrhythmia that is precipitated by an acute trigger, such as an ischemic event or electrolyte imbalance. The rhythm that is first recorded after the onset of cardiac arrest classified into three categories: (1) ventricular tachyarrhythmias, including pulseless ventricular tachycardia and VF (VT/VF); or (2) pulseless electrical activity (PEA); or (3) asystole.

Initial rhythm has a large impact on survival: published rates of survival after treatment of any initial rhythm range from 0% to greater than 20% among those with EMS-treated arrest and 0% to 45% for those with VF arrest.[11,19,60] Consistently, survival is greatest in patients with a first-recorded rhythm of VF.[61]

VF is characterized by rapid, ineffective, uncoordinated movement of the ventricles that does not produce a pulse. The ECG of VF shows measurable electrical activity with chaotic, irregular ventricular complexes. If untreated, the electrical organization of the ventricular fibrillation signal deteriorates into asystole over minutes.[62] Coronary ischemia is thought to be the primary precipitant of VT/VF, a correlation confirmed in recent studies.[46] The cause of PEA is diverse and related to a variety of factors, including hypoxia, hypovolemia, electrolyte imbalance, tamponade, pneumothorax, and thromboembolism.[46]

Historically, most out-of-hospital cardiac arrest cases documented VT/VF as the first recorded rhythm. The incidence of VF has declined steadily in regions that have tracked EMS data over 10 to 21 years.[16,63,64] The decline of VF may be attributed to treatment of cardiac risk factors, increasing rates of ICD placement, and increasing use of beta-blockers.[64–66] Another possibility is that multisystem organ failure is becoming more common and presenting frequently as non-VF cardiac arrest. This decline is of substantial importance for public health because survival rates are significantly less for PEA compared with VT/VF.[60]

COMMUNITY-LEVEL RISK FACTORS
Socioeconomic and Racial Differences

Disparities in the incidence of and survival from cardiac arrest are observed across socioeconomic gradients and between races.[33,67] In New York City, for example, a prospective study found that age-adjusted incidence of cardiac arrest was 10.1 per 10,000 for blacks and 5.8 per 10,000 for whites; survival to discharge was 1.4% for blacks and 3.4% for whites. However, after adjustment for socioeconomic factors, prior functional status, initial rhythm, and characteristics of the event, no significant racial differences were found.[68]

Environmental

There is temporal variability in cardiac arrest frequency, with cardiac arrest peaking in the morning and in the winter.[69] Underlying patient, EMS system, and environmental factors need to be explored to offer further insight into these observed patterns. Various physiologic processes have been proposed to explain the diurnal phenomenon, such as increased clotting or increased parasympathetic instability. Some researchers have suggested that part of the morning peak in cardiac arrest may be due to a reporting artifact (ie, when patients die during the night but are not discovered until early morning). Potential interventions to reduce periodic variation in unexpected cardiac death include resource allocation of EMS and hospital resources to match anticipated need.

A PUBLIC HEALTH APPROACH TO CARDIAC ARREST

Survival from cardiac arrest varies tremendously across communities. As noted above, this variation is associated with variation in prehospital emergency care. There are many ways to improve the chain of survival after cardiac arrest, including improved communications from citizens to EMS, delivery of care to the patient, delivery of the patient to the hospital, and delivery of cardiac and critical care. Yet few communities have been able to achieve sustained improvements in outcome.

There is only a twofold variation in outcome after care for the related disorder of acute myocardial infarction, but correlates of such variation have been better eluci-dated. These include geographic region,[70–72] hospital volume,[73,74] urban location,[75] teaching status,[72,76] and safety net status.[77] Variation in outcome does not seem to associate with large differences in protocols or processes of care, such as rapid response teams, clinical guidelines, use of hospitalists, and medication checks.[78] Instead, hospitals in the top or bottom tier of risk-standardized mortality after myocar-dial infarction differ substantially in terms of their organizational goals and values, senior management involvement, staff presence and expertise in care for patients with acute myocardial infarction, communication and coordination among relevant groups, and problem solving and learning. It has been suggested that such cultural differences are a major factor in regional variation in outcomes after cardiac arrest.[79]

SUMMARY

A cardiac resuscitation system is an interconnected community, EMS, and hospital response to out-of-hospital cardiac arrest.[80] A critical component of such a response is ongoing measurement and improvement of the process and outcome of care. Such regional systems of care have improved provider experience and patient outcome for other time-sensitive conditions, including ST-elevation myocardial infarction and life-threatening traumatic injury. The time has come for us to come together to implement such resuscitation systems of care in our communities. Interested physicians, EMS providers, and members of the lay public have begun this process in Arizona, Minne-sota, North Carolina, Pennsylvania, and Washington (www.heartrescueproject.com, accessed March 29, 2011). Ongoing efforts and evaluation are needed in these and other communities to ensure that public health is improved by reducing death and disability due to cardiac arrest.

REFERENCES

1. Jacobs I, Nadkarni V, Bahr J, et al. Cardiac arrest and cardiopulmonary resusci-tation outcome reports: update and simplification of the Utstein templates for resuscitation registries: a statement for healthcare professionals from a task force of the International Liaison Committee on Resuscitation (American Heart Associ-ation, European Resuscitation Council, Australian Resuscitation Council, New Zealand Resuscitation Council, Heart and Stroke Foundation of Canada,

InterAmerican Heart Foundation, Resuscitation Councils of Southern Africa). Circulation 2004;110(21):3385–97.

2. Zipes DP, Wellens HJ. Sudden cardiac death. Circulation 1998;98(21):2334–51.
3. Working Group on Ischemic Heart Disease Registers. WGoIHD. Report of a Working Group. Parts I and II. Copenhagen (Denmark): Regional Office for Europe, World Health Organization; 1969.
4. Fishman GI, Chugh SS, Dimarco JP, et al. Sudden cardiac death prediction and prevention: report from a National Heart, Lung, and Blood Institute and Heart Rhythm Society Workshop. Circulation 2010;122(22):2335–48.
5. Ziesche S, Rector TS, Cohn JN. Interobserver discordance in the classification of mechanisms of death in studies of heart failure. J Card Fail 1995;1(2):127–32.
6. Spaulding CM, Joly LM, Rosenberg A, et al. Immediate coronary angiography in survivors of out-of-hospital cardiac arrest. N Engl J Med 1997;336(23): 1629–33.
7. Adabag AS, Luepker RV, Roger VL, et al. Sudden cardiac death: epidemiology and risk factors. Nat Rev Cardiol 2010;7(4):216–25.
8. Zive D, Koprowicz K, Schmidt T, et al. Variation in out-of-hospital cardiac arrest resuscitation and transport practices in the Resuscitation Outcomes Consortium: ROC Epistry-Cardiac Arrest. Resuscitation 2011;82(3):277–84.
9. Morrison LJ, Nichol G, Rea TD, et al. Rationale, development and implementation of the Resuscitation Outcomes Consortium Epistry-Cardiac Arrest. Resuscitation 2008;78(2):161–9.
10. Nichol G, Thomas E, Callaway CW, et al. Regional variation in out-of-hospital cardiac arrest incidence and outcome. JAMA 2008;300(12):1423–31.
11. Rea TD, Eisenberg MS, Sinibaldi G, et al. Incidence of EMS-treated out-of-hospital cardiac arrest in the United States. Resuscitation 2004;63(1):17–24.
12. Chugh SS, Jui J, Gunson K, et al. Current burden of sudden cardiac death: multiple source surveillance versus retrospective death certificate-based review in a large U.S. community. J Am Coll Cardiol 2004;44(6):1268–75.
13. Atkins DL, Everson-Stewart S, Sears GK, et al. Epidemiology and outcomes from out-of-hospital cardiac arrest in children: the Resuscitation Outcomes Consortium Epistry-Cardiac Arrest. Circulation 2009;119(11):1484–91.
14. Zheng ZJ, Croft JB, Giles WH, et al. Sudden cardiac death in the United States, 1989 to 1998. Circulation 2001;104(18):2158–63.
15. Rea TD, Pearce RM, Raghunathan TE, et al. Incidence of out-of-hospital cardiac arrest. Am J Cardiol 2004;93(12):1455–60.
16. Cobb LA, Fahrenbruch CE, Olsufka M, et al. Changing incidence of out-of-hospital ventricular fibrillation, 1980-2000. JAMA 2002;288(23):3008–13.
17. Rea TD, Eisenberg MS, Becker LJ, et al. Temporal trends in sudden cardiac arrest: a 25-year emergency medical services perspective. Circulation 2003; 107(22):2780–5.
18. Sayre MR, Travers AH, Daya M, et al. Measuring survival rates from sudden cardiac arrest: the elusive definition. Resuscitation 2004;62(1):25–34.
19. Nichol G, Stiell IG, Laupacis A, et al. A cumulative meta-analysis of the effectiveness of defibrillator-capable emergency medical services for victims of out-of-hospital cardiac arrest. Ann Emerg Med 1999;34(4 Pt 1):517–25.
20. Rea TD, Cook AJ, Stiell IG, et al. Predicting survival after out-of-hospital cardiac arrest: role of the Utstein data elements. Ann Emerg Med 2010;55(3):249–57.
21. Fox CS, Evans JC, Larson MG, et al. Temporal trends in coronary heart disease mortality and sudden cardiac death from 1950 to 1999: the Framingham Heart Study. Circulation 2004;110(5):522–7.

22. Iwami T, Nichol G, Hiraide A, et al. Continuous improvements in "chain of survival" increased survival after out-of-hospital cardiac arrests: a large-scale population-based study. Circulation 2009;119(5):728–34.

23. Herlitz J, Bang A, Gunnarsson J, et al. Factors associated with survival to hospital discharge among patients hospitalised alive after out of hospital cardiac arrest: change in outcome over 20 years in the community of Goteborg, Sweden. Heart 2003;89(1):25–30.

24. Sasson C, Rogers MA, Dahl J, et al. Predictors of survival from out-of-hospital cardiac arrest: a systematic review and meta-analysis. Circ Cardiovasc Qual Outcomes 2010;3(1):63–81.

25. de Vreede-Swagemakers JJ, Gorgels AP, Dubois-Arbouw WI, et al. Out-of-hospital cardiac arrest in the 1990's: a population-based study in the Maastricht area on incidence, characteristics and survival. J Am Coll Cardiol 1997;30(6):1500–5.

26. McNally B, Stokes A, Crouch A, et al. CARES: Cardiac Arrest Registry to Enhance Survival. Ann Emerg Med 2009;54(5):674–683.e2.

27. Dawson DE. National Emergency Medical Services Information System (NEMSIS). Prehosp Emerg Care 2006;10(3):314–6.

28. Anonymous. Available at: www.americanheart.org/missionlifeline. Accessed February 14, 2010.

29. Nichol G, Steen P, Herlitz J, et al. International Resuscitation Network Registry: design, rationale and preliminary results. Resuscitation 2005;65(3):265–77.

30. Arrich J. Clinical application of mild therapeutic hypothermia after cardiac arrest. Crit Care Med 2007;35(4):1041–7.

31. Peberdy MA, Kaye W, Ornato JP, et al. Cardiopulmonary resuscitation of adults in the hospital: a report of 14,720 cardiac arrest from the National Registry of Cardiopulmonary Resuscitation. Resuscitation 2003;58:297–308.

32. Nadkarni VM, Larkin GL, Peberdy MA, et al. First documented rhythm and clinical outcome from in-hospital cardiac arrest among children and adults. JAMA 2006; 295(1):50–7.

33. Chan PS, Nichol G, Krumholz HM, et al. Racial differences in survival after in-hospital cardiac arrest. JAMA 2009;302(11):1195–201.

34. Chan PS, Nichol G, Krumholz HM, et al. Hospital variation in time to defibrillation after in-hospital cardiac arrest. Arch Intern Med 2009;169(14):1265–73.

35. Chugh SS, Reinier K, Teodorescu C, et al. Epidemiology of sudden cardiac death: clinical and research implications. Prog Cardiovasc Dis 2008;51(3): 213–28.

36. Mittleman MA, Maclure M, Tofler GH, et al. Triggering of acute myocardial infarction by heavy physical exertion. Protection against triggering by regular exertion. Determinants of Myocardial Infarction Onset Study Investigators. N Engl J Med 1993;329(23):1677–83.

37. Centers for Disease Control and Prevention (CDC). Smoking-attributable mortality, years of potential life lost, and productivity losses—United States, 2000–2004. MMWR Morb Mortal Wkly Rep 2008;57(45):1226–8.

38. Gaziano JM, Buring JE, Breslow JL, et al. Moderate alcohol intake, increased levels of high-density lipoprotein and its subfractions, and decreased risk of myocardial infarction. N Engl J Med 1993;329(25):1829–34.

39. Imhof A, Froehlich M, Brenner H, et al. Effect of alcohol consumption on systemic markers of inflammation. Lancet 2001;357(9258):763–7.

40. Siscovick DS, Lemaitre RN, Mozaffarian D. The fish story: a diet-heart hypothesis with clinical implications: n-3 polyunsaturated fatty acids, myocardial vulnerability, and sudden death. Circulation 2003;107(21):2632–4.

41. Jouven X, Desnos M, Guerot C, et al. Predicting sudden death in the population: the Paris Prospective Study I. Circulation 1999;99(15):1978–83.
42. Jouven X, Lemaitre RN, Rea TD, et al. Diabetes, glucose level, and risk of sudden cardiac death. Eur Heart J 2005;26(20):2142–7.
43. Veglio M, Chinaglia A, Cavallo Perin P. The clinical utility of QT interval assessment in diabetes. Diabetes Nutr Metab 2000;13(6):356–65.
44. Whang W, Manson JE, Hu FB, et al. Physical exertion, exercise, and sudden cardiac death in women. JAMA 2006;295(12):1399–403.
45. Reich P, DeSilva RA, Lown B, et al. Acute psychological disturbances preceding life-threatening ventricular arrhythmias. JAMA 1981;246(3):233–5.
46. Whang W, Kubzansky LD, Kawachi I, et al. Depression and risk of sudden cardiac death and coronary heart disease in women: results from the Nurses' Health Study. J Am Coll Cardiol 2009;53(11):950–8.
47. Gorgels AP, Gijsbers C, de Vreede-Swagemakers J, et al. Out-of-hospital cardiac arrest–the relevance of heart failure. The Maastricht Circulatory Arrest Registry. Eur Heart J 2003;24(13):1204–9.
48. Stecker EC, Vickers C, Waltz J, et al. Population-based analysis of sudden cardiac death with and without left ventricular systolic dysfunction: two-year findings from the Oregon Sudden Unexpected Death Study. J Am Coll Cardiol 2006; 47(6):1161–6.
49. Turakhia M, Tseng ZH. Sudden cardiac death: epidemiology, mechanisms, and therapy. Curr Probl Cardiol 2007;32(9):501–46.
50. Pell JP, Sirel JM, Marsden AK, et al. Presentation, management, and outcome of out of hospital cardiopulmonary arrest: comparison by underlying aetiology. Heart 2003;89(8):839–42.
51. Huikuri HV, Castellanos A, Myerburg RJ. Sudden death due to cardiac arrhythmias. N Engl J Med 2001;345(20):1473–82.
52. Silfvast T, Saarnivaara L. Comparison of alfentanil and morphine in the prehospital treatment of patients with acute ischaemic-type chest pain. Eur J Emerg Med 2001;8(4):275–8.
53. Davies MJ, Thomas A. Thrombosis and acute coronary-artery lesions in sudden cardiac ischemic death. N Engl J Med 1984;310(18):1137–40.
54. Dickinson MG, Ip JH, Olshansky B, et al. Statin use was associated with reduced mortality in both ischemic and nonischemic cardiomyopathy and in patients with implantable defibrillators: mortality data and mechanistic insights from the Sudden Cardiac Death in Heart Failure Trial (SCD-HeFT). Am Heart J 2007;153(4):573–8.
55. Goldberger JJ, Subacius H, Schaechter A, et al. Effects of statin therapy on arrhythmic events and survival in patients with nonischemic dilated cardiomyopathy. J Am Coll Cardiol 2006;48(6):1228–33.
56. Beri A, Contractor T, Khasnis A, et al. Statins and the reduction of sudden cardiac death: antiarrhythmic or anti-ischemic effect? Am J Cardiovasc Drugs 2010; 10(3):155–64.
57. Boriani G, Valzania C, Diemberger I, et al. Potential of non-antiarrhythmic drugs to provide an innovative upstream approach to the pharmacological prevention of sudden cardiac death. Expert Opin Investig Drugs 2007;16(5):605–23.
58. Yap YG, Camm AJ. Drug induced QT prolongation and torsades de pointes. Heart 2003;89(11):1363–72.
59. Chugh SS. Early identification of risk factors for sudden cardiac death. Nat Rev Cardiol 2010;7(6):318–26.
60. Atwood C, Eisenberg MS, Herlitz J, et al. Incidence of EMS-treated out-of-hospital cardiac arrest in Europe. Resuscitation 2005;67(1):75–80.

61. Nichol G, Detsky AS, Stiell IG, et al. Effectiveness of emergency medical services for victims of out-of-hospital cardiac arrest: a metaanalysis. Ann Emerg Med 1996;27(6):700–10.
62. Holmberg M, Holmberg S, Herlitz J. An alternative estimate of the disappearance rate of ventricular fibrillation in our-of-hospital cardiac arrest in Sweden. Resuscitation 2001;49(2):219–20.
63. Polentini MS, Pirrallo RG, McGill W. The changing incidence of ventricular fibrillation in Milwaukee, Wisconsin (1992-2002). Prehosp Emerg Care 2006;10(1):52–60.
64. Bunch TJ, White RD, Friedman PA, et al. Trends in treated ventricular fibrillation out-of-hospital cardiac arrest: a 17-year population-based study. Heart Rhythm 2004;1(3):255–9.
65. Bunch TJ, White RD. Trends in treated ventricular fibrillation in out-of-hospital cardiac arrest: ischemic compared to non-ischemic heart disease. Resuscitation 2005;67(1):51–4.
66. Youngquist ST, Kaji AH, Niemann JT. Beta-blocker use and the changing epidemiology of out-of-hospital cardiac arrest rhythms. Resuscitation 2008;76(3):376–80.
67. Gillum RF. Sudden cardiac death in Hispanic Americans and African Americans. Am J Public Health 1997;87(9):1461–6.
68. Galea S, Blaney S, Nandi A, et al. Explaining racial disparities in incidence of and survival from out-of-hospital cardiac arrest. Am J Epidemiol 2007;166(5):534–43.
69. Brooks SC, Schmicker RH, Rea TD, et al. Out-of-hospital cardiac arrest frequency and survival: evidence for temporal variability. Resuscitation 2010;81(2):175–81.
70. Krumholz HM, Chen J, Rathore SS, et al. Regional variation in the treatment and outcomes of myocardial infarction: investigating New England's advantage. Am Heart J 2003;146(2):242–9.
71. Normand ST, Glickman ME, Sharma RG, et al. Using admission characteristics to predict short-term mortality from myocardial infarction in elderly patients. Results from the Cooperative Cardiovascular Project. JAMA 1996;275(17):1322–8.
72. Krumholz HM, Merrill AR, Schone EM, et al. Patterns of hospital performance in acute myocardial infarction and heart failure 30-day mortality and readmission. Circ Cardiovasc Qual Outcomes 2009;2(5):407–13.
73. Ross JS, Normand SL, Wang Y, et al. Hospital volume and 30-day mortality for three common medical conditions. N Engl J Med 2010;362(12):1110–8.
74. Thiemann DR, Coresh J, Oetgen WJ, et al. The association between hospital volume and survival after acute myocardial infarction in elderly patients. N Engl J Med 1999;340(21):1640–8.
75. Baldwin LM, MacLehose RF, Hart LG, et al. Quality of care for acute myocardial infarction in rural and urban US hospitals. J Rural Health 2004;20(2):99–108.
76. Allison JJ, Kiefe CI, Weissman NW, et al. Relationship of hospital teaching status with quality of care and mortality for Medicare patients with acute MI. JAMA 2000; 284(10):1256–62.
77. Ross JS, Cha SS, Epstein AJ, et al. Quality of care for acute myocardial infarction at urban safety-net hospitals. Health Aff (Millwood) 2007;26(1):238–48.
78. Curry LA, Spatz E, Cherlin E, et al. What distinguishes top-performing hospitals in acute myocardial infarction mortality rates? A qualitative study. Ann Intern Med 2011;154(6):384–90.
79. Eisenberg M. Resuscitate! How Your Community Can Improve Survival from Sudden Cardiac Arrest. Seattle (WA): University of Washington; 2009.
80. Nichol G, Aufderheide TP, Eigel B, et al. Regional systems of care for out-of-hospital cardiac arrest: a policy statement from the American Heart Association. Circulation 2010;121(5):709–29.

Out-of-Hospital Cardiac Arrest

Tanner S. Boyd, MD[a],*, Debra G. Perina, MD[b]

KEYWORDS

- Prehospital • Out-of-hospital • Cardiac arrest • Resuscitation

ACCESS AND PRESENTATION

Emergency medical services (EMS) medical care has changed significantly since its inception. Initially, ambulances functioned merely as transport vehicles. Today, EMS has matured into an integrated part of the health care system, with the ability to provide advanced care en-route to a hospital. Regional dispatch centers now decide which resources should respond to an emergency call. EMS dispatchers are trained in emergency medical dispatch techniques and can provide prearrival instructions to bystanders, thereby expediting initial first aid and cardiopulmonary resuscitation (CPR).

Historically, much of the medical care provided by EMS grew out of traditional practice with little scientific basis. Today, in mature EMS systems, rigorous research studies are being completed and evidence-based medicine concepts used to determine proven benefit before introduction of new procedures, drugs, and adjuncts to out-of-hospital care. A research base for EMS practice now exists, a large component of which is related to out-of-hospital cardiac arrest (OHCA) techniques and therapies to improve survival. Current research is ongoing to evaluate the best treatment options for patients with OHCA.

Emphasis is placed on layperson education and all level of provider courses to rapidly access the emergency system in cases of OHCA to receive appropriate treatment. The patient (before arrest) or a witness or bystander must first recognize the problem and activate the EMS system. The more rapid this activation occurs, the more rapidly definitive care can arrive to the OHCA situation. Delays in arrival affect ultimate outcomes. Depending on the circumstances surrounding the presentation, delays can frequently occur. Cardiac arrests witnessed by bystanders or that which occur in a public area result in EMS being accessed more rapidly than in an unwitnessed event.[1] A Swedish study found that a period of activation of less than 4 minutes

The authors have nothing to disclose.

[a] Emergency Medicine Residency, Department of Emergency Medicine, University of Virginia School of Medicine, University of Virginia, PO Box 800699, Charlottesville, VA 22908, USA
[b] Division of Prehospital Care, Department of Emergency Medicine, University of Virginia School of Medicine, University of Virginia, PO Box 800699, Charlottesville, VA 22908, USA
* Corresponding author.
E-mail address: tanner.boyd@gmail.com

from time of cardiac arrest to EMS activation increased the 1-month survival rate from 2.8% to 6.9% (P<.0001).[2] Likewise, more rapid EMS response times[3] and shorter times to CPR initiation increase overall survival. The same conditions can also be extrapolated to traumatic cardiac arrests as well, although outcome in such settings is less optimal.

Delays in accessing care can also occur in patients with chest pain who are at high risk for OHCA or in a prearrest state. One of the largest randomized trials to date addressing delays in treatment to patients experiencing chest pain is the European Myocardial Infarction Project.[4] Collecting data from 15 European countries and Canada between 1988 and 1992, this study found the largest delays occurred in female patients, those older than 65 years, those who had experienced chest pain in the previous 24 hours, and those with pulmonary edema. Characteristics of patients with the shortest delay to summoning an ambulance included those with a history of previous myocardial infarction (MI), those in shock, and those experiencing ventricular fibrillation.

These factors associated with delays to EMS activation were also noted again in numerous smaller studies with the addition of other factors such as lower socioeconomic status, a family member being present at symptom onset, and the belief that symptoms were not severe enough to summon EMS. Some studies suggest increased frequency of atypical symptoms in women causing a larger time gap between onset of symptoms and access of care,[5] whereas others show no gender difference at all.[6] A large Swedish study reviewing demographics of patients with acute MI over 15 years found that before the age of 65 years, there was no gender difference in hospital delay. However, after 65 years of age, there was an increased time delay for women.[7]

Adding to delay in access to care, certain populations can present without chest pain at all and suddenly experience OHCA. Elderly and diabetic patients may have atypical presentations of acute MI with nonspecific symptoms such as dizziness, syncope, malaise, nausea, vomiting, or abdominal pain. Patients experiencing a significant cardiac or prearrest event may also present with congestive heart failure, hypotension, or severe respiratory distress. These presentations not only can cause delays in access of care but also may mislead health care personnel, causing a delay in recognition of the prearrest setting that can degenerate into OHCA if not properly recognized and treated promptly.

Ready access to automated external defibrillator (AED) devices that can rapidly analyze and deliver electrical shocks if indicated should also be part of the overall community strategy to decrease delays in access to care. Strategies for optimal survival of patients with OHCA include minimizing delays in accessing care, proper placement of AEDs in locations where patients with OHCA may be more likely encountered, and dispatch call centers staffed by trained emergency dispatchers who use prearrival instructions to begin bystander care and CPR before EMS arrival. Public awareness, lay provider education campaigns, CPR AED instruction, and encouragement to use the EMS system all play important roles in the ultimate reduction in the access to care.

DEMOGRAPHICS

It is estimated that more than 166,000 patients experience OHCA each year.[8] Several historical risk factors have been associated with OHCA. A diagnosis of congestive heart failure carried an OHCA incidence of 21.87 per 1000 subject years, whereas a history of diabetes mellitus, previous MI, smoking, and hypertension resulted in incidences of 13.80, 13.69, 9.18, and 7.54, respectively.[9] Cardiac arrests, along with MIs and unstable angina, seem to have a circadian variation, with a morning peak after the initiation of daily activities.[10] EMS response to patients with OHCA seems to be more frequent during this period as well.

A well-defined body of resuscitation literature has reported that survivors of cardiac arrest have a greater chance of successful resuscitation if the presenting rhythm is shockable and the least likelihood if the presenting rhythm is asystole. Patients with OHCA have been reported to have initial rhythms of ventricular tachycardia, ventricular fibrillation, or a shockable rhythm as determined by an AED 23% of the time. Another 9% of patients with OHCA had nonshockable rhythms per AED, with 40% showing asystole, 20% pulseless electrical activity (PEA), and the final 9% being unknown or undetermined rhythms.[11] OHCA research suffered from the lack of a consistent definition of cardiac arrest and poor reporting across EMS services until the creation and adoption of the uniform data collection and reporting criteria, Utstein criteria, which now allow researchers to nationally pool data and perform comparisons across services.[12] OHCA rates show a wide variation with the overall incidence calculated, using the uniform criteria, to be 95 per 100,000 subject-years.

OHCA OUTCOMES

It is estimated that more than 166,000 patients experience OHCA each year. This public health condition has defined a research agenda to identify effective treatments and strategies that could result in increased survival rates. Despite efforts, OHCA survival rates remain bleak. Before adoption of the Utstein criteria, outcomes in patients with OHCA were difficult to measure secondary to the lack of standardization of variables between EMS systems. Some of these variables included pulse presence on arrival to the emergency department (ED), general return of circulation, and definition of what constitutes patient survival. This inconsistency led to the 1995 adoption of uniform definitions, data collection sets, and reporting with the use of the Utstein criteria that has allowed greater standardization and comparison between research studies.[12] Despite this, comparison of research data is still hampered by differences in EMS systems, response times, patient downtimes, and bystander CPR and AED availability.

Despite research limitations, several factors seem to be associated with an increased chance of survival in OHCA. Bystander CPR, witnessed arrest, initial presenting rhythm of ventricular fibrillation, and short response times to defibrillation are all associated with increased survival rates.[13,14] Eisenburger and colleagues[15] also showed that having a cardiac arrest in a public place was an independent predictor of improved outcome. Immediate defibrillation of patients in ventricular fibrillation results in a pulse-generating rhythm and survival to hospital discharge in 56% of patients. This decreases, with each successive defibrillation attempt eventually reaching 6% by the third attempt. Survival rates have been shown to be at their highest if defibrillation occurs within the first 6 minutes of cardiac arrest, decreasing as the interval increases up to 11 minutes, and leveling off after that time.[15]

There is a large degree of variability reported in OHCA survival ranges, with a low of 6% and a high of 46%. However, the largest cumulative meta-analysis study to date documented a mean survival to hospital discharge for all rhythm groups of only 7.6% and a hospital admission rate of only 23.8%.[16] This outcome variability is attributable to the factors previously mentioned in addition to local population characteristics and other factors. Liu and colleagues[17] reported that younger age, nonwhite race, and male gender were associated with better outcomes. Time of EMS arrival is linked to higher survival rates, with even a 1-minute decrease in mean response times showing an approximate 1% (0.7%–2.1% range) absolute increase in survival. In addition to response times, decreasing overall pauses in CPR is associated with better results.[18] EMS-witnessed cardiac arrests seem to have the best outcomes followed by bystander-witnessed arrests with bystander CPR, bystander-witnessed arrests without bystander CPR, and unwitnessed arrests.[19]

The benefits of advanced life support (ALS) versus basic life support (BLS) on cardiac arrest outcomes have been questioned by some. The largest study to date, the Ontario Prehospital Advanced Life Support study, looked at the effects of multiple EMS variables on OHCA outcomes as ALS was phased into their EMS system. In phase 1 of this study, age, witnessed arrest, bystander CPR, CPR by fire or police, and short EMS response times were independently associated with survival in multivariate analysis.[20] In phase 2, a target of 8 minutes was set for the time from call receipt to response on scene with a defibrillator. Of the 1641 patients with cardiac arrest in the study, 90% of calls met this target with a 33% improvement in overall survival to discharge in all rhythm groups. This response time was estimated to save an additional 21 lives at a cost of $2400 per life.[14] When all patients were analyzed, there were a total of 1391 patients who were enrolled in the defibrillation plus BLS phase of the study and another 4247 patients enrolled in the advanced cardiac life support (ACLS) phase. The population with ACLS had greater return of spontaneous circulation (ROSC) rates (12.9% vs 18.0%, $P<.001$) and survival to hospital admission rates (10.9% vs 14.6%, $P<.001$), but hospital discharge rates were unchanged (5.0% vs 5.1%; $P = .83$). This rate led to an odds ratio of 1.1 for ACLS relative to BLS. This rate did not relate favorably to the odds ratios of 4.4, 3.7, and 3.4 for witnessed arrest, early CPR, and early defibrillation, respectively, in achieving meaningful impact of OHSA survival rates.[21]

Another study comparing prehospital ACLS in OHCA with and without intravenous (IV) medications found no difference in ROSC, survival to hospital admission, or hospital discharge among shockable rhythm groups. However, if the initial rhythm was PEA or asystole, the IV group had better rates of ROSC (29% vs 11%, $P<.001$) and survival to hospital admission (31% vs 16%, $P<.001$) but not to hospital discharge (2% vs 3%, $P = .65$).[22] This finding of lack of ALS impact on hospital discharge rates was not supported in a meta-analysis of 37 articles from 1999 describing 39 EMS systems and 33,124 patients. This study reported the odds ratio of survival to hospital discharge for BLS plus defibrillation systems to be 1.71 (95% confidence interval [CI], 1.09–2.70; $P = .01$) for ACLS, 1.47 (95% CI, 0.89–2.42; $P = .07$) for 2-tiered BLS and ALS systems, and 2.31 (95% CI, 1.47–3.62; $P<.01$) for 2-tiered BLS with defibrillation and ALS systems. This study was not sufficiently powered to demonstrate whether 1- or 2-tiered systems had better survival rates but was able to show that ALS is more effective than BLS plus defibrillation alone.[13] Regardless of whether one believes the data showing no benefit in hospital discharge with ACLS or favors the studies showing some improvement, both studies reported that ACLS improves survival to hospital admission and ROSC in the out-of-hospital setting.

Hospital destination for survivors of OHCA also seems to influence outcomes. Lui and colleagues[17] reported that hospital survival rates varied among hospitals from 29% to 42% despite identical EMS treatment. Another study also showed that outcomes at designated critical care medical centers are better.[23] Callaway and colleagues[24] found that hospitals with cardiac catheterization capability that come across at least 40 cardiac arrests per year have better outcomes, regardless of how many beds are in the hospital or whether it is considered a teaching hospital or not. Patients with cardiac arrests caused by ST elevation MIs who arrive at the ED with ROSC generally have better outcomes.[25] Surprisingly, higher survival rates are not limited to urban areas alone because rural locations have also documented neurologically intact survival to hospital discharge rates as high as 22%.

When to terminate out-of-hospital resuscitation efforts is still a topic of controversy with the wish to not prolong efforts beyond potential benefit along with the possibility of neurologic devastation weighed against the desire to not declare death prematurely. Concern for the safety and well-being of both EMS providers and the public because of the rate of ambulance accidents when running with lights and sirens, benched against the lack of proved benefit of transport of patients with OHCA without ROSC, has led to general acceptance of termination of resuscitation efforts in the field. Multiple rules have been validated for the termination of prehospital CPR, with the most popular one resulted from methodology that determined only 46% of cardiac arrests needed transportation.[26] This rule states that if there is no ROSC after 3 rounds of BLS with defibrillation pauses every 1 to 2 minutes, if no shock was delivered by an AED, and if the cardiac arrest was unwitnessed by an emergency medical technician or firefighter, then all resuscitation efforts may be terminated.[26] When validated, this rule had a sensitivity of 57.5% to 64.4%, a specificity of 90.2% to 100.0%, and a positive predictive value of 99.5% to 100.0%.[26,27] When neurologic status was factored in, this rule correctly identified 100% of those discharged with good neurologic outcome and 36% of those with poor neurologic outcome or who did not survive.[28] Although some EMS systems have enacted this, others prefer to make decisions on a per-case basis. Individual case factors that may lead to transportation despite this validated termination rule are airway difficulties, persistent ventricular dysrhythmias, excessively public location, family members who are unable to accept field termination, lack of IV cannulation, and cultural or language barriers. In addition, many emergency physicians do not feel comfortable pronouncing a PEA code in the field. Regardless of the decision to transport or terminate efforts at the scene, family members are generally accepting of termination in cases of unsuccessful out-of-hospital resuscitation efforts.

OHCAs can also be traumatic in origin. Patients with this condition have an extremely high mortality rate, with survivors having significant morbidity. However, as with medical cardiac arrests, research suggests that a small subset of these patients can potentially benefit from timely aggressive treatment. Studies looking at the impact of EMS care concluded that any intervention that delays a patient's hospital arrival has a negative impact on survival in the trauma patient. Although resuscitative thoracotomy is a possibility in the setting of traumatic cardiac arrests to allow for open cardiac massage, pericardiotomy for tamponade release, cardiac/aortic penetration occlusion, or descending aortic cross-clamping until definitive repair, this procedure only applies to a small subset of patients. These patients include those in arrest less than 4 minutes before ED arrival, those with signs of life on ED arrival, or those with suspected pericardial tamponade leading to arrest. Prognosis is dismal in those without signs of life on ED arrival and in patients with asystolic or bradyasystolic rhythms; resuscitative thoracotomy is generally not recommended.

RESPONSE SYSTEMS AND PROCESS

To improve cardiac arrest outcomes, each link in the chain of survival must be optimized. In the prehospital world, this optimization includes the prompt identification of a cardiac arrest, proper dispatch of care, rapid initiation of CPR, immediate defibrillation, high-quality CPR, and rapid transport to the most appropriate hospital. Public education campaigns continue to improve awareness of cardiac arrest signs and symptoms, but there is little that can be done to improve outcomes unless the emergency response system is activated.

The first person a caller speaks with when calling 911 is a trained dispatcher. Outcomes have been shown to be better when dispatchers receive more frequent cardiac arrest calls.[29] Unfortunately, any sign of breathing, including agonal breathing, decreases the chances that a dispatcher will recognize a cardiac arrest.[30] However, teaching dispatchers to recognize agonal breathing increases not only the detection of cardiac arrests[31] but also the frequency with which CPR instructions are given.[32] To help dispatchers, computer systems have been developed to assist in the detection of OHCA. The Medical Priority Dispatch System has been shown to have a sensitivity of 76.7% and a specificity of 99.2% at detecting a cardiac arrest.[33] Likewise, the Advanced Medical Priority Dispatch System increased the number of people accurately identified as being in cardiac arrest compared with dispatchers alone.[34] Despite these guides, it is clear that these computer systems continue to misidentify patients with OHCA, and, thus, there is still room for improvement in dispatcher detection of cardiac arrests.

Once a cardiac arrest is identified, dispatchers can then give CPR instructions to a bystander over the phone until further help arrives. Telephone instructions have been shown to increase the rates of bystander CPR[35] and enhance outcomes.[29] A simulation study showed that a lay volunteer, without any training in CPR, can do compressions just as well with phone instructions as a previously trained person without directions. This finding is easily extrapolated into the real world because some compressions are better than no compressions. Only 2% of witnesses to a cardiac arrest refuse to do CPR.[30] When receiving instructions, directions to put the phone down during chest compressions do not improve CPR quality.[36] With the advent of widespread cell phones, there is ongoing research using video calls to help dispatchers aid bystanders in CPR instructions.[37]

Studies have also shown that the time to initiation of chest compressions is more rapid if the caller is given hands-only instructions (ie, no rescue breaths) rather than standard CPR instructions.[38] Given the possibility that hands-only CPR could improve outcomes, 2 recent articles in the *New England Journal of Medicine* compared the new technique to standard CPR with ventilations. In one study, there was a trend, although not statistically significant, toward increased rates of survival to hospital discharge with hands-only CPR in the subgroups with a cardiac cause of OHCA (15.5% vs 12.3%, $P = .09$) and with a shockable rhythm (31.9% vs 25.7%, $P = .09$).[39] Another study reported a slightly more positive trend to hospital discharge (19.1% vs 14.7%, $P = .16$) but no change in 30-day mortality (8.7% vs 7.0%, $P = .26$).[40] With no apparent harm and possible benefit in providing hands-only CPR instructions, recently released American Heart Association guidelines call for compression-only CPR in the initial management of cardiac arrest. This recommendation is particularly relevant to dispatcher phone instructions because of the relative ease of remotely guiding someone through compression-only CPR.

As time to first defibrillation has been shown to positively affect outcomes in OHCA, a variety of methods have been developed to increase the speed with which someone in a shockable rhythm is defibrillated. The development of AEDs has given the lay public access to easy-to-use lifesaving interventions. AEDs have been widely placed in strategic locations, including public locations to facilitate more rapid defibrillation of the cardiac arrest patient. In addition, law enforcement officers, firefighters, and other first responders in many communities carry AEDs. Approximately 80% of police departments are used as first responders to medical events; of these law enforcement first responders, 39% carry AEDs. In general, 31% of police departments carry AEDs.[41]

High-quality uninterrupted chest compressions have been correlated with increased survival rates. Various devices have been created to increase the quality of compressions. Pressure-sensing devices placed between the chest and a provider's hands give real-time feedback to improve the quality of compressions. Mechanical devices that replace EMS providers may give more consistent compressions and free providers for other tasks in the resuscitation process.

Another innovation in methods of CPR is the concept of cardiocerebral resuscitation (CCR). CCR aims to improve outcomes through refocusing certain interventions in CPR to maximize myocardial and cerebral perfusion. In CCR, chest compressions are started immediately and continued for 200 continuous compressions. During this time, oxygen is given via a noninvasive airway (ie, no endotracheal intubation), and defibrillator pads are placed on the patient. The rhythm is analyzed, and, when appropriate, a shock is given followed immediately by another interval of 200 compressions without pulse check. Epinephrine is given early, and endotracheal intubation is delayed until after 3 rounds of chest compressions are completed.[42] Some have modified CCR by intubating earlier if the initial rhythm is not shockable.[43] Although much research is still underway regarding CCR, the early data is favorable. One study designed as a before-and-after intervention introducing CCR into an EMS system while all other factors remained constant reported that the rate of those who survived to discharge increased (47% vs 20%; P = not reported) and the total number of patients neurologically intact (39% vs 15%; P = not reported) increased.[44] Another study reported that the overall adjusted odds ratio of survival for CCR was 3.1 (95% CI, 1.96–4.76), with some age ranges improving more than others. All age ranges except for 70 to 79 years reached significance in their confidence intervals.[45] When the first 3 years of this data was presented in percentages, CCR showed a survival to hospital discharge increase of 5.4% versus 1.8% (P = not reported).[42] Despite much promise, this new method of CPR requires further ongoing study.

When ROSC occurs, it is vital to transport the patient to the most appropriate hospital rapidly. However, transport provides its own pitfalls to a pulseless patient still undergoing active resuscitation. Although compression quality en-route was equivalent in one study, hands-off time increased during transport when compared with on-scene resuscitation.[44] Another study showed that the efficiency of chest compressions, relative to being on scene, were 95% in a moving ambulance and 86% in a helicopter.[46] The rate and quality of chest compressions have been shown to increase as the speed of an ambulance increased.[47] Use of lights and sirens en-route to a hospital saved a mean of 2.62 minutes, yet only 4.5% of patients received time-critical interventions, none of which occurred during the specific time saved.[48] Given the risk of priority EMS transport to both providers and the public, consideration should be given to mitigate the use of lights as sirens unless absolutely necessary because minimal benefit has been shown by doing so. Longer transport times were not associated with increased survival, thereby calling for more research into bypassing smaller hospitals and taking patients directly to a regionally designated resuscitation hospital[49,50]; this issue is being thoroughly reviewed at this time with conflicting evidence noted for and against such transportation strategies. At present, patients who have undergone resuscitation are often taken to the closest hospital, stabilized, and then transferred to a larger more-specialized hospital. For these interfacility transports, specialized critical care ground or air transport units are often used that include a combination of advanced EMS providers, critical care nurses, or physicians. These services can provide specialized care options such as vasoactive drug administration, blood product transfusions, intra-aortic balloon pumps, ventilator management, and so forth. Despite the criticality of the patients transported, rearrest occurs while being transported to a tertiary care facility in a minority of patients with cardiac arrest who have undergone resuscitation.[51]

For those patients with ROSC, studies using therapeutic hypothermia have been promising. The definitive studies were conducted in Europe and Australia with therapeutic hypothermia showing benefit for those patients presenting with ventricular fibrillation, who remained in a coma, and who did not have persistent hypotension while being cooled to the target range within 4 hours of ROSC.[52] The current American Heart Association consensus guidelines call for such patients to be cooled as soon as possible but within 4 hours of ROSC to a core body temperature between 32°C and 34°C. This cooling can be accomplished on-scene or en-route by cooling of the patient with 2 L of ice-cold normal saline or lactated Ringer solution. No studies to date have shown that initiation of cooling by EMS improves either hospital discharge rates or neurologic function compared with cooling after arrival in the ED.[53] Further study is needed in this regard.

SUMMARY

Despite research and advances in cardiac arrest resuscitation, outcomes have not changed appreciably in nearly 3 decades, remaining dismal in most areas of the United States.[16] With a renewed focus on maximizing each link in the chain of survival, short-term outcomes (eg, ROSC and survival to hospital admission) are slowly increasing. Education is making the public more knowledgeable and able to recognize and provide prompt attention to patients in whom OHCA occurs. Studies bear out that improvements in EMS dispatch, response times, and more rapid defibrillation times have had an impact, albeit small, producing better outcomes. Standardization and use of the Utstein criteria have allowed higher-quality research to be conducted on patients with OHCA. Continued advancement in ACLS care gives us the hope of further improving outcomes. Regardless, further study is needed in all aspects of OHCA treatments if we are to meaningfully improve survival of such patients. There is still opportunity to improve each link in the OHCA chain of survival.

REFERENCES

1. Swor RA, Compton S, Domeier R, et al. Delay prior to calling 9-1-1 is associated with increased mortality after out-of-hospital cardiac arrest. Prehosp Emerg Care 2008;12(3):333–8.
2. Herlitz J, Engdahl J, Svensson L, et al. A short delay from out of hospital cardiac arrest to call for ambulance increases survival. Eur Heart J 2003;24(19):1750–5.
3. Vukmir RB. Survival from prehospital cardiac arrest is critically dependent upon response time. Resuscitation 2006;69(2):229–34.
4. Leizorovicz A, Haugh MC, Mercier C, et al. Pre-hospital and hospital time delays in thrombolytic treatment in patients with suspected acute myocardial infarction. Analysis of data from the EMIP study. European Myocardial Infarction Project. Eur Heart J 1997;18(2):248–53.
5. Ottesen MM, Dixen U, Torp-Pedersen C, et al. Prehospital delay in acute coronary syndrome—an analysis of the components of delay. Int J Cardiol 2004;96(1):97–103.
6. Moser DK, McKinley S, Dracup K, et al. Gender differences in reasons patients delay in seeking treatment for acute myocardial infarction symptoms. Patient Educ Couns 2005;56(1):45–54.
7. Isaksson RM, Holmgren L, Lundblad D, et al. Time trends in symptoms and prehospital delay time in women vs. men with myocardial infarction over a 15-year period. The Northern Sweden MONICA Study. Eur J Cardiovasc Nurs 2008;7(2):152–8.

8. Rosamond W, Flegal K, Furie K, et al. Heart disease and stroke statistics—2008 update: report from the American Heart Association Statistics Committee and Strokes Statistics Subcommittee. Circulation 2008;117(4):e25–146.
9. Rea TD, Pearce RM, Raghunathan TE, et al. Incidence of out-of-hospital cardiac arrest. Am J Cardiol 2004;93(12):1455–60.
10. Muller JE. Circadian variation in cardiovascular events. Am J Hypertens 1999; 12(2 Pt 2):35S–42S.
11. Lindholm DJ, Campbell JP. Predicting survival from out-of-hospital cardiac arrest. Prehosp Disaster Med 1998;12(2–4):51–4.
12. Spaite D, Benoit R, Brown D, et al. Uniform prehospital data elements and definitions: a report from the uniform prehospital emergency medical services data conference. Ann Emerg Med 1995;25(4):525–34.
13. Nichol G, Stiell IG, Laupacis A, et al. A cumulative meta-analysis of the effectiveness of defibrillator-capable emergency medical services for victims of out-of-hospital cardiac arrest. Ann Emerg Med 1999;34(4 Pt 1):517–25.
14. Stiell IG, Wells GA, Field BJ, et al. Improved out-of-hospital cardiac arrest survival through the inexpensive optimization of an existing defibrillation program: OPALS study phase II. Ontario Prehospital Advanced Life Support. JAMA 1999;281(13): 1175–81.
15. Eisenburger P, Sterz F, Haugk M, et al. Cardiac arrest in public locations—an independent predictor for better outcome? Resuscitation 2006;70(3):395–403.
16. Sasson C, Rogers MA, Dahl J, et al. Predictors of survival from out-of-hospital cardiac arrest: a systematic review and meta-analysis. Circ Cardiovasc Qual Outcomes 2010;3(1):63–81.
17. Liu JM, Yang Q, Pirrallo RG, et al. Hospital variability of out-of-hospital cardiac arrest survival. Prehosp Emerg Care 2008;12(3):339–46.
18. Lund-Kordahl I, Olasveengen TM, Lorem T, et al. Improving outcome after out-of-hospital cardiac arrest by strengthening weak links of the local Chain of Survival; quality of advanced life support and post-resuscitation care. Resuscitation 2010; 81(4):422–6.
19. Hostler D, Thomas EG, Emerson SS, et al. Increased survival after EMS witnessed cardiac arrest. Observations from the Resuscitation Outcomes Consortium (ROC) Epistry-Cardiac arrest. Resuscitation 2010;81(7):826–30.
20. Stiell IG, Wells GA, DeMaio VJ, et al. Modifiable factors associated with improved cardiac arrest survival in a multicenter basic life support/defibrillation system: OPALS Study Phase I results. Ontario Prehospital Advanced Life Support. Ann Emerg Med 1999;33(1):44–50.
21. Stiell IG, Wells GA, Field B, et al. Advanced cardiac life support in out-of-hospital cardiac arrest. N Engl J Med 2004;351(7):647–56.
22. Olasveengen TM, Sunde K, Brunborg C, et al. Intravenous drug administration during out-of-hospital cardiac arrest: a randomized trial. JAMA 2009;302(20): 2222–9.
23. Kajino K, Iwami T, Daya M, et al. Impact of transport to critical care medical centers on outcomes after out-of-hospital cardiac arrest. Resuscitation 2010; 81(5):549–54.
24. Callaway CW, Schmicker R, Kampmeyer M, et al. Receiving hospital characteristics associated with survival after out-of-hospital cardiac arrest. Resuscitation 2010;81(5):524–9.
25. Pleskot M, Hazukova R, Stritecka H, et al. Long-term prognosis after out-of-hospital cardiac arrest with/without ST elevation myocardial infarction. Resuscitation 2009;80(7):795–804.

26. Morrison LJ, Verbeek PR, Zhan C, et al. Validation of a universal prehospital termination of resuscitation clinical prediction rule for advanced and basic life support providers. Resuscitation 2009;80(3):324–8.
27. Morrison LJ, Visentin LM, Kiss A, et al. Validation of a rule for termination of resuscitation in out-of-hospital cardiac arrest. N Engl J Med 2006;355(5):478–87.
28. Ruygrok ML, Byyny RL, Haukoos JS, et al. Validation of 3 termination of resuscitation criteria for good neurologic survival after out-of-hospital cardiac arrest. Ann Emerg Med 2009;54(2):239–47.
29. Kuisma M, Boyd J, Vayrynen T, et al. Emergency call processing and survival from out-of-hospital ventricular fibrillation. Resuscitation 2005;67(1):89–93.
30. Bohm K, Rosenqvist M, Hollenberg J, et al. Dispatcher-assisted telephone-guided cardiopulmonary resuscitation: an underused lifesaving system. Eur J Emerg Med 2007;14(5):256–9.
31. Roppolo LP, Westfall A, Pepe PE, et al. Dispatcher assessments for agonal breathing improve detection of cardiac arrest. Resuscitation 2009;80(7):769–72.
32. Bohm K, Stalhandske B, Rosenqvist M, et al. Tuition of emergency medical dispatchers in the recognition of agonal respiration increases the use of telephone assisted CPR. Resuscitation 2009;80(9):1025–8.
33. Flynn J, Archer F, Morgans A. Sensitivity and specificity of the medical priority dispatch system in detecting cardiac arrest emergency calls in Melbourne. Prehosp Disaster Med 2006;21(2):72–6.
34. Heward A, Damiani M, Hartley-Sharpe C. Does the use of the advanced medical priority dispatch system affect cardiac arrest detection? Emerg Med J 2004;21(1):115–8.
35. Vaillancourt C, Verma A, Trickett J, et al. Evaluating the effectiveness of dispatch-assisted cardiopulmonary resuscitation instructions. Acad Emerg Med 2007;14(10):877–83.
36. Brown TB, Saini D, Pepper T, et al. Instructions to "put the phone down" do not improve the quality of bystander initiated dispatcher-assisted cardiopulmonary resuscitation. Resuscitation 2008;76(2):249–55.
37. Johnsen E, Bolle SR. To see or not to see—better dispatcher-assisted CPR with video-calls? A qualitative study based on simulated trials. Resuscitation 2008;78(3):320–6.
38. Dorph E, Wik L, Steen PA. Dispatcher-assisted cardiopulmonary resuscitation. An evaluation of efficacy amongst elderly. Resuscitation 2003;56(3):265–73.
39. Rea TD, Fahrenbruch C, Culley L, et al. CPR with chest compression alone or with rescue breathing. N Engl J Med 2010;363(5):423–33.
40. Svensson L, Bohm K, Castren M, et al. Compression-only CPR or standard CPR in out-of-hospital cardiac arrest. N Engl J Med 2010;363(5):434–42.
41. Hawkins SC, Shapiro AH, Sever AE, et al. The role of law enforcement agencies in out-of-hospital emergency care. Resuscitation 2007;72(3):386–93.
42. Bobrow BJ, Clark LL, Ewy GA, et al. Minimally interrupted cardiac resuscitation by emergency medical services for out-of-hospital cardiac arrest. JAMA 2008;299(10):1158–65.
43. Kellum MJ, Kennedy KW, Barney R, et al. Cardiocerebral resuscitation improves neurologically intact survival of patients with out-of-hospital cardiac arrest. Ann Emerg Med 2008;52(3):244–52.
44. Olasveengen TM, Wik L, Steen PA. Quality of cardiopulmonary resuscitation before and during transport in out-of-hospital cardiac arrest. Resuscitation 2008;76(2):185–90.

45. Mosier J, Itty A, Sanders A, et al. Cardiocerebral resuscitation is associated with improved survival and neurologic outcome from out-of-hospital cardiac arrest in elders. Acad Emerg Med 2010;17(3):269–75.
46. Havel C, Schreiber W, Trimmel H, et al. Quality of closed chest compression on a manikin in ambulance vehicles and flying helicopters with a real time automated feedback. Resuscitation 2010;81(1):59–64.
47. Chung TN, Kim SW, Cho YS, et al. Effect of vehicle speed on the quality of closed-chest compression during ambulance transport. Resuscitation 2010;81(7):841–7.
48. Marques-Baptista A, Ohman-Strickland P, Baldino KT, et al. Utilization of warning lights and siren based on hospital time-critical interventions. Prehosp Disaster Med 2010;25(4):335–9.
49. Spaite DW, Bobrow BJ, Vadeboncoeur TF, et al. The impact of prehospital transport interval on survival in out-of-hospital cardiac arrest: implications for regionalization of post-resuscitation care. Resuscitation 2008;79(1):61–6.
50. Spaite DW, Stiell IG, Bobrow BJ, et al. Effect of transport interval on out-of-hospital cardiac arrest survival in the OPALS study: implications for triaging patients to specialized cardiac arrest centers. Ann Emerg Med 2009;54(2): 248–55.
51. Hartke A, Mumma BE, Rittenberger JC, et al. Incidence of re-arrest and critical events during prolonged transport of post-cardiac arrest patients. Resuscitation 2010;81(8):938–42.
52. Nolan JP, Morley T, Vanden Hoek TL, et al. Therapeutic hypothermia after cardiac arrest. Circulation 2003;108:118–21.
53. Bernard SA, Smith K, Cameron P, et al. Induction of therapeutic hypothermia by paramedics after resuscitation from out-of-hospital ventricular fibrillation cardiac arrest: a randomized controlled trial. Circulation 2010;122(7):737–42.

In-Hospital Cardiac Arrest

Peter P. Monteleone, MD[a],*, Christine M. Lin, MD[b]

KEYWORDS

- Sudden cardiac arrest • Hospital
- In-hospital sudden cardiac arrest
- Cardiopulmonary resuscitation

Cardiopulmonary resuscitation (CPR) developed in different environments from the inpatient setting; out-of-hospital medical and traumatic cardiac arrest victims are different from patients hospitalized with cardiac arrests, but much of the early literature focused on these outpatients.[1–5] Resuscitation was often targeted at select populations and implemented with only specific tools and interventions. As an often-cited 1985 JAMA editorial stated, "In some ways we have wandered from treating sudden expected death to practicing universal resuscitation."[6] As resuscitation has grown and developed over decades, the patients treated, and the processes used, have grown more complex. This complexity is shown in in-hospital sudden cardiac arrest (IHSCA), because revolutions in modern medical practice have provided more advanced means of treating cardiopulmonary arrest and have led to the survival of more ill, more complicated, and more rigorously analyzed patients.

DEMOGRAPHICS

Epidemiologic analysis of sudden cardiac death is challenging. In the out-of-hospital arena, the challenges of data derived from death-certificates, lack of rescuer experience in diagnosis, and lack of access to pre-event and postevent data are obvious. However, when cardiac arrest occurs in the hospital, periarrest monitoring makes epidemiologic analysis more straightforward. However, the many distinct hospital types, patient presentations, and types of periarrest care further complicate this analysis for the inpatient.

Consider also the variable definition of sudden cardiac arrest (SCA) itself. Is SCA defined as pulselessness developed within 2 hours of development of symptoms leading to arrest? Twenty-four hours? What of the patient in long-term intensive care who requires increasing doses of vasoactive medications and who develops

a Department of Medicine, University of Virginia, PO Box 800136, Charlottesville, VA 22908-0136, USA
b Department of Medicine, University of Virginia, Charlottesville, VA 22908, USA
* Corresponding author.
E-mail address: ppm4u@Virginia.EDU

Emerg Med Clin N Am 30 (2012) 25–34
doi:10.1016/j.emc.2011.09.005
0733-8627/12/$ – see front matter © 2012 Published by Elsevier Inc.

pulselessness requiring CPR; is this patient experiencing SCA? Different studies have included many different definitions ranging from patients being pulseless and apneic to patients for whom a cardiac arrest form was filled out.[7] Thus, the hospital-based definition of SCA has many variables.

A annual rate of 370,000 and 750,000 in-hospital resuscitation attempts performed in the United States is often cited in the literature.[8,9] Although quoted frequently, this number appears first as a contractor estimate provided in 1987,[10] which highlights the paucity of reliable data in the epidemiology of IHSCA. In 2003, the National Registry of Cardiopulmonary Resuscitation (NRCPR) was developed as an American Heart Association–sponsored, prospective, multisite observational study of in-hospital cardiac arrest (IHCA).[11] Analysis of this dataset in 2003 reported an incidence of 0.17 (±0.09) cardiac arrest events per bed per year. This rate did not vary significantly between teaching (0.17) and nonteaching hospitals.

As of most recent analysis, in March 2010, the NRCPR has documented 49,130 pulseless cardiac arrests in all patients, visitors, employees, and staff within 366 facilities (including ambulatory care areas).[12] They included in their analyses all patients developing pulseless events warranting CPR. Mean duration of hospitalization before an event was 151.9 hours; 31.9% (15,675) of patients had the event within 24 hours of admission; and 23% (11,440) of patients experienced the event greater than 1 week after hospitalization.

In this dataset, most IHSCA were experienced in men (57.5%) who were white (69%). Mean age was 66.7 years, which does not mean that white men are at highest risk of cardiac arrest, but only that, in the study population, IHSCA was more common in this population (potentially because these white male patients at higher risk of cardiac arrest were more likely to be hospitalized at the time of arrest). Forty-seven percent (23,337) of IHSCAs occurred in intensive care units (ICUs), 2.3% (1117) in the postanesthetic care unit/operating room, 33.9% (16,636) in general inpatient areas, 10.7% (5254) in emergency departments, and 4% (1951) in diagnostic intervention areas. Ninety-two percent (45,216) of arrest events occurred in patients who had experienced a prior arrest. Patients in this analysis were often heavily monitored at the time of IHSCA. Seventy-seven percent (38,180) had telemetric monitoring in place at the time of arrest, 58.1% (28,529) had pulse oximetry monitoring, 8.4% (4133) had intra-arterial catheter monitoring, and 5.0% (2428) had a pulmonary artery catheter in place.

This analysis also shows the complexity of the IHSCA population. Thirty-one percent (15,170) of patients in the analysis had an invasive airway in place at the time of arrest; 24.9% (12,221) of the patients were on vasoactive medications; 24% (11,904) of patients carried a diagnosis of heart failure; 42.5% (20,854) of patients had respiratory insufficiency requiring oxygen supplementation; 32% (15,963) of patients had renal insufficiency; and 13.1% (6,429) of patients had documented evidence of infection. Despite the algorithmic foundation of treatments of OOHSCA and IHSCA being the same, the two populations are different and the phenomenon of IHSCA and the treatment of the in-hospital SCA patient must be approached accordingly.

PATHOPHYSIOLOGY

Patients admitted to a hospital often suffer from multiorgan injury or multiorgan failure, so the pathophysiology of IHSCA in these patients can be extremely complicated. The frequency of severe pulmonary disease in admitted patients frequently leads to a primary pulmonary cause of SCA that is not frequently seen in OOHSCA. A large British trial characterized 11% of IHSCA as primary respiratory, 56% primary cardiac, and 18% combined.[13] In these patients, hypoxia or hypercarbia secondary to pulmonary failure precipitated cardiac arrest rather than it being a primary cardiac event. This pathophysiology is important because, in addition to acute cardiac life support being provided, urgent work must also be done to correct the underlying pulmonary pathophysiology to address the underlying respiratory process. Short of pulmonary embolism and drowning victims, this primary respiratory cause of SCA is seen less frequently in the OOHSCA population.

Even when the cause of SCA is primarily cardiac, the pathophysiology of IHSCA can be complex secondary to the multiorgan dysfunction of many inpatients. In OOHSCA, approximately 70% of primary cardiac arrest is thought to be secondary to coronary heart disease.[14] This percentage is an imperfect statistic secondary to the inability to perfectly characterize cause of death in this patient population. Nonetheless, it shows that a large percentage of OOHSCA is secondary to myocardial ischemia. Trauma, primary dysrhythmia, and pulmonary embolism make up a large portion of the other causes of OOHSCA.

In IHSCA, the frequency of multiorgan dysfunction in the inpatient population raises a multitude of other possible causes. The distinct pathophysiologies of cardiac arrest includes the dysrhythmia of pulseless ventricular tachycardia (VT) and ventricular fibrillation (VF), the complete electrical failure of asystole, and the electromechanical dissociation of pulseless electrical activity. In IHSCA, ventricular ectopy can be precipitated iatrogenically by medications or therapies, by renal dysfunction and electrolyte disarray, by hypoxia or hypoglycemia and myocyte irritability, by the catecholaminergic state of sepsis, and so forth. Asystole can represent the end state of any of these conditions or result from overwhelming insult to the cardiac conduction system. Electromechanical dissociation can be precipitated by pulmonary embolism, massive myocardial infarction, progressive severe heart failure, metabolic disarray, and so forth.

These variable comorbid conditions in individuals experiencing IHSCA are extremely common. Shown repeatedly in series analyzing IHSCA, including the NRCPR dataset as well as recent work assessing IHSCA defibrillation, are rates of respiratory insufficiency approaching 36%, renal insufficiency approaching 33%, hepatic insufficiency 7%, metabolic derangement 17%, diabetes mellitus 33%, acute stroke 4%, sepsis 11%, and malignancy 10%. This high rate of comorbidity shows the complex population of IHSCA victims.[4,12]

PREDICTION

As discussed later, the mortality and morbidity of IHSCA is extremely high. In the IHSCA population, the opportunity for intensive evaluation exists before an arrest occurs. A major goal is thus to predict which admitted patients will experience IHSCA so therapy can be designed to prevent it. As shown by data on inpatient telemetry use, physicians are not good at predicting which inpatients will arrest. One large study in a 5-year period at a tertiary care Toronto hospital showed that only 20 ISCHAs occurred in telemetrically monitored patients of the 367 cardiac arrests that occurred in 357 patients.[15] Although this dataset is imperfect evidence that the 95% of non–telemetrically monitored patients with IHSCA were not predicted to be at high risk of IHSCA, it nonetheless shows that there is room for improvement for health care personnel in predicting which patients are at highest risk of IHSCA. Furthermore, among certain populations (most notably women), the classic predictors of risk for SCA (coronary disease, structural heart disease, and so forth) may be even less reliable for prediction.[16]

Furthermore, improved prediction of mortality resulting from IHSCA would not only allow for therapeutic efforts in prevention but also in death planning when limited therapeutic options exist. The therapeutic as well as social benefit of improved mortality prediction for both patients and patients' families would thus be enormous. However, IHSCA mortality predictions based on clinical gestalt are no better than chance alone.[17] Multiple attempts at using multivariate analysis to develop prediction models for mortality resulting from IHSCA have thus been developed. Perhaps the most robust grew from the NRCPR dataset.[12] This work showed that advanced age, black race, noncardiac/nonsurgical illness, preexisting malignancy, acute stroke, trauma, septicemia, hepatic insufficiency, patient location on a general floor or in the emergency department, and prearrest use of vasopressors or assisted/mechanical ventilation were independently predictive of in-hospital mortality. It also showed that cardiac monitoring and shockable initial pulseless rhythms were strongly associated with survival.

In general, the duration of arrest, primary rhythm, time to CPR/resuscitation, and primary mode of arrest (respiratory vs cardiac) are the key factors that have repeatedly been shown to influence survival after inpatient hospital cardiac arrests.[18] The van Walraven criteria for predicting patients unlikely to be discharged from hospital after cardiopulmonary arrest were unwitnessed arrest, initial rhythm other than VF/VT, and duration of resuscitation of more than 10 minutes.[19] This collection of clinical features has been shown in smaller institutional studies as well.[20,21] However, the most commonly cited score for predicting survival is the prearrest morbidity index,[22] which lists hypotension, renal insufficiency, and age as the greatest risk factors for poor outcome.[22] In contrast, a retrospective chart review by Dancui and colleagues[23] showed that length of hospitalization before the arrest event as well as increased body mass index (BMI) were significantly correlated with survival. For patients in that study, renal insufficiency was associated with better outcome, which was thought to be secondary to electrolyte abnormalities being recognized sooner with appropriate interventions made in a timely manner; a rapidly identified and correctable cause. However, clinicians are unable to reliably predict which individuals are likely to have a favorable outcome in a postarrest situation.

PRESENTATION

With thorough evaluation and monitoring of inpatients, as well as with the performance of frequent assessments by nurses, physicians, and medical assistants, the ways in which IHSCA is discovered are variable. In the NRCPR dataset, the onset of the IHSCA was witnessed in 79.2% of instances. Pulselessness at the time of the need for CPR being established was present 90.7% of the time and thus almost 10% of the time a pulse was being assessed at the time of development of pulselessness.[12]

Equally interesting is the time of cardiac arrest occurrence during hospitalization. The NRCPR dataset shows that approximately 32% of events occurred within 24 hours of admission, 34% of events occurred within 1 week of admission, and 23% occurred more than 1 week after admission.[12] This distribution of arrest occurrence shows how variable the presentation of IHSCA can be, from the acute arrest of the newly admitted patient about whom little is known and to whom little intervention has been performed, to the patient in long-term admission who has often undergone a multitude of tests and interventions and has nonetheless suffered IHSCA. This fact alone speaks to the wide variety of IHSCA.

With the use of inpatient telemetry, electrophysiologic change precipitating arrest can cause an alert even if the patient is alone. However, the question often arises about how useful telemetric monitoring is toward early identification, and thus treatment, of IHSCA. Schull and Redelmeier[15] assessed the impact of telemetric monitoring on mortality. Of 8932 patients admitted to telemetrically monitored inpatient beds over 5 years, 20 suffered cardiac arrest. Of those arrests, only 56% of the patients monitored by electrocardiogram were recognized from abnormal signaling by the monitor. Of arresting patients, 3 survived to discharge; only 2 of these survivors had monitor-signaled events. Among all 8932 patients evaluated, approximately 1 in 5000 were survivors of monitor-noted cardiac arrests. This finding suggests that physicians are not accurate at predicting who will arrest and thus who should have telemetric monitoring. It also suggests that, despite the use of telemetry monitoring, such surveillance often does not rapidly identify IHSCA. In addition, when telemetry does detect the onset of IHSCA, it does not seem to favorably affect mortality. Thus, although inpatient telemetry may be useful for many elements of medical care, it does not seem to play an important role in identification and treatment of IHSCA, or affect its outcome.

Regarding the electrocardiographic rhythm in which IHSCA presents, in the NRCPR dataset, the first documented rhythm in patients with IHCA was asystole in 36.2% (17,772), pulseless electrical activity (PEA) in 33.4% (16,409), VF in 13.5% (6633), and pulseless VT in 8.5% (4198); the rhythm was not documented in 8.4% (4110) of cases.[12] Thus, in this broad analysis, 22% (10,831) of patients presented with pulseless VT or VF (ie, a rhythm warranting defibrillation). This trend has also been shown in several smaller studies.[23,24] Recent analysis of OOHSCA initial rhythms found that 26% (3336 of 12,930 patients) were found to have an initial rhythm of VF or pulseless VT.[25]

RESPONSE SYSTEMS AND PROCESS

In any given institution, sudden and unexpected cardiopulmonary arrests are managed by health care teams, rather than individual health care workers. Hospitals can be thought of as contained emergency response systems, where the chain of survival that is critical to out-of-hospital arrests can be applied to an inpatient setting. In hospitals, cardiac arrest is a common event, with some variation resulting from the various institutions' particular inpatient populations. In general, inpatient cardiac arrests seem to be more associated with progressive respiratory failure, circulatory shock, or both, rather than an acute coronary event or myocardial ischemia.[26] In out-of-hospital arrests, citizen CPR and early defibrillation have been consistently shown as the most effective interventions to increase survival.[27] However, as detailed later, arrests that take place in the in-hospital setting have their own unique challenges to overcome. Despite modern CPR having existed for more than 40 years, the overall survival rate from in-hospital arrests remains poor. Although approximately 45% to 50% of those who suffer an arrest have return of spontaneous circulation (ROSC),[11] combined studies in more than 40,000 patients show a survival rate to discharge of only approximately 15%.[11,23]

Cardiac arrest teams (CATs) often comprise trained medical, nursing, and respiratory therapy staff. Depending on the location (teaching vs urban or rural/community hospitals), both the physician and ancillary staff can be highly variable. Some institutions require that the CAT comprise individuals trained and continually recertified in advance cardiac life support (ACLS) at regular intervals; other institutions only require basic life support (BLS) knowledge for team members. Even the physical structure of an institution can affect the structure of the CAT; if an institution has multiple buildings, the CAT leader may be the one who mainly practices in an outpatient setting.[28] In addition, rural hospitals may not have equipment or medication readily available (eg, automated external defibrillator/defibrillator) that may be needed in a cardiopulmonary arrest.[20] In these situations, the arrest often more closely follows an out-of-hospital scenario than a true IHCA.

Because teaching hospitals comprise a large number of institutions and serve a large patient population, trainees (resident physicians) with varying levels of medical or surgical knowledge often function as team leaders on CATs. Leadership, team management, and resource allocation are key components when managing high-risk situations such as cardiopulmonary arrest.[29] However, a recent survey of internal medicine residents has shown that almost half (48%) thought that standard training was inadequate to effectively lead a CAT.[30] In addition, ACLS training focuses on algorithms, not team management. The same survey reported that postevent feedback was rare; qualitative studies have shown that postevent debriefing allows residents to focus and reflect on items that may have led to improved performance[30,31] with better rates of ROSC in patients. However, when teams incorporate real-time audiovisual feedback, quality of CPR and time to ROSC improved.[32] In addition, during a cardiac arrest, rhythm interpretation is often done by the physician leader; however, the likelihood of an inappropriate shock is greater when performed manually and the proportion of inappropriate manual shocks was higher for resident physicians in IHCAs than for paramedics in out-of-hospital cardiac arrests.[32]

Even within nonteaching institutions, there is a wide variability in physician leadership. A simulation study has shown that, comparing teams led by general practitioners versus hospitalists, general practitioners showed a significant difference in the time to defibrillation and administration of the first dose of epinephrine, and had lower compression rates than those who primarily worked in a hospital setting.[33] Overall, it seems that experience is a key factor, as shown by a study that showed that inexperienced providers (those who experienced <5 cardiac arrests events per year) who were CAT leaders were less likely to have ROSC or have the patient survive until discharge.[28]

It is also recognized that, even if a dedicated CAT exists within an institution, such teams are usually not immediately available and most medical emergencies must be managed by ad-hoc teams. It has been postulated that survival after inpatient cardiac arrests depends more on first responders (as in the community) than on CATs,[34] which, in turn, affects outcomes because, compared with preformed teams (in which members are familiar with and work with one another), ad-hoc teams had less hands-on CPR time in the first 3 minutes of an event and delayed their first defibrillation with a shockable rhythm,[33] which are the 2 variables that have been proved to improve mortality in out-of-hospital arrest situations. In addition, after-hours cardiac arrests (evening and weekends) are associated with twice the mortality of office-hour arrests, which is thought to be a result of both the availability and the experience of staff.[35]

In recent years, several institutions have developed a pre–cardiac arrest team, or a rapid response team (RRT). An RRT is typically a multidisciplinary team of medical, nursing, and respiratory staff charged with the prompt evaluation, triage, and treatment of patients with signs of clinical deterioration who are not currently being treated in an ICU. The development of RRTs (see the article by McCURDY and colleagues elsewhere in this issue for further exploration of this topic) has grown and reflects an increasing interest in hospital quality outcomes. Launched in 2006, the Institute for Healthcare Improvement's 100,000 Lives Campaign has recommended that hospitals implement RRTs as a possible strategy to reduce preventable in-hospital deaths.[36] However, despite widespread adoption, the results of studies examining RRTs and their effect on patient outcomes and mortality are contradictory. Some studies indicate that the presence of RRTs decreases the activation of CATs, but not the incidence of cardiac arrest events, unplanned ICU admissions, or unexpected deaths.[37] A recent meta-analysis performed in 2010 looked at 18 studies that involved nearly 1.3 million hospital admissions; implementation of an RRT was associated with a 33.8% reduction in the rate of cardiopulmonary arrest outside the ICU but was not associated with a lower mortality. In the past decade, the effect of RRT implementation on hospital mortality has shifted toward the null,[38] suggesting that there may have been early bias in the literature toward the benefit of these teams. Also, although RRT intervention may prevent cases of cardiopulmonary arrest, it may only represent a short-term impact in these severely ill patients and not affect long-term mortality. However, respiratory failure and hemodynamic instability (which are often triggers for RRTs) should be recognized by CAT team members as common antecedents to IHCAs.

OUTCOMES

Multiple studies have shown institutional variation in survival after inpatient cardiac arrest.[39,40] The literature has consistently shown a high mortality (60%–70%)[41–43] of IHCA, although it has been shown to be lower in urban, teaching, and large hospitals.[41,44] This difference in outcome is thought to be secondary to postarrest ICU care.

Nonetheless, the low survival rate to discharge is offset by most patients tending to have good neurologic recovery. In most studies of patients after arrest, the American Heart Association's Cerebral Performance Score (CPC) is often used to assess a patient's neurologic status. A CPC score of 1 corresponds with a normal life in which an individual is conscious and alert, but may have some minor psychological or neurologic deficits. A CPC score of 2 is also considered a good neurologic outcome, with which people can function in a sheltered environment and are able to perform independent activities of daily living (IADL). NRCPR data from approximately 14,000 patients has shown that most (86%) patients with a CPC score of 1 at the time of admission had a postarrest CPC score of 1 at the time of discharge.[11]

A later, prospective analysis of 36,902 patients showed that 73% had a good neurologic outcome with a CPC score of 1 or 2. In addition, a favorable neurologic outcome was significantly associated with interventions in place before arrest, witnessed/monitored status, time to defibrillation, and duration of CPR.[45] One small German study of 354 patients found that almost one-third of patients who had cardiac arrests and who survived to ICU admission were still alive 5 years after discharge.[46] Given the concerns about the rapidly aging population, a study of 956 patients at a United States teaching hospital showed that IHCAs in octogenarians had a similar discharge rate (11%),[47] suggesting that survival after an IHCA tends to have a favorable and sustained outcome in these patients.

SUMMARY

In 1960, in a landmark article published in the *Journal of the American Medical Association*, Kowenhoven and colleagues[48] wrote, "Cardiac resuscitation after cardiac arrest or ventricular fibrillation has been limited by the need for open thoracotomy and direct cardiac massage. As a result of exhaustive animal experimentation … immediate resuscitative measures can now be initiated to give … adequate cardiac massage without thoracotomy. Anyone, anywhere, can now initiate cardiac resuscitative procedures. All that is needed are two hands." Since that time, resuscitation, which was never originally recommended for all patients, has grown into a common medical treatment.

Resuscitation from IHSCA has grown increasingly complex as a result of medicine's ability to sustain very ill patients as well as the range of interventions available to the practitioner.

REFERENCES

1. Eftestol T, Sunde K, Steen PA. Effects of interrupting precordial compressions on the calculated probability of defibrillation success during out-of-hospital cardiac arrest. Circulation 2002;105(19):2270–3.

2. Andreka P, Frenneaux MP. Haemodynamics of cardiac arrest and resuscitation. Curr Opin Crit Care 2006;12(3):198–203.
3. Field JM, Hazinski MF, Sayre MR, et al. Part 1: Executive summary: 2010 American Heart Association guidelines for cardiopulmonary resuscitation and emergency cardiovascular care. Circulation 2010;122(18 Suppl 3):S640–56.
4. Chan PS, Krumholz HM, Nichol G, et al. Delayed time to defibrillation after in-hospital cardiac arrest. N Engl J Med 2008;358(1):9–17.
5. Cooper JA, Cooper JD, Cooper JM. Cardiopulmonary resuscitation: history, current practice, and future direction. Circulation 2006;114(25):2839–49.
6. Haynes BE, Niemann JT. Letting go: DNR orders in prehospital care. JAMA 1985; 254(4):532–3.
7. Ballew KA, Philbrick JT. Causes of variation in reported in-hospital CPR survival: a critical review. Resuscitation 1995;30(3):203–15.
8. Sandroni C, Nolan J, Cavallaro F, et al. In-hospital cardiac arrest: incidence, prognosis and possible measures to improve survival. Intensive Care Med 2007;33(2): 237–45.
9. Eisenberg MS, Mengert TJ. Cardiac resuscitation. N Engl J Med 2001;344(17): 1304–13.
10. US Congress, Office of Technology Assessment. Life-sustaining technologies and the elderly. 1987. p. 11.
11. Peberdy MA, Kaye W, Ornato JP, et al. Cardiopulmonary resuscitation of adults in the hospital: a report of 14720 cardiac arrests from the National Registry of Cardiopulmonary Resuscitation. Resuscitation 2003;58(3):297–308.
12. Larkin GL, Copes WS, Nathanson BH, et al. Pre-resuscitation factors associated with mortality in 49,130 cases of in-hospital cardiac arrest: a report from the National Registry for Cardiopulmonary Resuscitation. Resuscitation 2010;81(3): 302–11.
13. Tunstall-Pedoe H, Bailey L, Chamberlain DA, et al. Survey of 3765 cardiopulmonary resuscitations in British hospitals (the BRESUS study): Methods and overall results. BMJ 1992;304(6838):1347–51.
14. CDC. State-specific mortality from sudden cardiac death-1999. MMWR Morb Mortal Wkly Rep 2002;51:123–6.
15. Schull MJ, Redelmeier DA. Continuous electrocardiographic monitoring and cardiac arrest outcomes in 8,932 telemetry ward patients. Acad Emerg Med 2000;7(6):647–52.
16. Chugh SS, Uy-Evanado A, Teodorescu C, et al. Women have a lower prevalence of structural heart disease as a precursor to sudden cardiac arrest: The Ore-SUDS (Oregon Sudden Unexpected Death Study). J Am Coll Cardiol 2009; 54(22):2006–11.
17. Ebell MH, Bergus GR, Warbasse L, et al. The inability of physicians to predict the outcome of in-hospital resuscitation. J Gen Intern Med 1996;11(1):16–22.
18. Cooper S, Cade J. Predicting survival, in-hospital cardiac arrests: resuscitation survival variables and training effectiveness. Resuscitation 1997;35(1):17–22.
19. van Walraven C, Forster AJ, Parish DC, et al. Validation of a clinical decision aid to discontinue in-hospital cardiac arrest resuscitations. JAMA 2001;285(12): 1602–6.
20. Brindley PG, Markland DM, Mayers I, et al. Predictors of survival following in-hospital adult cardiopulmonary resuscitation. CMAJ 2002;167(4):343–8.
21. Sandroni C, Ferro G, Santangelo S, et al. In-hospital cardiac arrest: survival depends mainly on the effectiveness of the emergency response. Resuscitation 2004;62(3):291–7.

22. George AL Jr, Folk BP 3rd, Crecelius PL, et al. Pre-arrest morbidity and other correlates of survival after in-hospital cardiopulmonary arrest. Am J Med 1989; 87(1):28–34.
23. Danciu SC, Klein L, Hosseini MM, et al. A predictive model for survival after in-hospital cardiopulmonary arrest. Resuscitation 2004;62(1):35–42.
24. Aldawood A. The outcomes of patients admitted to the intensive care unit following cardiac arrest at a tertiary hospital in Saudi Arabia. Pol Arch Med Wewn 2007;117(11–12):497–501.
25. Weisfeldt ML, Everson-Stewart S, Sitlani C, et al. Ventricular tachyarrhythmias after cardiac arrest in public versus at home. N Engl J Med 2011;364(4):313–21.
26. Weil MH, Fries M. In-hospital cardiac arrest. Crit Care Med 2005;33(12):2825–30.
27. Stiell IG, Wells GA, Field B, et al. Advanced cardiac life support in out-of-hospital cardiac arrest. N Engl J Med 2004;351(7):647–56.
28. Hou SK, Chern CH, How CK, et al. Is ward experience in resuscitation effort related to the prognosis of unexpected cardiac arrest? J Chin Med Assoc 2007;70(9):385–91.
29. Lighthall GK, Barr J, Howard SK, et al. Use of a fully simulated intensive care unit environment for critical event management training for internal medicine residents. Crit Care Med 2003;31(10):2437–43.
30. Hayes CW, Rhee A, Detsky ME, et al. Residents feel unprepared and unsupervised as leaders of cardiac arrest teams in teaching hospitals: a survey of internal medicine residents. Crit Care Med 2007;35(7):1668–72.
31. O'Brien G, Haughton A, Flanagan B. Interns' perceptions of performance and confidence in participating in and managing simulated and real cardiac arrest situations. Med Teach 2001;23(4):389–95.
32. Edelson DP, Litzinger B, Arora V, et al. Improving in-hospital cardiac arrest process and outcomes with performance debriefing. Arch Intern Med 2008; 168(10):1063–9.
33. Hunziker S, Tschan F, Semmer NK, et al. Hands-on time during cardiopulmonary resuscitation is affected by the process of teambuilding: a prospective randomised simulator-based trial. BMC Emerg Med 2009;9:3.
34. Soar J, McKay U. A revised role for the hospital cardiac arrest team? Resuscitation 1998;38(3):145–9.
35. Herlitz J, Bang A, Alsen B, et al. Characteristics and outcome among patients suffering from in hospital cardiac arrest in relation to whether the arrest took place during office hours. Resuscitation 2002;53(2):127–33.
36. Berwick DM, Calkins DR, McCannon CJ, et al. The 100,000 lives campaign: setting a goal and a deadline for improving health care quality. JAMA 2006; 295(3):324–7.
37. Dichtwald S, Matot I, Einav S. Improving the outcome of in-hospital cardiac arrest: the importance of being EARNEST. Semin Cardiothorac Vasc Anesth 2009;13(1): 19–30.
38. Chan PS, Jain R, Nallmothu BK, et al. Rapid response teams: a systematic review and meta-analysis. Arch Intern Med 2010;170(1):18–26.
39. Ballew KA, Philbrick JT, Caven DE, et al. Differences in case definitions as a cause of variation in reported in-hospital CPR survival. J Gen Intern Med 1994;9(5):283–5.
40. Blackhall LJ, Ziogas A, Azen SP. Low survival rate after cardiopulmonary resuscitation in a county hospital. Arch Intern Med 1992;152(10):2045–8.
41. Carr BG, Goyal M, Band RA, et al. A national analysis of the relationship between hospital factors and post-cardiac arrest mortality. Intensive Care Med 2009;35(3): 505–11.

42. Keenan SP, Dodek P, Martin C, et al. Variation in length of intensive care unit stay after cardiac arrest: where you are is as important as who you are. Crit Care Med 2007;35(3):836–41.
43. Nolan JP, Laver SR, Welch CA, et al. Outcome following admission to UK intensive care units after cardiac arrest: a secondary analysis of the ICNARC case mix programme database. Anaesthesia 2007;62(12):1207–16.
44. Carr BG, Kahn JM, Merchant RM, et al. Inter-hospital variability in post-cardiac arrest mortality. Resuscitation 2009;80(1):30–4.
45. Nadkarni VM, Larkin GL, Peberdy MA, et al. First documented rhythm and clinical outcome from in-hospital cardiac arrest among children and adults. JAMA 2006; 295(1):50–7.
46. Graf J, Muhlhoff C, Doig GS, et al. Health care costs, long-term survival, and quality of life following intensive care unit admission after cardiac arrest. Crit Care 2008;12(4):R92.
47. Paniagua D, Lopez-Jimenez F, Londono JC, et al. Outcome and cost-effectiveness of cardiopulmonary resuscitation after in-hospital cardiac arrest in octogenarians. Cardiology 2002;97(1):6–11.
48. Kouwenhoven WB, Jude JR, Knickerbocker GG. Closed-chest cardiac massage. JAMA 1960;173:1064–7.

Cardiopulmonary Resuscitation Update

Joshua C. Reynolds, MD[a], Michael C. Bond, MD[b],*,
Sanober Shaikh, MD[a]

KEYWORDS

- Cardiopulmonary resuscitation • Cardiac arrest
- Chest compression

Based on extensive research into means of lowering the morbidity and mortality associated with cardiac arrest, the American Heart Association (AHA) drastically revised its guidelines for cardiopulmonary resuscitation (CPR) and emergency cardiovascular care in 2010. The AHA no longer recommends rescue breathing or pulse checks by untrained laypeople or, for trained responders, the interruption of chest compressions to check the victim's pulse. Instead, emphasis is placed on the delivery of high-quality chest compressions and early defibrillation. Even medications (eg, epinephrine and atropine) are no longer emphasized, because they have not been shown to improve outcomes. This article summarizes the AHA 2010 guidelines for CPR and emergency cardiovascular care with a discussion of the science supporting these recommendations; in certain instances, additional recommendations beyond that of the AHA are made (**Table 1**).

The old mantra of "A-B-C" (airway, breathing, and circulation) has been replaced by "C-A-B" (circulation, airway, and breathing). Delay in the start of chest compressions is minimized by placing circulation first. Individuals who are fearful of performing rescue breathing are more likely to start the resuscitation process if they only have to do chest compressions.[1] The "C" in "CAB" is further delineated by the four "Cs" of cardiac arrest care: (1) chest compressions; (2) cardioversion and defibrillation; (3) cooling (ie, postarrest therapeutic hypothermia); and (4) catheterization (ie, early catheterization for all patients who have had a cardiac arrest, regardless of whether ST segment elevation is evident on their electrocardiogram).

CIRCULATION

Circulation, specifically, high-quality chest compressions, is the most critical portion of CPR. Chest compressions augment the cardiocerebral circulation, and any interruption in them decreases the likelihood of favorable neurologic outcomes. Cardiocerebral

[a] Department of Emergency Medicine, University of Maryland Medical Center, Baltimore, MD, USA
[b] Department of Emergency Medicine, University of Maryland School of Medicine, Baltimore, MD, USA
* Corresponding author. 110 South Paca Street, Suite 200, 6th Floor, Baltimore, MD 21201.
E-mail address: mbond@smail.umaryland.edu

Emerg Med Clin N Am 30 (2012) 35–49
doi:10.1016/j.emc.2011.09.006
0733-8627/12/$ – see front matter © 2012 Elsevier Inc. All rights reserved.

emed.theclinics.com

Table 1
Major changes of the 2010 AHA cardiopulmonary resuscitation guidelines

BLS

Change	Explanation
No pulse checks	If the patient is unresponsive and has no breathing or abnormal breathing, chest compressions should be performed.
"ABC" becomes "CAB"	Circulation is to be addressed first with the initiation of chest compressions. Compression:ventilation ratio of 30:2 should be maintained after the first round of 30 chest compressions.
Push Hard, Push Fast (high-quality CPR is emphasized)	100 compressions/min at a depth of at least 2 inches.
Hands-only CPR for the untrained lay rescuer	Hands-only CPR is easier to perform for those with no training and eliminates the reluctance that individuals may have with rescue breathing.

ACLS

Should follow all of the BLS recommendations listed above.

Atropine removed from asystole/PEA	Atropine is no longer recommended for routine use in the management of asystole and PEA arrest.
End-tidal carbon dioxide monitoring of all intubated patients	A new Class 1 recommendation for all adults who are intubated is that they have continuous quantitative waveform capnography for confirmation and monitoring of endotracheal tube placement.
Cricoid pressure is no longer recommended for routine use	The routine use of cricoid pressure during the placement of an endotracheal tube is no longer recommended. Instead, it should be used only to improve visualization of the vocal cords.
Routine use of chronotropic drugs is recommended for bradycardia.	For symptomatic or unstable bradycardia, intravenous infusion of chronotropic drugs is now recommended as an equally effective alternative to external pacing when atropine is not effective.
Postresuscitation therapeutic hypothermia	Postcardiac arrest care in those who have not returned to a normal mental status should include the initiation of therapeutic hypothermia to optimize neurologic recovery.
Cardiac catheterization	Patients with return of spontaneous circulation should be considered for urgent cardiac catheterization regardless of whether there is ST-segment elevation on their postresuscitation electrocardiogram. In the field, patients suspected of having acute coronary syndrome should be transported to a facility with reperfusion capabilities.

resuscitation represents a comprehensive strategy to maximize circulation. It emphasizes chest compressions over ventilation in patients thought to have had an arrest from a cardiac cause.[2–5] In patients who have experienced a primary pulmonary arrest, rescue breathing should commence as soon as possible, but this scenario is not common in adults. Hyperventilation and pauses in compressions to administer rescue breathing impair cardiocerebral blood flow and are associated with increased morbidity and mortality rates (discussed later).[6]

Pulse Check

Assessment of circulation traditionally begins with a pulse check. For many years, emergency care providers have been trained to check for a carotid or femoral pulse, because those pulses are closest to the central circulation and should be palpable at lower arterial blood pressures. Even seasoned healthcare providers have difficulty reliably discerning the presence of a pulse,[7–16] and the search can become a lengthy process.[5,9,12] Laypersons are now instructed not to check for a pulse but to focus instead on evaluating the person for other signs of life. They should assume that a person is in cardiac arrest if he or she is unresponsive and breathing abnormally. Healthcare providers should spend a maximum of 10 seconds searching for a pulse; if a definitive and reliable pulse is not detected, they should begin chest compressions immediately.[17,18]

Compression Technique

Chest compressions restore partial circulation to the heart and brain by building up and maintaining coronary and cerebral perfusion pressure.[18,19] The perfusion of these two organs is critical to short-term and meaningful long-term survival. Chest compressions are deceptively difficult to deliver correctly,[5,20,21] but it is imperative that they be performed with the highest degree of perfection possible. The ideal components of effective chest compressions and alternative methods of delivering them are discussed next.

Proper positioning of the patient and rescuer is fundamental to proper compression delivery. The recommended position in out-of-hospital scenarios is to kneel perpendicular beside the patient's torso.[22] For in-hospital cardiac arrest response, the rescuer should stand beside the bed at the level of the patient's torso. Patients who have an in-hospital cardiac arrest are usually on a bed or stretcher, and the mattress absorbs a significant amount of the force delivered. Placing a firm backboard between the patient and the mattress minimizes this loss.[23–26] If possible, air-filled mattresses should be deflated before starting compressions.[27,28]

Place the heel of one hand on the lower half of the sternum, with the heel of the opposite hand over top of the first.[29–32] In adults, depress the sternum at least 2 inches[33–36] and allow proper recoil before the next compression. Compression time and recoil time should be equal, and the chest should re-expand completely before the next compression.[37–41] During the upstroke of compressions, the hands should be slightly removed from the chest wall. This technique helps ensure adequate recoil. Inadequate recoil results in higher intrathoracic pressure and an impaired hemodynamic profile (ie, decreased coronary perfusion pressure, cardiac index, myocardial blood flow, and cerebral perfusion).[39,42]

The recommended raw rate for compression delivery is at least 100 compressions per minute. Matlock demonstrated that singing, humming, or listening to the Bee Gees' song "Stayin' Alive" improved compliance with the 100-compressions-per-minute recommendation.[43] The total number of compressions per minute is a predictor of return of spontaneous circulation (ROSC) and neurologically intact survival.[44,45]

The best outcomes have been achieved in patients who received 68 to 89 compressions per minute after out-of-hospital arrest and at least 80 compressions per minute after in-hospital cardiac arrest.[44]

The recommended compression-to-ventilation ratio is based on expert consensus and one case series.[46–50] The general guideline is a ratio of 30:2 (compressions:ventilations) in adults.[51–56] If an advanced airway management device is in place, then two providers can perform a combination of uninterrupted compressions and intermittent ventilations. However, an advanced airway device should be inserted and used to provide ventilations only after the patient has received 2 to 3 minutes of chest compressions and attempted defibrillation, if appropriate.

Barriers to Delivering Effective Chest Compressions

Every effort should be made to minimize interruptions in chest compressions.[2,57–60] Interruptions are common and can consume 24% to 57% of the total resuscitation time.[5,20,21,44] Even a brief pause in compressions results in a dramatic drop-off in coronary and cerebral perfusion pressures.[61] Adequate coronary perfusion washes out inflammatory mediators and renews myocardial energy substrates. Chest compressions restore adequate coronary perfusion pressure, but they must be truly continuous if they are to reach a threshold for successful defibrillation and resuscitation.[62,63] Maintaining perfusion pressure to cerebral tissue is also vital because of the brain's extreme sensitivity to ischemic injury.

Typical advanced cardiac life support (ACLS) interventions result in numerous pauses in chest compressions. Advanced airway management accounts for almost 25% of all interruptions, with a median duration of almost 2 minutes.[64] Pulse checks should be limited to 10 seconds. Compressions should not be stopped to check the patient's pulse unless there is some other evidence of ROSC, such as an increase in the patient's oxygenation level, as measured by pulse oximetry or end tidal carbon dioxide ($EtCO_2$) measurement. Pokorna and colleagues[65] showed that individuals with ROSC had a mean increase of 10 mm Hg on $EtCO_2$ readings compared with cardiac arrest victims who did not survive ($P<.001$). Measuring $EtCO_2$ is an easy, noninvasive way to monitor for ROSC without the need to interrupt chest compressions.

Chest compressions should be continued through defibrillation or resumed immediately afterward without a postshock pulse check, because ROSC is not instantaneous, even after successful defibrillation.[2,57–60] Even the interruption in compressions while preparing for defibrillation results in a drop-off of coronary perfusion pressure, so every effort should be made to transition seamlessly into defibrillation.[61] Edelson and colleagues[66] reported that the traditional method of stopping compressions, analyzing the heart rhythm, charging the defibrillator, and then delivering the shock to the patient resulted in an average hands-off time of 14.8 seconds. When compressions were stopped only during the rhythm analysis and shock delivery, as recommended by the current AHA guidelines, the average hands-off time was 11.5 seconds. In accordance with the AHA guidelines, compressions were continued while the defibrillator was charging. However, if the defibrillator was charged in anticipation of shocking the patient, and then compressions were held for rhythm analysis and immediate shock delivery, the average hands-off time was only 3.9 seconds. This time could be further reduced if the providers immediately resumed compressions after rhythm analysis. Several studies have shown that it is completely safe for a rescuer wearing standard examination gloves to continue chest compressions during use of a biphasic defibrillator with self-adhesive pads.[67,68] Lloyd and colleagues[67] reported that the average and maximal current leakages were 280 and 900 μA, respectively, which are far less than the occupational and medical electrical safety standards for medical equipment. Yu and colleagues[68] demonstrated that these currents can be reduced further by the use of a resuscitation blanket. The fear of rescuers being shocked dates back to the use of older monophasic defibrillators; recent studies demonstrate that this risk is not present with the newer biphasic defibrillators.

Rescuer fatigue is another pitfall in delivering high-quality, continuous chest compressions. After just 1 minute of performing CPR, the depth of compressions is compromised. Rescuers tend not to recognize their own fatigue until after approximately 5 minutes of CPR.[69] A shallow depth not only fails to generate adequate coronary perfusion pressure but also leads to inadequate chest recoil. Incomplete recoil further compromises coronary perfusion pressure and adversely increases intrathoracic pressure.[40,70] Providers delivering chest compressions should rotate every 2 minutes to minimize the effects of rescuer fatigue, and the switch should take less than 5 seconds. One technique to minimize the interruption is to position a rescuer on either side of the patient for more seamless transitions.

Hands-only CPR

Minimizing interruptions in chest compressions is paramount to restoring circulation to the heart and brain. Hands-only CPR removes many of the barriers to delivering effective chest compressions.[71] The performance of hands-only CPR allows the rescuer to focus solely on compression technique. Ventilations are often not necessary during the first few minutes of resuscitation, because blood oxygen levels usually remain adequate for several minutes after a cardiac arrest from a nonrespiratory cause.[1] The acceptable duration is not known. Agonal gasping and chest wall recoil may provide some amount of passive ventilation and oxygenation during hands-only CPR.

This simplified version of conventional CPR is easier for laypersons, who are often reluctant to perform mouth-to-mouth resuscitation for fear of acquiring a communicable disease.[72,73] Hands-only CPR has better patient outcomes than no CPR and outcomes similar to those achieved with conventional CPR.[74–78]

Alternative CPR Techniques

Many alternative techniques of CPR have been documented in the literature, with mixed evidence of effectiveness. High-frequency chest compressions are delivered at a rate exceeding 120 per minute but are otherwise similar to conventional chest compressions.[79] Two clinical trials demonstrated improved hemodynamic profiles generated by rapid compressions but not improved patient outcome.[80,81] There is insufficient evidence to recommend the routine use of this technique.

Open-chest CPR with direct cardiac massage is typically used after cardiac arrest from a traumatic chest injury. Case series of open-chest CPR for nontraumatic cardiac arrest in inpatients after cardiac surgery[82–84] and out-of-hospital cardiac arrest[83–86] revealed improved coronary perfusion pressure and ROSC compared with conventional (closed-chest) CPR. There is insufficient evidence to recommend routine use of this technique, but it may be used if the chest is already open (ie, intraoperatively) or cardiac arrest occurs soon after thoracotomy or laporatomy.

Interposed abdominal compression (IAC) is another strategy that has been proposed to increase cardiocerebral perfusion. IAC requires three providers and involves alternating chest compressions with abdominal compressions.[85] The first provider performs conventional chest compressions, while the second compresses the abdomen with similar hand position and depth midway between the xiphoid process and umbilicus during chest wall recoil. The third provider delivers intermittent ventilation, typically via an advanced airway management device. IAC improves the diastolic aortic pressure and venous return, which results in higher coronary perfusion pressure. Two randomized controlled trials (by the same author) of in-hospital cardiac arrest demonstrated improved survival compared with conventional CPR,[86,87] but a randomized controlled trial of out-of-hospital cardiac arrest patients showed no benefit with this technique.[88] The only published complication of IAC CPR is traumatic pancreatitis in a child.[89] This technique could be considered for victims of in-hospital cardiac arrest if a sufficient number of trained providers are present. An external study to validate the findings of the two original studies is needed before this technique can be recommended for routine use.

A precordial thump is a forceful striking of the anterior chest wall, which is used to mechanically stun the myocardium to convert a ventricular tachyarrhythmia into a perfusable rhythm.[90] Case reports and case series demonstrate mixed effectiveness for this maneuver.[90–100] It has been associated with sternum fracture, osteomyelitis, stroke, and adverse arrhythmias.[98–100] The precordial thump technique is not recommended for unwitnessed cardiac arrests, but it may be considered for witnessed, monitored, unstable ventricular tachycardia (VT) if a defibrillator is not immediately available and if it does not delay conventional resuscitation.[1]

Percussion pacing, an extension of the precordial thump, is essentially rhythmic percussion of the chest wall with a fist to pace the myocardium. Several case reports and small case series have documented successful resuscitation with this technique, but there is insufficient evidence to support its routine use.[101–107]

DEFIBRILLATION

Early defibrillation is critical to survival after sudden cardiac arrest (SCA). The most frequent initial rhythm in out-of-hospital witnessed SCA is ventricular fibrillation (VF), and the chance of successful defibrillation diminishes rapidly over time.[108–110] ACLS protocols continue to stress the importance of early defibrillation for the unstable rhythms of VF and pulseless VT.[111]

CPR Before Defibrillation

The rate of survival-to-hospital discharge is higher among patients who experienced an unwitnessed SCA and received 1.5 to 3 minutes of CPR followed by defibrillation.[112,113] In witnessed SCA, early defibrillation is imperative; CPR should be performed while the defibrillator is being prepared. Chest compressions increase the myocardial readiness for the defibrillation by delivering oxygen and metabolic substrates.[20] Patients who receive early defibrillation have a higher likelihood of survival and of return to their prearrest quality of life.[114] Every minute that a patient remains in VF/pulseless VT arrest decreases the chance of survival by 10%.[115]

Hands-on Defibrillation

Minimizing interruptions during chest compressions improves the likelihood of ROSC. In the past, hands-off time during defibrillation was thought to be unavoidable, given the need to prevent electrocution of the rescuer during shock delivery. However, studies have affirmed that it is extremely safe to continue compressions during defibrillation when a biphasic defibrillator is used with self-adhesive electrodes and the rescuer wears standard examination gloves.[67,68] The simulated rescuers in these studies perceived no electrical charge, despite voltage delivery during the compressions. Therefore, uninterrupted manual chest compressions are feasible during shock delivery, without risk of harm to the rescuer. The AHA did not adopt this practice in the

2010 guidelines, but future iterations might recommend interruption of chest compressions solely for the purpose of rhythm analysis.

Pulse Check After Defibrillation

Compressions should be resumed immediately after defibrillation. The patient's rhythm and pulse should not be checked after defibrillation. Even if the patient is successfully converted out of VF/VT, the myocardium is probably stunned and unable to generate adequate perfusion pressures. The pulse and rhythm can be checked at the next 2-minute interval. Ideally, compressions should be continued throughout the defibrillation and stopped only to relieve a tired rescuer or for a rhythm check before the next defibrillation attempt. Compressions support and maintain adequate perfusion.

AIRWAY AND BREATHING

The current AHA basic life support and ACLS guidelines have repositioned airway and breathing below circulation for individuals who have experienced SCA from a cardiac cause. In this scenario, the oxygen reserve tends to be adequate, so giving priority to ventilation lowers the survival rate. In the early stages of SCA, poor cardiocerebral oxygenation is caused by decreased perfusion, not decreased ventilation or oxygenation. However, for patients who have experienced SCA from a pulmonary cause (eg, drowning, choking, or respiratory failure), in whom oxygen reserve is likely depleted, the airway and breathing should be restored as quickly as possible.

Details about airway management in the cardiac arrest patient are beyond the scope of this article but are presented elsewhere in this issue. Relevant AHA recommendations are summarized next[116]:

1. It is unknown whether administration of 100% inspired oxygen is beneficial to people who have sustained SCA; however, there is no evidence that it causes harm in short-term resuscitation. Therefore, the use of 100% oxygen is reasonable during initial resuscitative efforts.
2. Chest compressions cause air to be expelled during the compression phase and oxygen to be passively drawn into the chest during the recoil phase. Therefore, the passive inhalation of oxygen via a nonrebreather facemask is likely to be sufficient for several minutes after the onset of SCA in patients who have a patent airway.
3. Bag-mask ventilation can be challenging to perform correctly and is best done by two trained rescuers. If this technique is used, it is recommended that a tidal volume of approximately 600 mL be delivered over 1 second at a rate of 8 to 10 times per minute.
4. The routine use of cricoid pressure is no longer recommended. The application of this pressure does not decrease the risk of aspiration[117–119] and impedes ventilation.[120–123] Cricoid pressure should be reserved for helping to visualize the vocal cords during endotracheal intubation.
5. If advanced airway placement interrupts chest compressions, insertion of the airway can be delayed until the patient fails to respond to initial CPR or defibrillation attempts or demonstrates ROSC.
6. Continuous waveform capnography, in addition to clinical assessment, is the most reliable method of confirming and monitoring correct placement of an endotracheal tube. Capnography also has the benefit of alerting the providers to ROSC, as evidenced by an increase of more than 10 mm Hg in the patient's $EtCO_2$ level.[65]
7. Ventilations should be provided every 6 to 8 seconds (8–10 breaths per minute). Higher ventilations rates, which are common during resuscitation, can increase

intrathoracic pressure, resulting in diminished venous return and reduced cardiac output.[6,124] High ventilation rates can also cause gastric inflation, which increases the risk of aspiration and can impede ventilation further by elevating the diaphragm and restricting lung expansion.

SUMMARY

The 2010 AHA guidelines for CPR and emergency cardiovascular care present a significant change from how most people have learned adult CPR. The mantra is no longer "A-B-C" (airway, breathing, and circulation) but instead "C-A-B" (circulation, airway, and breathing). High-quality chest compressions (100 per minute at a depth of at least 2 in) should be started as soon as possible and continued with minimal interruptions. Interruptions should be limited to rhythm checks or the exchange of providers performing compressions. Defibrillation should be delayed until at least 30 chest compressions have been done. After a patient has been resuscitated, the focus of the providers needs to shift to postresuscitation care, which emphases the maintenance of cardiocerebral perfusion pressure, achieving therapeutic hypothermia, and considering the patient for early cardiac catheterization. The four C's of CPR (compressions, cardioversion, cooling, and catheterization) are the only interventions that have been shown to improve long-term outcomes.

ACKNOWLEDGMENTS

The manuscript was copyedited by Linda J. Kesselring, MS, ELS, the technical editor and writer in the Department of Emergency Medicine at the University of Maryland School of Medicine.

REFERENCES

1. Berg RA, Hemphill R, Abella BS, et al. Part 5: adult basic life support: 2010 American Heart Association guidelines for cardiopulmonary resuscitation and emergency cardiovascular care. Circulation 2010;122:S685–705.
2. Bobrow BJ, Clark LL, Ewy GA, et al. Minimally interrupted cardiac resuscitation by emergency medical services for out-of-hospital cardiac arrest. JAMA 2008; 299:1158–65.
3. Ewy GA, Kern KB, Sanders AB, et al. Cardiocerebral resuscitation for cardiac arrest. Am J Med 2006;119:6.
4. Kern KB, Hilwig RW, Berg RA, et al. Efficacy of chest compression-only BLS CPR in the presence of an occluded airway. Resuscitation 1998;39:179–88.
5. Valenzuela TD, Kern KB, Clark LL, et al. Interruptions of chest compressions during emergency medical systems resuscitation. Circulation 2005;112: 1259–65.
6. Aufderheide TP, Sigurdsson G, Pirrallo RG, et al. Hyperventilation-induced hypotension during cardiopulmonary resuscitation. Circulation 2004;109: 1960–5.
7. Bahr J, Klingler H, Panzer W, et al. Skills of lay people in checking the carotid pulse. Resuscitation 1997;35:23–6.
8. Brennan RT, Braslow A. Skill mastery in public CPR classes. Am J Emerg Med 1998;16:653–7.
9. Chamberlain D, Smith A, Woollard M, et al. Trials of teaching methods in basic life support (3): comparison of simulated CPR performance after first training

and at 6 months, with a note on the value of re-training. Resuscitation 2002;53: 179–87.

10. Eberle B, Dick WF, Schneider T, et al. Checking the carotid pulse check: diagnostic accuracy of first responders in patients with and without a pulse. Resuscitation 1996;33:107–16.

11. Frederick K, Bixby E, Orzel MN, et al. Will changing the emphasis from "pulseless" to "no signs of circulation" improve the recall scores for effective life support skills in children? Resuscitation 2002;55:255–61.

12. Lapostolle F, Le Toumelin P, Agostinucci JM, et al. Basic cardiac life support providers checking the carotid pulse: performance, degree of conviction, and influencing factors. Acad Emerg Med 2004;11:878–80.

13. Moule P. Checking the carotid pulse: diagnostic accuracy in students of the healthcare professions. Resuscitation 2000;44:195–201.

14. Nyman J, Sihvonen M. Cardiopulmonary resuscitation skills in nurses and nursing students. Resuscitation 2000;47:179–84.

15. Owen CJ, Wyllie JP. Determination of heart rate in the baby at birth. Resuscitation 2004;60:213–7.

16. Sarti A, Savron F, Ronfani L, et al. Comparison of three sites to check the pulse and count heart rate in hypotensive infants. Paediatr Anaesth 2006;16: 394–8.

17. Mather C, O'Kelly S. The palpation of pulses. Anaesthesia 1996;51:189–91.

18. Ochoa FJ, Ramalle-Gomara E, Carpintero JM, et al. Competence of health professionals to check the carotid pulse. Resuscitation 1998;37:173–5.

19. Frenneaux M. Cardiopulmonary resuscitation-some physiological considerations. Resuscitation 2003;58:259–65.

20. Abella BS, Alvarado JP, Myklebust H, et al. Quality of cardiopulmonary resuscitation during in-hospital cardiac arrest. JAMA 2005;293:305–10.

21. Wik L, Kramer-Johansen J, Myklebust H, et al. Quality of cardiopulmonary resuscitation during out-of-hospital cardiac arrest. JAMA 2005;293:299–304.

22. Handley AJ, Handley JA. Performing chest compressions in a confined space. Resuscitation 2004;61:55–61.

23. Andersen LO, Isbye DL, Rasmussen LS. Increasing compression depth during manikin CPR using a simple backboard. Acta Anaesthesiol Scand Suppl 2007; 51:747–50.

24. Noordergraaf GJ, Paulussen IW, Venema A, et al. The impact of compliant surfaces on in-hospital chest compressions: effects of common mattresses and a backboard. Resuscitation 2009;80:546–52.

25. Perkins GD, Kocierz L, Smith SC, et al. Compression feedback devices over estimate chest compression depth when performed on a bed. Resuscitation 2009;80:79–82.

26. Perkins GD, Smith CM, Augre C, et al. Effects of a backboard, bed height, and operator position on compression depth during simulated resuscitation. Intensive Care Med 2006;32:1632–5.

27. Perkins GD, Benny R, Giles S, et al. Do different mattresses affect the quality of cardiopulmonary resuscitation? Intensive Care Med 2003;29:2330–5.

28. Delvaux AB, Trombley MT, Rivet CJ, et al. Design and development of a cardiopulmonary resuscitation mattress. J Intensive Care Med 2009;24:195–9.

29. Kundra P, Dey S, Ravishankar M. Role of dominant hand position during external cardiac compression. Br J Anaesth 2000;84:491–3.

30. Kusunoki S, Tanigawa K, Kondo T, et al. Safety of the inter-nipple line hand position landmark for chest compression. Resuscitation 2009;80:1175–80.

31. Nikandish R, Shahbazi S, Golabi S, et al. Role of dominant versus non-dominant hand position during uninterrupted chest compression CPR by novice rescuers: a randomized double-blind crossover study. Resuscitation 2008;76:256–60.
32. Shin J, Rhee JE, Kim K. Is the inter-nipple line the correct hand position for effective chest compression in adult cardiopulmonary resuscitation? Resuscitation 2007;75:305–10.
33. Babbs CF, Kemeny AE, Quan W, et al. A new paradigm for human resuscitation research using intelligent devices. Resuscitation 2008;77:306–15.
34. Edelson DP, Abella BS, Kramer-Johansen J, et al. Effects of compression depth and pre-shock pauses predict defibrillation failure during cardiac arrest. Resuscitation 2006;71:137–45.
35. Edelson DP, Litzinger B, Arora V, et al. Improving in-hospital cardiac arrest process and outcomes with performance debriefing. Arch Intern Med 2008; 168:1063–9.
36. Kramer-Johansen J, Myklebust H, Wik L, et al. Quality of out-of-hospital cardiopulmonary resuscitation with real time automated feedback: a prospective interventional study. Resuscitation 2006;71:283–92.
37. Aufderheide TP, Pirrallo RG, Yannopoulos D, et al. Incomplete chest wall decompression: a clinical evaluation of CPR performance by trained laypersons and an assessment of alternative manual chest compression-decompression techniques. Resuscitation 2006;71:341–51.
38. Niles D, Nysaether J, Sutton R, et al. Leaning is common during in-hospital pediatric CPR, and decreased with automated corrective feedback. Resuscitation 2009;80:553–7.
39. Yannopoulos D, McKnite S, Aufderheide TP, et al. Effects of incomplete chest wall decompression during cardiopulmonary resuscitation on coronary and cerebral perfusion pressures in a porcine model of cardiac arrest. Resuscitation 2005;64:363–72.
40. Sutton RM, Maltese MR, Niles D, et al. Quantitative analysis of chest compression interruptions during in-hospital resuscitation of older children and adolescents. Resuscitation 2009;80:1259–63.
41. Sutton RM, Niles D, Nysaether J, et al. Quantitative analysis of CPR quality during in-hospital resuscitation of older children and adolescents. Pediatrics 2009;124:494–9.
42. Zuercher M, Hilwig RW, Ranger-Moore J, et al. Leaning during chest compressions impairs cardiac output and left ventricular myocardial blood flow in piglet cardiac arrest. Crit Care Med 2010;38:1141–6.
43. Lloyd J. Pop song "Stayin' Alive" helps people perform chest compressions for CPR [press release]. American College of Emergency Physicians; 2008. Available at: http://www.acep.org/content.aspx?id=45601. Accessed February 10, 2010.
44. Abella BS, Sandbo N, Vassilatos P, et al. Chest compression rates during cardiopulmonary resuscitation are suboptimal: a prospective study during in-hospital cardiac arrest. Circulation 2005;111:428–34.
45. Christenson J, Andrusiek D, Everson-Stewart S, et al. Chest compression fraction determines survival in patients with out-of-hospital ventricular fibrillation. Circulation 2009;120:1241–7.
46. Aufderheide TP, Yannopoulos D, Lick CJ, et al. Implementing the 2005 American Heart Association Guidelines improves outcomes after out-of-hospital cardiac arrest. Heart Rhythm 2010;7:1357–62.

47. Hinchey PR, Myers JB, Lewis R, et al. Improved out-of-hospital cardiac arrest survival after the sequential implementation of 2005 AHA guidelines for compressions, ventilations, and induced hypothermia: the Wake County experience. Ann Emerg Med 2010;56:348–57.
48. Rea TD, Helbock M, Perry S, et al. Increasing use of cardiopulmonary resuscitation during out-of-hospital ventricular fibrillation arrest: survival implications of guideline changes. Circulation 2006;114:2760–5.
49. Sayre MR, Cantrell SA, White LJ, et al. Impact of the 2005 American Heart Association cardiopulmonary resuscitation and emergency cardiovascular care guidelines on out-of-hospital cardiac arrest survival. Prehosp Emerg Care 2009;13:469–77.
50. Steinmetz J, Barnung S, Nielsen SL, et al. Improved survival after an out-of-hospital cardiac arrest using new guidelines. Acta Anaesthesiol Scand Suppl 2008;52:908–13.
51. Babbs CF, Kern KB. Optimum compression to ventilation ratios in CPR under realistic, practical conditions: a physiological and mathematical analysis. Resuscitation 2002;54:147–57.
52. Berg RA, Hilwig RW, Kern KB, et al. "Bystander" chest compressions and assisted ventilation independently improve outcome from piglet asphyxial pulseless "cardiac arrest." Circulation 2000;101:1743–8.
53. Berg RA, Kern KB, Hilwig RW, et al. Assisted ventilation does not improve outcome in a porcine model of single-rescuer bystander cardiopulmonary resuscitation. Circulation 1997;95:1635–41.
54. Berg RA, Kern KB, Hilwig RW, et al. Assisted ventilation during "bystander" CPR in a swine acute myocardial infarction model does not improve outcome. Circulation 1997;96:4364–71.
55. Berg RA, Sanders AB, Kern KB, et al. Adverse hemodynamic effects of interrupting chest compressions for rescue breathing during cardiopulmonary resuscitation for ventricular fibrillation cardiac arrest. Circulation 2001;104:2465–70.
56. Dorph E, Wik L, Stromme TA, et al. Oxygen delivery and return of spontaneous circulation with ventilation:compression ratio 2:30 versus chest compressions only CPR in pigs. Resuscitation 2004;60:309–18.
57. Berg RA, Hilwig RW, Berg MD, et al. Immediate post-shock chest compressions improve outcome from prolonged ventricular fibrillation. Resuscitation 2008;78:71–6.
58. Garza AG, Gratton MC, Salomone JA, et al. Improved patient survival using a modified resuscitation protocol for out-of-hospital cardiac arrest. Circulation 2009;119:2597–605.
59. Kellum MJ, Kennedy KW, Barney R, et al. Cardiocerebral resuscitation improves neurologically intact survival of patients with out-of-hospital cardiac arrest. Ann Emerg Med 2008;52:244–52.
60. Tang W, Snyder D, Wang J, et al. One-shock versus three-shock defibrillation protocol significantly improves outcome in a porcine model of prolonged ventricular fibrillation cardiac arrest. Circulation 2006;113:2683–9.
61. Mader TJ, Paquette AT, Salcido DD, et al. The effect of the preshock pause on coronary perfusion pressure decay and rescue shock outcome in porcine ventricular fibrillation. Prehosp Emerg Care 2009;13:487–94.
62. Paradis NA, Martin GB, Rivers EP, et al. Coronary perfusion pressure and the return of spontaneous circulation in human cardiopulmonary resuscitation. JAMA 1990;263:1106–13.

63. Reynolds JC, Salcido DD, Menegazzi JJ. Coronary perfusion pressure and return of spontaneous circulation after prolonged cardiac arrest. Prehosp Emerg Care 2010;14:78–84.

64. Wang HE, Simeone SJ, Weaver MD, et al. Interruptions in cardiopulmonary resuscitation from paramedic endotracheal intubation. Ann Emerg Med 2009; 54:645.e1–52.e1.

65. Pokorna M, Necas E, Kratochvil J, et al. A sudden increase in partial pressure end-tidal carbon dioxide ($PEtCO_2$) at the moment of return of spontaneous circulation. J Emerg Med 2010;38:614–21.

66. Edelson DP, Robertson-Dick BJ, Yuen TC, et al. Safety and efficacy of defibrillator charging during ongoing chest compressions: a multi-center study. Resuscitation 2010;81:1521–6.

67. Lloyd MS, Heeke B, Walter PF, et al. Hands-on defibrillation: an analysis of electrical current flow through rescuers in direct contact with patients during biphasic external defibrillation. Circulation 2008;117:2510–4.

68. Yu T, Ristagno G, Li Y, et al. The resuscitation blanket: a useful tool for "hands-on" defibrillation. Resuscitation 2010;81:230–5.

69. Manders S, Geijsel FE. Alternating providers during continuous chest compressions for cardiac arrest: every minute or every two minutes? Resuscitation 2009; 80:1015–8.

70. Aufderheide TP, Pirrallo RG, Yannopoulos D, et al. Incomplete chest wall decompression: a clinical evaluation of CPR performance by EMS personnel and assessment of alternative manual chest compression-decompression techniques. Resuscitation 2005;64:353–62.

71. Olasveengen TM, Wik L, Steen PA. Standard basic life support vs. continuous chest compressions only in out-of-hospital cardiac arrest. Acta Anaesthesiol Scand Suppl 2008;52:914–9.

72. Hew P, Brenner B, Kaufman J. Reluctance of paramedics and emergency medical technicians to perform mouth-to-mouth resuscitation. J Emerg Med 1997;15:279–84.

73. Sirbaugh PE, Pepe PE, Shook JE, et al. A prospective, population-based study of the demographics, epidemiology, management, and outcome of out-of-hospital pediatric cardiopulmonary arrest. Ann Emerg Med 1999;33: 174–84.

74. SOS-KANTO study group. Cardiopulmonary resuscitation by bystanders with chest compression only (SOS-KANTO): an observational study. Lancet 2007; 369:920–6.

75. Bohm K, Rosenqvist M, Herlitz J, et al. Survival is similar after standard treatment and chest compression only in out-of-hospital bystander cardiopulmonary resuscitation. Circulation 2007;116:2908–12.

76. Iwami T, Kawamura T, Hiraide A, et al. Effectiveness of bystander-initiated cardiac-only resuscitation for patients with out-of-hospital cardiac arrest. Circulation 2007;116:2900–7.

77. Ong ME, Ng FS, Anushia P, et al. Comparison of chest compression only and standard cardiopulmonary resuscitation for out-of-hospital cardiac arrest in Singapore. Resuscitation 2008;78:119–26.

78. Sayre MR, Berg RA, Cave DM, et al. Hands-only (compression-only) cardiopulmonary resuscitation: a call to action for bystander response to adults who experience out-of-hospital sudden cardiac arrest: a science advisory for the public from the American Heart Association Emergency Cardiovascular Care Committee. Circulation 2008;117:2162–7.

79. Ornato JP, Gonzalez ER, Garnett AR, et al. Effect of cardiopulmonary resuscitation compression rate on end-tidal carbon dioxide concentration and arterial pressure in man. Crit Care Med 1988;16:241–5.
80. Kern KB, Sanders AB, Raife J, et al. A study of chest compression rates during cardiopulmonary resuscitation in humans. The importance of rate-directed chest compressions. Arch Intern Med 1992;152:145–9.
81. Swenson RD, Weaver WD, Niskanen RA, et al. Hemodynamics in humans during conventional and experimental methods of cardiopulmonary resuscitation. Circulation 1988;78:630–9.
82. Anthi A, Tzelepis GE, Alivizatos P, et al. Unexpected cardiac arrest after cardiac surgery: incidence, predisposing causes, and outcome of open chest cardiopulmonary resuscitation. Chest 1998;113:15–9.
83. Pottle A, Bullock I, Thomas J, et al. Survival to discharge following open chest cardiac compression (OCCC). A 4-year retrospective audit in a cardiothoracic specialist centre–Royal Brompton and Harefield NHS Trust, United Kingdom. Resuscitation 2002;52:269–72.
84. Raman J, Saldanha RF, Branch JM, et al. Open cardiac compression in the postoperative cardiac intensive care unit. Anaesth Intensive Care 1989;17: 129–35.
85. Babbs CF. Interposed abdominal compression CPR: a comprehensive evidence based review. Resuscitation 2003;59:71–82.
86. Sack JB, Kesselbrenner MB, Bregman D. Survival from in-hospital cardiac arrest with interposed abdominal counterpulsation during cardiopulmonary resuscitation. JAMA 1992;267:379–85.
87. Sack JB, Kesselbrenner MB, Jarrad A. Interposed abdominal compression-cardiopulmonary resuscitation and resuscitation outcome during asystole and electromechanical dissociation. Circulation 1992;86:1692–700.
88. Mateer JR, Stueven HA, Thompson BM, et al. Pre-hospital IAC-CPR versus standard CPR: paramedic resuscitation of cardiac arrests. Am J Emerg Med 1985;3: 143–6.
89. Waldman PJ, Walters BL, Grunau CF. Pancreatic injury associated with interposed abdominal compressions in pediatric cardiopulmonary resuscitation. Am J Emerg Med 1984;2:510–2.
90. Pellis T, Kette F, Lovisa D, et al. Utility of pre-cordial thump for treatment of out of hospital cardiac arrest: a prospective study. Resuscitation 2009;80: 17–23.
91. Amir O, Schliamser JE, Nemer S, et al. Ineffectiveness of precordial thump for cardioversion of malignant ventricular tachyarrhythmias. Pacing Clin Electrophysiol 2007;30:153–6.
92. De Maio VJ, Stiell IG, Spaite DW, et al. CPR-only survivors of out-of-hospital cardiac arrest: implications for out-of-hospital care and cardiac arrest research methodology. Ann Emerg Med 2001;37:602–8.
93. Haman L, Parizek P, Vojacek J. Precordial thump efficacy in termination of induced ventricular arrhythmias. Resuscitation 2009;80:14–6.
94. Dale KM, Lertsburapa K, Kluger J, et al. Moxifloxacin and torsade de pointes. Ann Pharmacother 2007;41:336–40.
95. Pennington JE, Taylor J, Lown B. Chest thump for reverting ventricular tachycardia. N Engl J Med 1970;283:1192–5.
96. Bornemann C, Scherf D. Electrocardiogram of the month. Paroxysmal ventricular tachycardia abolished by a blow to the precordium. Dis Chest 1969;56: 83–4.

97. Rahner E, Zeh E. Regulation of ventricular tachycardia with precordial fist blow. Med Welt 1978;29:1659–63.

98. Ahmar W, Morley P, Marasco S, et al. Sternal fracture and osteomyelitis: an unusual complication of a precordial thump. Resuscitation 2007;75:540–2.

99. Miller J, Tresch D, Horwitz L, et al. The precordial thump. Ann Emerg Med 1984; 13:791–4.

100. Muller GI, Ulmer HE, Bauer JA. Complications of chest thump for termination of supraventricular tachycardia in children. Eur J Pediatr 1992;151:12–4.

101. Chan L, Reid C, Taylor B. Effect of three emergency pacing modalities on cardiac output in cardiac arrest due to ventricular asystole. Resuscitation 2002;52:117–9.

102. Dowdle JR. Ventricular standstill and cardiac percussion. Resuscitation 1996; 32:31–2.

103. Eich C, Bleckmann A, Paul T. Percussion pacing in a three-year-old girl with complete heart block during cardiac catheterization. Br J Anaesth 2005;95: 465–7.

104. Eich C, Bleckmann A, Schwarz SK. Percussion pacing: an almost forgotten procedure for haemodynamically unstable bradycardias? A report of three case studies and review of the literature. Br J Anaesth 2007;98:429–33.

105. Iseri LT, Allen BJ, Baron K, et al. Fist pacing, a forgotten procedure in bradyasystolic cardiac arrest. Am Heart J 1987;113:1545–50.

106. Tucker KJ, Shaburihvili TS, Gedevanishvili AT. Manual external (fist) pacing during high-degree atrioventricular block: a lifesaving intervention. Am J Emerg Med 1995;13:53–4.

107. Zeh E, Rahner E. The manual extrathoracal stimulation of the heart. Technique and effect of the precordial thump (author's transl). Z Kardiol 1978;67:299–304.

108. Holmberg M, Holmberg S, Herlitz J. Incidence, duration and survival of ventricular fibrillation in out-of-hospital cardiac arrest patients in Sweden. Resuscitation 2000;44:7–17.

109. Larsen MP, Eisenberg MS, Cummins RO, et al. Predicting survival from out-of-hospital cardiac arrest: a graphic model. Ann Emerg Med 1993;22:1652–8.

110. Valenzuela TD, Roe DJ, Cretin S, et al. Estimating effectiveness of cardiac arrest interventions: a logistic regression survival model. Circulation 1997;96:3308–13.

111. Link MS, Atkins DL, Passman RS, et al. Part 6: Electrical therapies: automated external defibrillators, defibrillation, cardioversion, and pacing: 2010 American Heart Association Guidelines for Cardiopulmonary Resuscitation and Emergency Cardiovascular Care. Circulation 2010;122:S706–19.

112. Cobb LA, Fahrenbruch CE, Walsh TR, et al. Influence of cardiopulmonary resuscitation prior to defibrillation in patients with out-of-hospital ventricular fibrillation. JAMA 1999;281:1182–8.

113. Wik L, Hansen TB, Fylling F, et al. Delaying defibrillation to give basic cardiopulmonary resuscitation to patients with out-of-hospital ventricular fibrillation: a randomized trial. JAMA 2003;289:1389–95.

114. Bunch TJ, White RD, Gersh BJ, et al. Long-term outcomes of out-of-hospital cardiac arrest after successful early defibrillation. N Engl J Med 2003;348: 2626–33.

115. Hayakawa M, Gando S, Okamoto H, et al. Shortening of cardiopulmonary resuscitation time before the defibrillation worsens the outcome in out-of-hospital VF patients. Am J Emerg Med 2009;27:470–4.

116. Neumar RW, Otto CW, Link MS, et al. Part 8: Adult advanced cardiovascular life support: 2010 American Heart Association Guidelines for Cardiopulmonary

Resuscitation and Emergency Cardiovascular Care. Circulation 2010;122: S729–67.

117. Lawes EG, Campbell I, Mercer D. Inflation pressure, gastric insufflation and rapid sequence induction. Br J Anaesth 1987;59:315–8.

118. Petito SP, Russell WJ. The prevention of gastric inflation: a neglected benefit of cricoid pressure. Anaesth Intensive Care 1988;16:139–43.

119. Salem MR, Wong AY, Mani M, et al. Efficacy of cricoid pressure in preventing gastric inflation during bag-mask ventilation in pediatric patients. Anesthesiology 1974;40:96–8.

120. Asai T, Goy RW, Liu EH. Cricoid pressure prevents placement of the laryngeal tube and laryngeal tube-suction II. Br J Anaesth 2007;99:282–5.

121. Brimacombe J, White A, Berry A. Effect of cricoid pressure on ease of insertion of the laryngeal mask airway. Br J Anaesth 1993;71:800–2.

122. McNelis U, Syndercombe A, Harper I, et al. The effect of cricoid pressure on intubation facilitated by the gum elastic bougie. Anaesthesia 2007;62:456–9.

123. Turgeon AF, Nicole PC, Trepanier CA, et al. Cricoid pressure does not increase the rate of failed intubation by direct laryngoscopy in adults. Anesthesiology 2005;102:315–9.

124. O'Neill JF, Deakin CD. Do we hyperventilate cardiac arrest patients? Resuscitation 2007;73:82.

Electrical Therapies in Cardiac Arrest

Peter P. Monteleone, MD[a], Heather A. Borek, MD[b],*,
Seth O. Althoff, MD[c]

KEYWORDS

- Cardiac arrest • Automated external defibrillator
- Cardiac pacing • Defibrillation

With the clinical updates made in the 2010 American Heart Association (AHA) Advanced Cardiac Life Support Guidelines, the focus of resuscitation from cardiac arrest has returned to an emphasis on the basics.[1] Although much importance is placed on performance of high-quality, uninterrupted cardiopulmonary resuscitation (CPR), many forget that emphasis should also be placed on early and appropriate use of defibrillation to treat ventricular fibrillation (VF) or pulseless ventricular tachycardia (VT).

Electricity as a therapeutic modality is a science with a long history going all the way back to the Leyden jar. Developed in 1745, this was the first glass capacitor capable of storing electricity. Soon after its discovery, it was used to study electricity's clinical effects.[2] By 1775, there were descriptions of an apparent accidental cardiac defibrillation by Peter Abildgaard "when having shocked a single chicken into lifelessness... on repeating the shock, the bird took off and eluded further experimentation."[3–5] As early as 1788, Charles Kite described, in his "Essay on the Recovery of the Apparently Dead," what may have been the first successful intentional defibrillation, that of a 3-year-old girl who was successfully defibrillated after a fall.[6,7]

As knowledge of the dysrhythmias underlying sudden cardiac death grew, Jean-Louis Prevost and Frederic Battelli noted in 1899 that after inducing VF with electricity, a second larger shock delivered to an animal brought the animal back into sinus rhythm.[8] At the turn of the twentieth century, interest in the science skyrocketed when the Consolidated Edison Electric Company of New York City made the transition from direct to alternating current on their electric lines. While performing the switch, multiple linemen working on the project died of electrocution. These deaths led

---

The authors have nothing to disclose.

[a] Department of Medicine, University of Virginia, PO Box 800136, Charlottesville, VA 22908-0136, USA

[b] Department of Emergency Medicine, University of Virginia, PO Box 800774, Charlottesville, VA 22908–0774, USA

[c] Department of Emergency Medicine, Bridgeport Hospital, 267 Grant Street, Bridgeport, CT 06610, USA

* Corresponding author.

E-mail address: hab2t@virginia.edu

to the company's funding of multiple research initiatives studying the lethality of electricity and how it could potentially be used therapeutically. The resulting work of William Kouwenhoven and Guy Knickerbocker at Johns Hopkins highlighted results similar to those of Prevost and Battelli, that after a single shock induces VF, a second "counter-shock" could restore sinus rhythm in dogs.[9]

It was with this foundation that Claude Beck, a cardiothoracic surgeon at Western Reserve University/University Hospitals of Cleveland, made the decision to undertake what became the first documented successful intentional defibrillation of an exposed human heart after a 14-year-old patient developed cardiac arrest and documented VF. The first shock failed to defibrillate the heart, the second shock succeeded, allowing a sinus rhythm to recapture the myocardium and gaining dramatic support for defibrillation as a treatment of cardiac arrest.[2,10]

The science of electrical therapy in cardiac arrest has considerably evolved to investigate multiple modes of cardiac defibrillation and cardiac pacing. Historic work done around the globe has resulted in what currently is a fairly simple science, the termination of a dysrhythmia with an overwhelming current. Elegant and simple, it is a clinical act fundamental to the modern treatment of sudden cardiac arrest. This article focuses on the use of electrical therapies, including defibrillation, cardiac pacing, and automated external defibrillators in cardiac arrest.

DEFIBRILLATION

The first step to successful use of defibrillation is rapid and accurate identification of the rhythms warranting defibrillation. With regards to current AHA Advanced Cardiac Life Support algorithms, defibrillation is warranted to treat pulseless VT or VF. These rhythms are incapable of sustaining a perfusing blood pressure and thus warrant defibrillation to break the dysrhythmia and allow a pulse-sustaining rhythm to resume.

The mechanism by which defibrillation "breaks the dysrhythmia" remains controversial. In general, it is thought that defibrillation alters the cardiac cellular transmembrane electrical potentials making cardiac cells temporarily unexcitable by a wave of depolarization.[11] The disorganized waves of VF and the organized wavefronts of VT are thus left unable to excite the myocardium. The resultant absence of VT- or VF-induced depolarization allows normal cardiac excitation pathways and resultant contraction to resume.[12] As new technology has developed, so too has understanding of the varied and complex effects of defibrillation on the heart at the cellular, tissue, and organ-specific levels. However, it is important to remember that although much is known about clinical outcomes from different types of defibrillation, there is much to learn about how these outcomes are mediated physiologically.

To understand the basics of defibrillation, it is important to review the basics of electrical energy. Voltage is a measure of electrical potential difference measured in volts. In the defibrillation model, voltage is the stored electrical potential difference created by the defibrillator device between the two defibrillator pads. Current is the flow of electric charge through a medium and is what actually defibrillates the heart. Current is expressed as voltage/impedance and is measured in amperes. Impedance is a measure of resistance to the flow of current and is measured in ohms. In the defibrillator model, impedance is created by the electrical circuit itself and by the patient's body. Impedance is affected by patient body mass, temperature, skin moisture, types of defibrillator pads, attachment of the pads to the patient's body, and so forth. Energy is the amount of work associated with the passage of one amp of current through one ohm of resistance for one second. Energy is measured in Joules and is expressed in the following equation: voltage × current × time. Although the current is what actually induces defibrillation, what is selected on the device by a clinician is the energy (in Joules). Selecting an energy in Joules essentially alters what current is supplied during defibrillation.

Monophasic Versus Biphasic Defibrillation

Although the terms "monophasic" and "biphasic" and the resultant discussion of waveform shape can often be daunting, the principle underlying the difference between these types of defibrillation is actually quite straightforward. Essentially, monophasic devices send current in a single direction across the defibrillation pads (from pad A to pad B). Biphasic devices send a defibrillatory current initially in one direction for a specified duration (from pad A to pad B) and then the current is reversed and flows in the opposite direction (from pad B to pad A) for the remainder of the defibrillation.

There are many distinct types of biphasic waveforms used by the many varieties of biphasic defibrillators. They use different energy settings and can distribute voltage and current differently among these settings. Some can also vary the duration of the shock and the voltage to adapt to high-impedance patients. As demonstrated in the ORBIT and TIMBER trials, there do not seem to be major differences in clinical outcomes, including rate of return of spontaneous circulation or survival to discharge in patients treated with monophasic versus biphasic defibrillation.[13,14] One exception was the ORCA trial, which demonstrated an improvement in neurologic outcomes after discharge with the use of biphasic current.[15]

Despite little data demonstrating a clinical outcome difference, biphasic waveforms do seem to defibrillate more effectively and with lower energies compared with monophasic waveforms. This observation has been demonstrated in animal and human studies.[13–17] Although the exact physiologic explanation remains unclear, it seems likely that the nature of the biphasic current allows more myocardium to be effectively depolarized, and thus defibrillated, with less energy. These features collectively avoid the high energies sometimes required by monophasic current, which can result in higher rates of damage to myocardial tissue and damage to surface tissue, including burns.[18]

In summarizing these data, the 2010 AHA guidelines state "...over the last decade, biphasic waveforms have been shown to be more effective than monophasic waveforms in cardioversion and defibrillation."[1] There are no recommendations against the use of monophasic defibrillators in these guidelines and, indeed, recommendations targeted to monophasic devices (regarding how to escalate energy in these devices) are provided in the same guidelines. However, in light of the general expert consensus support of biphasic devices, the growing trend across institutions has been transition from monophasic to biphasic devices.

Single Versus Stacked Shocks

As a general rule "stacked shocks" for refractory VF or VT have fallen out of favor. Before the 2005 AHA guidelines, shocks stacked in groups of three before initiation of CPR were deemed appropriate on the grounds that the efficacy of the first shock to defibrillate a monomorphic dysrhythmia was low. The improving efficacy of immediately repeated, or stacked, shocks was thought to be caused by the theoretical decrease in transthoracic impedance, or TTI, after each shock.[19,20] Emerging data show that this theoretical improvement of stacking shocks does not seem to improve the success of defibrillation or clinical outcomes.[19,21] Stacking shocks leads to decreased quality and quantity of CPR, potentially worsening outcome. Also, as stated in the 2010 AHA guidelines, after a single shock "intervening chest compressions may improve oxygen and substrate delivery to the myocardium, making the subsequent shock more likely to result in defibrillation."[1] As a result, stacked shocks in true pulseless arrest are no longer recommended, although some debate continues regarding the use of shock stacking in experienced hands, in certain situations.

Fixed Versus Escalating Energy

During defibrillation, a large amount of current is dissipated away from the heart to the various structures of the chest, including the bony chest wall and the lungs. Work with dogs calculating the ratio of transcardiac to transthoracic threshold currents determined that only approximately 4% of current applied by defibrillation actually reaches the heart.[22] With such a limited percentage of current reaching the muscle to be defibrillated, the idea of increasing defibrillation energy to defibrillate myocardium is an important consideration. This notion was particularly important when the use of monophasic current was standard.

Monophasic defibrillators do not compensate for impedance and simply create a monophasic energy waveform that is also degraded in the face of high impedance. These two facts made a strong case for using escalating energies for defibrillation failure, which suggested that transthoracic impedance was likely too high for successful defibrillation. However, newer biphasic defibrillators use a biphasic truncated exponential waveform, a technology originally developed for implantable cardioverter-defibrillators (ICDs). The benefit of the biphasic truncated exponential waveform is that it does not degrade in the face of high impedance. Also, many of the new biphasic defibrillators include technology capable of adjusting the biphasic waveform to compensate for high impedance. Therefore, the importance of a routine algorithm of energy dose escalation has become less important since the dawn of the biphasic defibrillator. The notion that higher energy levels may succeed where lower energy levels have failed, however, does remain, resulting in the following statement in the 2010 AHA Guidelines: "if higher energy levels are available in the device at hand, they may be considered if initial shocks are unsuccessful in terminating the arrhythmia."[1]

Time to Defibrillation

The initial rhythm in prehospital witnessed cardiac arrest is not uncommonly VF.[23] It has been well documented that the time to both CPR and defibrillation are critically important in cardiac arrest. Survival rates decrease by approximately 7% to 10% for every minute that passes from the time of arrest to defibrillation if no CPR is provided.[23-26] VF eventually deteriorates to asystole over time.[27] CPR can prolong the period of VF and increase the time when defibrillation may be successful.[27-30] Because delays to both CPR and defibrillation decrease survival in witnessed cardiac arrest, the current AHA guidelines recommend that the rescuer immediately start CPR and use the automatic electronic defibrillator (AED)/defibrillator as soon as possible.[31]

In cases where there is an unwitnessed arrest, it is unclear whether initiating CPR before defibrillation or immediate defibrillation provides better outcomes. Several studies have attempted to answer this question with varying results. Two studies demonstrated improved outcomes in patients receiving delayed defibrillation after CPR by emergency medical services (EMS) providers where EMS call-to-arrival intervals were 4 minutes or longer.[32,33] However, several other randomized controlled trials assessing delayed defibrillation did not demonstrate any improvement in return of spontaneous circulation or survival to discharge regardless of EMS response interval.[34,35] Although these results are contradictory, it has been demonstrated that CPR before defibrillation, in cases where VF has been present for more than a few minutes, may increase oxygen delivery and important metabolic substrates required for successful termination of VF.[36] The current recommendation suggests that clinicians determine, based on an analysis of their patient, the most appropriate time to defibrillate the individual.

CARDIAC PACING

The estimated incidence of out-of-hospital, EMS-treated cardiac arrest in North America is 52.1 per 100,000 people.[37] For cardiac arrest in the pediatric population, the presenting rhythm is generally asystole or idioventricular bradycardia. In adult cardiac arrest victims, the true prevalence of bradyasystole is unknown, although some studies suggest the incidence may be as high as 25% to 56%.[38] Bradyasystole is generally defined as a cardiac rhythm with a ventricular rate less than 60 beats per minute (in adults), periods of asystole, or both. There may be an absence or presence of a pulse, which may or may not be adequately perfusing.

In the setting of asystolic cardiac arrest, there have been attempts to return circulation by external pacing. Intuitively, it would be thought that capturing a heartbeat with electrical energy would improve patient survival; however, the available studies are unconvincing. Cardiac pacing can be performed either transcutaneously or transvenously. In the emergency setting, transcutaneous pacing is rapidly available to prehospital and in-hospital personnel. Studies evaluating the use of pacing in cardiac arrest have primarily evaluated trancutaneous pacing. Studies have assessed both prehospital and in-hospital use of pacing in cardiac arrest. In studies of prehospital asystolic arrest, little benefit in survival to hospital admission or hospital discharge has been found with transcutaneous pacing versus standard resuscitation alone.

In a study of prehospital asystolic cardiac arrest, Hedges and colleagues[39] found no benefit in overall admission to the hospital or to hospital discharge when transcutaneous pacing was used versus standard medical resuscitation alone. However, in this study the mean estimated time to pacing was 21.8 minutes. Barthell and colleagues[40] conducted a study evaluating the efficacy of prehospital pacing in asystolic cardiac arrest and pulseless electrical activity arrest. This study investigated 226 pulseless patients and found no benefit in survival for paced patients. Similarly, in a larger study by Cummins and colleagues,[41] no benefit was found in survival to hospital admission or survival to hospital discharge despite a mean time to pacing in this study of only 9 minutes. In addition, analysis of those patients with a mean collapse-to-pacing time of less than 9 minutes with those with a collapse-to-pacing time of greater than 9 minutes found no difference in survival to hospital admission.[41]

Similarly, evaluation of pacing for in-hospital cardiac arrest offers little available evidence. In an examination of in-hospital asystole and bradycardia, Knowlton and Falk[42] found no difference in survival between paced patients and those receiving standard pharmacotherapy. A limitation of this study was the small sample size, including only 58 patients. Dalsey and colleagues[43] performed a small study in which 52 patients initially received transcutaneous pacing after aystolic cardiac arrest, pulseless electrical activity arrest, or hemodynamically compromised bradycardia. Pacing was initiated after failure of standard medical resuscitation. No patient in the series survived to hospital discharge. In a more recent evaluation, a systematic review of the literature by Sherbino and colleagues[44] found no benefit from transcutaneous pacing in either in-hospital or prehospital asystolic arrest. Although evidence is limited, based on the few available studies it seems that emergency cardiac pacing in the asystolic patient has little value; there is no evidence that pacing is more beneficial than standard resuscitation alone. Accordingly, the 2010 AHA guidelines do not support the use of pacing in asystolic cardiac arrest.[45]

Emergent cardiac pacing has historically been recommended for symptomatic bradydysrhythmias and is a consideration for patients who are unresponsive to pharmacologic therapy. For example, in one study of 170 patients with symptomatic bradycardia 54 were refractory to pharmacologic management and received external cardiac pacing.[46] Unfortunately, as in asystolic cardiac arrest, there is limited evidence that cardiac pacing results in improved outcomes in the bradycardic, hemodynamically compromised patient.

In the prehospital setting, a study of symptomatic bradycardia by Hedges and colleagues[47] found a trend toward improved survival to hospital discharge for transcutaneously paced patients versus nonpaced patients. Survival to hospital discharge was 15% in the paced group versus 0% in the nonpaced group. However, this study had multiple limitations and only included 51 individuals with only 27 paced. The P value missed significance at 0.07. A prospective, controlled study by Barthell and colleagues[40] showed a significant improvement in resuscitation and survival to hospital discharge in the transcutaneously paced group compared with controls for symptomatic bradycardia. However, again in this study the sample size was small (total of 13 patients) and there were inequalities between control and treatment groups in terms of isoproterenol administration. In an interhospital study (patients being transferred from hospital to hospital) by Vukov and Johnson,[48] 23 patients in a series of 297 required transcutaneous or transvenous pacing for symptomatic bradycardia that was unresponsive to atropine; of these 23 patients, 12 survived. Sherbino and coworkers[44] reviewed the literature of transcutaneous pacing in the prehospital setting in patients with symptomatic bradycardia or bradyasystolic arrest and found only seven studies, all of which were rated as having poor methodology by reviewers. For symptomatic bradycardia this review seems to show no benefit in the prehospital setting, although there may be a benefit for transcutaneous pacing in the in-hospital setting.[44,48] Sherbino and coworkers[44] suggested that prehospital transcutaneous pacing for symptomatic bradycardia be given a class indeterminate recommendation. Because the data for the use of pacing for symptomatic bradycardia in the in-hospital setting are more robust the AHA recommends transcutaneous pacing as a second-line therapy, to be considered when pharmacologic (atropine) management fails.[45,49] Transcutaneous pacing may also be considered in patients presenting with unstable bradycardia who have no intravenous access.[49]

A final indication for emergent cardiac pacing is overdrive pacing for torsades de pointes (TdP). TdP may be either congenital or acquired. Congenital forms are caused by inherited gene mutations encoding ion channels (sodium or potassium) involved in cardiac action potential repolarization.[50–53] Acquired QT prolongation occurs most commonly because of medications and toxins and electrolyte imbalances.[50,53,54] Medication-induced QT prolongation is most commonly generated by potassium efflux channel blockade.[55,56]

Refractory TdP can be treated by cardiac pacing, either chemical or electrical. Pacing can be used prophylactically to suppress frequent, self-limited runs of TdP or to override refractory, persistent TdP with a pulse before degeneration to VF. Any patient with pulseless VT or VF must be treated with direct current cardioversion and standard advanced resuscitation protocols. Isoproterenol is a β-adrenergic receptor agonist that causes positive inotropic and chronotropic effects, and is a chemical means of overdrive pacing. Isoproterenol, however, may increase the risk of dysrhythmia in patients with congenital long QT syndrome and, therefore, should be reserved for those patients with acquired long QT syndrome.[53,57]

There are few studies evaluating the efficacy of electrical overdrive pacing for the treatment of TdP. Although limited, these studies seem to show effective termination of TdP when appropriately paced.[58,59] Current AHA guidelines list overdrive pacing as an option for polymorphic VT associated with familial long QT syndrome. It may also be considered for acquired long QT syndrome when it seems to be pause induced or associated with bradycardia.[60]

AUTOMATED EXTERNAL DEFIBRILLATORS

AEDs were created to decrease the time between cardiac arrest and defibrillation in the out-of-hospital setting, although in-hospital applications are now not uncommon. AEDs execute two important functions: they perform a cardiac rhythm analysis and provide a shock delivery system. Manual defibrillation requires extensive training because the operator is required to analyze the rhythm and determine the appropriate treatment. The operator must also determine the amount of energy they wish to use for defibrillation. AEDs simplify this process by internally analyzing the rhythm and, if required, administering a shock of a predetermined, device-specific amount of energy.

AEDs are classified as automatic and semiautomatic. Fully automatic machines only require the operator to turn on the machine and appropriately place the electrode pads. The machine then analyzes the rhythm and automatically delivers a shock, if required. Semiautomatic machines analyze the rhythm and charge, but require the operator to discharge the machine. As an additional function, AEDs often prompt rescuers to provide CPR; some of the newer devices even give feedback regarding the adequacy of the chest compressions being given.

The amount of energy received by the heart during defibrillation depends on the amount of transthoracic impedance, which can be affected by such things as hair, body weight, chest size, and pad size. The higher the impedance, the lower the amount of energy and current generated, which may be insufficient to achieve defibrillation. AED pads are nonpolarized so either pad can be placed in various positions without complications. There are four acceptable and equally effective positions to place the pads: (1) anteriolateral, (2) anteroposterior, (3) anterior-left infrascapular, and (4) anterior-right infrascapular.[61-65] Pads come in different sizes, ranging from pediatric sizes of 24 cm^2 up to the adult sizes of 8 to 12 cm in length. The larger 12-cm pads decrease transthoracic impedance and may achieve higher defibrillation success rates than smaller pads.[21,66] Also, briefly shaving any excess body hair or wiping off any perspiration or water more accurately guarantees that the desired energy is received.

The first AEDs delivered a monophasic current during defibrillation. Almost all modern AEDs generate a biphasic current that requires less energy to achieve a successful defibrillation, which has led to the ability to produce smaller units. Commercially available AEDs can provide either a fixed or escalating amount of energy for subsequent shocks. For AEDs, AHA guidelines do not give specific recommendations for the amount of biphasic energy for the first shock, but state each additional shock should be at least as strong as the initial shock, and energy may be increased for additional shocks.[31]

AEDs automatically perform rhythm analysis using complex algorithms; QRS rate, amplitude, slope, and morphology are just a few aspects of the electrocardiogram that are evaluated. There are various algorithms that AED manufacturers use for their specific machines. For this reason, the AHA has specific recommendations regarding the specificity and sensitivity for each of the various rhythms. Manufacturers are recommended to report the performance of their algorithms using a standard format to the Food and Drug Administration.[31]

In rhythm analysis, the most difficult challenge is differentiating fine VF from asystole or artifact. Amplitude settings have to be set low enough to adequately detect VF and high enough to exclude unnecessary shocks for asystole or artifact. Artifacts can be caused by CPR, agonal respirations, transport of the patient, seizures, pacemaker spikes, tremor and other rhythmic body motions, and electrostatic fields. Ideally, each AED should have 100% specificity for detecting asystole or artifact. However, because there are differences in the data acquisition algorithms for each different machine, compiling a common test bank is impractical. To ensure integrity, each manufacturer should provide their performance report and explain how the testing was completed.

There are a few unique circumstances to consider when using an AED. AED use is not contraindicated in patients who have an ICD. Occasionally, there may be some discrepancies in rhythm analysis between the ICD and AED. If the ICD has a pacing function, this may also interfere with the ability of the AED to appropriately detect VF.[67] If the ICD is delivering shocks, it is recommended to wait up to 1 minute before attaching the AED. When placing the electrode pads for those patients with ICDs, the anteroposterior and anterolateral locations are acceptable positions. It is not recommended to place the pads directly over the device.[31] Patients who have transdermal medication patches should have those removed before pad placement. The patch may impede the energy delivery of the shock or cause burns to the patient's skin.[68] Patients who are extremely diaphoretic or found lying in water should be removed from the water source and have their chest wiped off before pad placement.[31]

Cardiac arrest in children also poses a unique situation. Unlike adults, VF is relatively uncommon and only observed in 5% to 15% of pediatric and adolescent arrests.[69–73] In those circumstances, defibrillation may improve outcomes; however, the lowest effective energy dose is unknown.[73,74] Most AED devices come with pediatric-sized pads and a pediatric dose-attenuator cord. In children 1 to 8 years, it is recommended to use the dose-attenuator system. For children less than 1 years of age, manual defibrillation is preferred; if that is not available, however, the pediatric dose-attenuator system should be implemented. In circumstances where neither manual defibrillation nor the pediatric dose-attenuator system are available, an adult AED should be used.[31] Some form of early defibrillation in infants and children is preferable to either delayed or no such intervention.

Since 1995, the AHA has been instrumental in the development of the lay rescuer AED or public access defibrillation programs. The goal of these programs was to shorten the time interval between cardiac arrest and the initiation of CPR and defibrillation. A large prospective trial demonstrated a twofold increase in the number of survivors of out-of-hospital cardiac arrest when early AED use was compared with early EMS call.[75] These programs emphasize placing an AED in public locations; however, roughly 60% to 80% of out-of-hospital arrests occur in private or residential areas. When studies evaluated residential use of AEDs, there was no significant difference demonstrated comparing early AED use with CPR alone.[76,77] Both AED use and CPR are vital to the potential survival of patients who have cardiac arrest. The mere presence of an AED does not ensure proper use. When evaluating areas with established AED programs, one study demonstrated that the AED was only used in 34% of arrested patients.[75] As these programs evolve, it is extremely important to have quality improvement measures and continual training of those first-responders to achieve the maximum benefits that are capable with AEDs.

Several studies have considered the use of AEDs in the hospital setting. Four studies demonstrated improved survival rates to hospital discharge, whereas one study did not demonstrate increased rates of survival or return of spontaneous circulation.[78–82] These studies primarily evaluated the use of AEDs by nursing staff or medical emergency teams on non–intensive care unit patients experiencing cardiac arrest. In these instances AEDs may decrease length of time between VT or VF cardiac arrest and defibrillation. Patients who may most benefit from in-hospital AEDs are those in unmonitored or non–intensive care unit beds or those in outpatient and diagnostic facilities. Although limited data are available, as with other studies evaluating early AED use, increased access to AEDs at outpatient healthcare facilities is expected to improve patient outcome. The goal of decreasing the time from cardiac arrest to defibrillation is the same for both in-hospital and out-of-hospital settings.

SUMMARY

Recognition and appropriate treatment of VF or pulseless VT is an essential skill for healthcare providers. Appropriate defibrillation can improve survival and benefit patient outcome. Similarly, increased public access to AEDs has been shown to improve out-of-hospital survival for cardiac arrest. When combined with high-quality CPR, electrical therapies are an important aspect of resuscitation in the patient with cardiac arrest.

REFERENCES

1. Field JM, Hazinski MF, Sayre MR, et al. Part 1: executive summary: 2010 American Heart Association guidelines for cardiopulmonary resuscitation and emergency cardiovascular care. Circulation 2010;122:s640–56.
2. Cakulev I, Efimov IR, Waldo AL. Cardioversion: past, present, and future. Circulation 2009;120:1623–32.
3. Abildgaard PC. Tentamina electrica in animalibus instituta. Societatis Medicae Havniensis Colectanea 1775;2:157.
4. Lown B. Defibrillation and cardioversion. Cardiovasc Res 2002;55:220–4.
5. Cooper JA, Cooper JD, Cooper JM. Cardiopulmonary resuscitation: history, current practice, and future direction. Circulation 2006;114:2839–49.
6. Eisenberg MS. Charles Kite's essay on the recovery of the apparently dead: the first scientific study of sudden death. Ann Emerg Med 1994;23:1049–53.
7. The Royal Humane Society for the recovery of the apparently drowned. Annual Reports 1774:1–31.
8. Prevost JL, Battelli F. Le mort par les descharges electrique. J Physiol 1899;1: 1085–100.
9. Kouwenhoven WB. Current flowing through heart under conditions of electric shock. Am J Physiol 1932;100:344–50.
10. Beck CS, Pritchard WH, Feil HS. Ventricular fibrillation of long duration abolished by electrical shock. JAMA 1947;135:985–6.
11. Adgey AA, Walsh SJ. Theory and practice of defibrillation: (1) atrial fibrillation and DC conversion. Heart 2004;90:1493–8.
12. Dosdall DJ, Fast VG, Ideker RE. Mechanisms of defibrillation. Annu Rev Biomed Eng 2010;12:233–58.
13. Morrison LJ, Dorian P, Long J, et al, Steering Committee, Central Validation Committee, Safety and Efficacy Committee. Out-of-hospital cardiac arrest rectilinear biphasic to monophasic damped sine defibrillation waveforms with advanced life support intervention trial (ORBIT). Resuscitation 2005;66:149–57.
14. Kudenchuk PJ, Cobb LA, Copass MK, et al. Transthoracic Incremental Monophasic Versus Biphasic Defibrillation By Emergency Responders (TIMBER): a randomized comparison of monophasic with biphasic waveform ascending

energy defibrillation for the resuscitation of out-of-hospital cardiac arrest due to ventricular fibrillation. Circulation 2006;114:2010–8.

15. Schneider T, Martens PR, Paschen H, et al. Multicenter, randomized, controlled trial of 150-J biphasic shocks compared with 200 to 360J monophasic shocks in the resuscitation of out-of-hospital cardiac arrest victims. Optimized Response to Cardiac Arrest (ORCA) investigators. Circulation 2000;102:1780–7.

16. Leng CT, Paradis NA, Calkins H, et al. Resuscitation after prolonged ventricular fibrillation with use of monophasic and biphasic waveform pulses for external defibrillation. Circulation 2000;101:2968–74.

17. Jones JL, Jones RE. Improved defibrillator waveform safety factor with biphasic waveforms. Am J Physiol 1983;245:H60–5.

18. Niebauer MJ, Brewer JE, Chung MK, et al. Comparison of the rectilinear biphasic waveform with the monophasic damped sine waveform for external cardioversion of atrial fibrillation and flutter. Am J Cardiol 2004;93:1495–9.

19. Niemann JT, Garner D, Lewis RJ. Transthoracic impedance does not decrease with rapidly repeated countershocks in a swine cardiac arrest model. Resuscitation 2003;56:91–5.

20. Rea TD, Helbock M, Perry S, et al. Increasing use of cardiopulmonary resuscitation during out-of-hospital ventricular fibrillation arrest: survival implications of guideline changes. Circulation 2006;114:2760–5.

21. Kerber RE, Grayzel J, Hoyt R, et al. Transthoracic resistance in human defibrillation. Influence of body weight, chest size, serial shocks, paddle size and paddle contact pressure. Circulation 1981;63:676–82.

22. Deale OC, Lerman BB. Intrathoracic current flow during transthoracic defibrillation in dogs. Transcardiac current fraction. Circ Res 1990;67:1405–19.

23. Valenzuela TD, Roe DJ, Cretin S, et al. Estimating effectiveness of cardiac arrest interventions: a logistic regression survival model. Circulation 1997;96:3308–13.

24. Larsen MP, Eisenberg MS, Cummins RO, et al. Predicting survival from out-of-hospital cardiac arrest: a graphic model. Ann Emerg Med 1993;22:1652–8.

25. Chan PS, Krumholz HM, Nichol G, et al. Delayed time to defibrillation after in-hospital cardiac arrest. N Engl J Med 2008;358:9–17.

26. Stiell IG, Wells GA, Field B, et al. Advanced cardiac life support in out-of-hospital cardiac arrest. N Engl J Med 2004;351:647–56.

27. Kudenchuk PJ. Electrical therapies. In: Field JM, Kudenchuk JP, O'Conner RE, et al, editors. The textbook of emergency cardiovascular care and CPR. Philadelphia: Lippincott Williams & Wilkins; 2008. p. 362–78.

28. Cummins RO, Eisenberg MS, Hallstrom AP, et al. Survival of out-of-hospital cardiac arrest with early initiation of cardiopulmonary resuscitation. Am J Emerg Med 1985;3:114–9.

29. Holmberg M, Holmberg S, Herlitz J. Effect of bystander cardiopulmonary resuscitation in out-of-hospital cardiac arrest patients in Sweden. Resuscitation 2000; 47:59–70.

30. Waalewijn RA, Tijssen JG, Koster RW. Bystander initiated actions in out-of-hospital cardiopulmonary resuscitation: results from the Amsterdam Resuscitation Study (ARRESUST). Resuscitation 2001;50:273–9.

31. Kerber RE, Becker LB, Bourland JD, et al. Automatic external defibrillators for public access defibrillation: recommendations for specifying and reporting arrhythmia analysis algorithm performance, incorporating new waveforms, and enhancing safety. A Statement for Health Professionals From the American Heart Association Task Force on Automatic External Defibrillation, Subcommittee on AED Safety and Efficacy. Circulation 1997;95:1677–82.

32. Wik L, Hansen TB, Fylling F, et al. Delaying defibrillation to give basic cardiopulmonary resuscitation to patients with out-of-hospital ventricular fibrillation: a randomized trial. JAMA 2003;289:1389–95.
33. Cobb LA, Fahrenbruch CE, Walsh TR, et al. Influence of cardiopulmonary resuscitation prior to defibrillation in patients with out-of-hospital ventricular fibrillation. JAMA 1999;281:1182–8.
34. Baker PW, Conway J, Cotton C, et al. Defibrillation or cardiopulmonary resuscitation first for patients with out-of-hospital cardiac arrests found by paramedics to be in ventricular fibrillation? A randomized control trial. Resuscitation 2008;79:424–31.
35. Jacobs IG, Finn JC, Oxer HF, et al. CPR before defibrillation in out-of-hospital cardiac arrest: a randomized trial. Emerg Med Australas 2005;17:39–45.
36. Eftestol T, Wik L, Sunde K, et al. Effects of cardiopulmonary resuscitation on predictors of ventricular fibrillation defibrillation success during out-of-hospital cardiac arrest. Circulation 2004;110:10–5.
37. Brooks SC, Schmicker RH, Rea TD, et al. Out-of-hospital cardiac arrest frequency and survival: evidence for temporal variability. Resuscitation 2010;81:175.
38. Ornato JP, Peberdy MA. The mystery of bradyasystole during cardiac arrest. Ann Emerg Med 1996;27:567–87.
39. Hedges JR, Syverud SA, Dalsey WC, et al. Prehospital trial of emergency transcutaneous cardiac pacing. Circulation 1987;76:1337–43.
40. Barthell E, Troiano P, Olson D, et al. Prehospital external cardiac pacing: a prospective, controlled clinical trial. Ann Emerg Med 1988;17:1221–6.
41. Cummins RO, Graves JR, Larsen MP, et al. Out-of-hospital transcutaneous pacing by emergency medical technicians in patients with asystolic cardiac arrest. N Engl J Med 1991;328:1377–82.
42. Knowlton AA, Falk RH. External cardiac pacing during in-hospital cardiac arrest. Am J Cardiol 1986;57:1295–8.
43. Dalsey WC, Syverud SA, Hedges JR. Emergency department use of transcutaneous pacing for cardiac arrests. Crit Care Med 1985;3:399–401.
44. Sherbino J, Verbeek PR, MacDonald RD, et al. Prehospital transcutaneous cardiac pacing for symptomatic bradycardia or bradyasystolic cardiac arrest: a systematic review. Resuscitation 2006;70:193–200.
45. Link MS, Atkins DL, Passman RS, et al. Part 6: electrical therapies: automated external defibrillators, defibrillation, cardioversion, and pacing: 2010 American Heart Association Guidelines for Cardiopulmonary Resuscitation and Emergency Cardiovascular Care. Circulation 2010;122:s706–16.
46. Sodeck GH, Domanovits H, Meron G, et al. Compromising bradycardia: management in the emergency department. Resuscitation 2007;73:96–102.
47. Hedges JR, Feero S, Shultz B, et al. Prehospital transcutaneous cardiac pacing for symptomatic bradycardia. Pacing Clin Electrophysiol 1991;14:1473–8.
48. Vukov LF, Johnson DQ. External transcutaneous pacemakers in interhospital transport of cardiac patients. Ann Emerg Med 1989;18:738–40.
49. Neumar RW, Otto CW, Link MS, et al. Part 8: adult advanced cardiovascular life support: 2010 American Heart Association Guidelines for Cardiopulmonary Resuscitation and Emergency Cardiovascular Care. Circulation 2010;122:s729–67.
50. Gowda RM, Khan IA, Wilbur SL, et al. Torsade de pointes: the clinical considerations. Int J Cardiol 2004;96:1–6.
51. Khan IA, Gowda RM. Novel therapeutics for treatment of long-QT syndrome and torsade de pointes. Int J Cardiol 2004;95:1–6.

52. Chiang CE. Congenital and acquired long QT syndrome: current concepts and management. Cardiol Rev 2004;12:222–34.
53. Viskin S. Long QT syndromes and torsade de pointes. Lancet 1999;354:1625–33.
54. Mancuso EM, Brady WJ, Harrigan RA, et al. Electrocardiographic manifestations: long QT syndrome. J Emerg Med 2004;27:385–93.
55. Viskin S, Justo D, Halkin A, et al. Long QT syndrome caused by noncardiac drugs. Prog Cardiovasc Dis 2003;45:415–27.
56. Kao LW, Furbee RB. Drug-induced Q-T prolongation. Med Clin North Am 2005; 89:1125–44.
57. Gupta A, Lawrence AT, Krishnan K, et al. Current concepts in the mechanisms and management of drug-induced QT prolongation and torsade de pointes. Am Heart J 2007;153:891–9.
58. Stern S, Keren A, Tzivoni D. Torsades de pointes: definitions, causative factors, and therapy: experience with sixteen patients. Ann N Y Acad Sci 1984;427: 234–40.
59. Nguyen PT, Scheinman MM, Seger J. Polymorphous ventricular tachycardia: clinical characterization, therapy, and the QT interval. Circulation 1986;74:340–9.
60. Morrison LJ, Deakin CD, Morley PT, et al. Part 8: advanced life support: 2010 International Consensus on Cardiopulmonary Resuscitation and Emergency Cardiovascular Care Science with Treatment Recommendations. Circulation 2010;122:s345–421.
61. England H, Hoffman C, Hodgman T, et al. Effectiveness of automated external defibrillators in high schools in greater Boston. Am J Cardiol 2005;95:1484–6.
62. Boodhoo L, Mitchell AR, Bordoli G, et al. DC cardioversion of persistent atrial fibrillation: a comparison of two protocols. Int J Cardiol 2007;114:16–21.
63. Brazdzionyte J, Babarskiene RM, Stanaitiene G. Anterior-posterior versus anterior-lateral electrode position for biphasic cardioversion of atrial fibrillation. Medicina (Kaunas) 2006;42:994–8.
64. Chen CJ, Guo GB. External cardioversion in patients with persistent atrial fibrillation: a reappraisal of the effects of electrode pad position and transthoracic impedance on cardioversion success. Jpn Heart J 2003;44:921–32.
65. Stanaitiene G, Babarskiene RM. Impact of electrical shock waveform and paddle positions on efficacy of direct current cardioversion for atrial fibrillation. Medicina (Kaunas) 2008;44:665–72 [in Lithuanian].
66. Hoyt R, Grayzel J, Kerber RE. Determinants of intracardiac current in defibrillation. Experimental studies in dogs. Circulation 1981;64:818–23.
67. Monsieurs KG, Conraads VM, Goethals MP, et al. Semi-automatic external defibrillation and implanted cardiac pacemakers: understanding the interactions during resuscitation. Resuscitation 1995;30:127–31.
68. Panacek EA, Munger MA, Rutherford WF, et al. Report of nitropatch explosions complicating defibrillation. Am J Emerg Med 1992;10:128–9.
69. Hickey RW, Cohen DM, Strausbaugh S, et al. Pediatric patients requiring CPR in the prehospital setting. Ann Emerg Med 1995;25:495–501.
70. Appleton GO, Cummins RO, Larson MP, et al. CPR and the single rescuer: at what age should you "call first" rather than "call fast"? Ann Emerg Med 1995; 25:492–4.
71. Ronco R, King W, Donley DK, et al. Outcome and cost at a children's hospital following resuscitation for out-of-hospital cardiopulmonary arrest. Arch Pediatr Adolesc Med 1995;149:210–4.
72. Losek JD, Hennes H, Glaeser P, et al. Prehospital care of the pulseless, nonbreathing pediatric patient. Am J Emerg Med 1987;5:370–4.

73. Mogayzel C, Quan L, Graves JR, et al. Out-of-hospital ventricular fibrillation in children and adolescents: causes and outcomes. Ann Emerg Med 1995;25: 484–91.
74. Safranek DJ, Eisenberg MS, Larsen MP. The epidemiology of cardiac arrest in young adults. Ann Emerg Med 1992;21:1102–6.
75. Hallstrom AP, Ornatao JP, Weisfeldt M, et al, The Public Access Defibrillation Trial Investigators. Public-access defibrillation and survival after out-of-hospital cardiac arrest. N Engl J Med 2004;351:637–46.
76. Becker L, Eisenberg M, Fahrenbruch C, et al. Public locations of cardiac arrest: implications for public access defibrillation. Circulation 1998;97:2106–9.
77. Bardy GH, Lee KL, Mark DB, et al. Home use of automated external defibrillators for sudden cardiac arrest. N Engl J Med 2008;358:1793–804.
78. Zafari AM, Zarter SK, Heggen V, et al. A program encouraging early defibrillation results in improved in-hospital resuscitation efficacy. J Am Coll Cardiol 2004;44: 846–52.
79. Destro A, Marzaloni M, Sermasi S, et al. Automatic external defibrillators in the hospital as well? Resuscitation 1996;31:39–43.
80. Gombotz H, Weh B, Mitterndorfer W, et al. In-hospital cardiac resuscitation outside the ICU by nursing staff equipped with automated external defibrillators—the first 500 cases. Resuscitation 2006;70:416–22.
81. Hanefeld C, Lichte C, Mentges-Schroter I, et al. Hospital-wide first-responder automated external defibrillator programme: 1 year experience. Resuscitation 2005;66:167–70.
82. Smith M. Service is improving everywhere. But what about EMS? EMS Mag 2009; 38:26.

The Impact of the Code Drugs: Cardioactive Medications in Cardiac Arrest Resuscitation

Kelly Williamson, MD[a], Meghan Breed, BA, EMT-I[b,c],
Kostas Alibertis, BA, CCEMT-P[d,e,f], William J. Brady, MD[c,d,g,h],*

KEYWORDS

- Cardiac arrest • Anti-arrhythmic agent • Vasopressor

Approximately 325,000 cardiac arrests occur each year in the United States; primary cardiac events represent the precipitating cause in 75% of all episodes of sudden death. Most of these cardiac arrests (250,000) occur outside of a hospital annually. Despite innumerable advancements in medical treatments and technology, survival of individuals after an out-of-hospital cardiac arrest remains low, averaging less than 7%.[1]

The human circulatory system is a complex vascular network, and dysfunction rapidly leads to impaired oxygen delivery, progressive cellular dysfunction, organ failure, and ultimately patient death. Therefore, interventions for victims of cardiac arrest must be performed rapidly and efficiently to maximize the chance of a favorable cardiac and neurologic outcome. In an attempt to address this dysfunction and

[a] Department of Emergency Medicine, Northwestern University, Chicago, IL 60611, USA
[b] Department of Emergency Medicine, University of Virginia, Charlottesville, VA 22908, USA
[c] Charlottesville-Albemarle Rescue Squad, Charlottesville, VA 22901, USA
[d] Center for Emergency Preparedness and Response, University of Virginia, Charlottesville, VA 22908, USA
[e] Western Albemarle Rescue Squad, Crozet, VA 22932, USA
[f] American Heart Association, Committee for Emergency for Cardiovascular Care, Dallas, TX 75231, USA
[g] Departments of Emergency Medicine and Medicine, University of Virginia School of Medicine, Charlottesville, VA 22908, USA
[h] Albemarle County Fire Rescue, Charlottesville, VA 22901, USA
* Corresponding author. Departments of Emergency Medicine and Medicine, University of Virginia School of Medicine. Charlottesville, VA 22908.
E-mail address: WB4Z@hscmail.mcc.virginia.edu

Emerg Med Clin N Am 30 (2012) 65–75
doi:10.1016/j.emc.2011.09.008
0733-8627/12/$ – see front matter © 2012 Elsevier Inc. All rights reserved.

alter its natural history, the American Heart Association (AHA) has proposed a 4-step chain of survival to improve the outcomes of patients who experience an out-of-hospital cardiac arrest. The survival benefit of the first 3 steps, which include early access to medical care, early initiation of cardiopulmonary resuscitation (CPR), and early defibrillation, have been established in the literature and are discussed elsewhere in this issue. The incremental benefit of the fourth step in the chain of survival, which is early access to advanced care including airway management and the use of cardioactive intravenous (IV) medications, has not yet been well established, and there have been few advances in the pharmacologic component of the chain of survival.

The impact of advanced care has been questioned. Stiell and colleagues[2] concluded that the use of cardioactive medications during cardiac arrest does not improve survival to hospital discharge or the resulting neurologic status despite an increase in the return of spontaneous circulation (ROSC) and survival to hospital admission. The OPALS (Ontario Prehospital Advanced Life Support) trial examined the incremental effect on the rate of survival of individuals after cardiac arrest of adding advanced life support to an already present rapid defibrillation program. The multicenter, controlled, clinical trial reviewed the cases of 5638 patients. The investigators concluded that although the addition of cardioactive medications increased survival to hospital admission, it did not affect survival to hospital discharge. Further work by Stiell and colleagues[3] examined the relative importance of interventions in cardiac arrest with the determination of the value added by these therapies; selected odds ratios supporting survival from cardiac arrest include the following: witnessed arrest (4.4), any form of bystander CPR (3.7), electrical defibrillation less than 8 minutes into arrest (3.4), and advanced life support with cardioactive medications (1.1). This data set does not suggest that the advanced interventions offer significant benefit when compared with the basic therapies such as CPR and defibrillation. Furthermore, medication administration should not interfere with other lifesaving interventions such as chest compressions and defibrillation.

Despite this less-than-impressive database supporting their use, the various cardioactive medications, or code drugs, remain prominently placed in the AHA's Advanced Cardiac Life Support (ACLS) Guidelines 2010 (G2010).[4] There are several categories of medications used during cardiac arrest: vasopressor medications (epinephrine, vasopressin, and atropine), antiarrhythmic medications (amiodarone and lidocaine), and adjunct medications (sodium bicarbonate, calcium, magnesium, and fibrinolytics). This review discusses the evidence for their use and notes their current position in the AHA G2010.[4]

VASOPRESSOR MEDICATIONS

Vasopressors, namely epinephrine and vasopressin, are routinely administered during cardiac arrest, and there is evidence to suggest that this usage positively affects ROSC. There are, however, no published placebo-controlled clinical trials demonstrating that the administration of any vasopressor medication at any stage in the management of pulseless ventricular tachycardia (VT), ventricular fibrillation (VF), pulseless electrical activity (PEA), or asystole increases the rate of neurologically intact survival to hospital discharge.[4]

Epinephrine is one of the most widely used drugs in the ACLS regimen, indicated for VF, pulseless VT, PEA, and asystolic arrests. Epinephrine is a sympathomimetic agent that serves as a potent adrenergic agonist stimulating both α and β receptors. Stimulation of the α_1 and α_2 receptors causes arterial vasoconstriction, which is deemed beneficial because such vasoconstriction promotes higher perfusion pressures of the coronary and cerebral vascular beds and increases the aortic diastolic pressure during CPR. Stimulation of β_1 receptor increases heart rate and myocardial contractility, which may be helpful in the immediate postresuscitation period, but these effects are often considered detrimental because they lead to increased myocardial oxygen consumption and may impair subendocardial perfusion. In addition, β_2 receptor stimulation causes vascular and respiratory smooth muscle relaxation, thereby diminishing coronary and cerebral perfusion pressures.

There has been much research surrounding the use of epinephrine for cardiac arrests. In general, the prognosis of patients who require epinephrine, the so-called shock-resistant patients, during cardiac arrest remains extremely poor. These patients are candidates for vasopressor therapy in that they have not responded favorably to electrical defibrillation, thus the shock resistance notation. For instance, a retrospective analysis by Herlitz and colleagues[5] examined 1360 patients who experienced a VF arrest. Epinephrine was given in 417 cases (35%), and those who received the medication experienced ROSC more frequently and had a statistically significant improvement for survival to hospital admission compared with those who did not receive this therapy. The rate of hospital discharge, however, did not differ between the 2 groups. The investigators concluded that although patients receiving epinephrine had a more favorable initial outcome, the final outcome was not significantly affected.

Several studies have compared the standard dose of epinephrine with escalating doses as well as a high-dose strategy. Callaham and colleagues[6] published a randomized, prospective, clinical trial that compared standard-dose and high-dose epinephrine for the initial treatment of prehospital arrest. A total of 816 patients were enrolled. In this study, 13% of patients receiving high-dose epinephrine (15 mg IV) had ROSC compared with 8% receiving standard-dose epinephrine (1 mg IV); furthermore, more patients in the high-dose group survived to hospital admission. However, there was no statistically significant difference in the occurrence of either survival to hospital discharge or neurologically intact survival. A second prospective randomized study published by Gueugniaud and colleagues[7] also compared repeated high doses of epinephrine with repeated doses of standard-dose (ie, 1 mg) epinephrine for out-of-hospital cardiac arrest. Although patients in the high-dose group had higher rates of ROSC and survival to hospital admission, no differences in survival to hospital discharge or neurologic status in the treatment groups were observed. Brown and colleagues[8] conducted a prospective multicenter trial also comparing standard-dose epinephrine with high-dose epinephrine and concluded that there were no differences in the overall rate of ROSC, survival to hospital admission, survival to hospital discharge, or neurologic outcome between the 2 groups. As a result of these studies, high-dose epinephrine is not currently recommended in the treatment of cardiac arrest.

The other primary bolus-dose vasopressor, vasopressin, is a peptide hormone that is normally released from the posterior pituitary gland in response to physiologic demands related to either significant hypovolemia and/or systemic hypoperfusion. Endogenous vasopressin levels have been found to be significantly higher when measured in patients who survived a cardiac arrest compared with those who died.[9] Synthetic vasopressin serves as a nonadrenergic vasopressor with pronounced peripheral vasoconstriction by actions on the V1 receptors of the endothelium. Different from epinephrine, however, vasopressin has no direct effect on cardiac contractility and thereby does not increase myocardial and cerebral oxygen demand. Animal studies have suggested that vasopressin increases blood flow in vital organs, enhances cerebral oxygen delivery, and improves short-term survival and favorable neurologic outcome. Lindner and colleagues[9] also demonstrated such findings in the cardiac arrest scenario; these investigators noted that vasopressin not only increased arterial and coronary pressures but also enhanced myocardial and cerebral blood flows compared with standard doses of epinephrine in animal models of cardiac arrest.

Human studies demonstrate less-than-convincing results when compared with animal studies using vasopressin as a 1-time alternative to epinephrine as the first or second vasopressor administered during cardiac arrest. Stiell and colleagues[10] studied 200 inpatients who had a cardiac arrest. In this study, the patients were randomized to receive either 1 mg of epinephrine or 40 units of vasopressin IV as the initial vasopressor following cardiac arrest, with additional doses of epinephrine then used as a rescue medication at the discretion of the resuscitation team. The investigators noted that there was no survival advantage for vasopressin over epinephrine. Guyette and colleagues[11] examined the outcomes of patients receiving epinephrine only, a combination of vasopressin and epinephrine, or no vasopressor medications in cardiac arrest management. They concluded that ROSC was associated with witnessed collapse, bystander CPR, and initial cardiac rhythm of VF or pulseless VT. The subjects who received vasopressin and epinephrine were more likely to have a ROSC during the resuscitation and survive to hospital arrival than those treated with epinephrine alone, although they do not comment on survival rates to hospital discharge. This study was not constructed to determine ultimate patient outcome, which is unfortunate with regard to a meaningful contribution to the resuscitation literature.

In 2004, Wenzel and colleagues[12] published a study that concluded administration of vasopressin did not change VT, VF, or PEA outcomes, although there was a more frequent ROSC at the time of the event as well as a trend toward a better, although still dismal, initial outcome for patients in asystole. In this study of 1219 patients, vasopressin had outcomes similar to those of epinephrine for patients who had VF or VT during cardiac arrest but was demonstrated to be superior in patients with asystole because these patients were 40% more likely to reach the hospital alive. Once again, the ultimate outcome was not altered. Additional investigation of this topic includes a randomized clinical trial in which 1442 patients received epinephrine and vasopressin during the cardiac arrest and 1452 received epinephrine alone. There were no significant differences in ROSC, survival to hospital admission, survival to hospital discharge, 1-year survival, or neurologic recovery at hospital discharge.[13]

Although there is no demonstrated benefit of vasopressin over epinephrine, there is no evidence of harm either. Although large populations of cardiac arrest patients do not benefit significantly from either vasopressor, it is conceivable that certain individuals do experience an advantage as a consequence of the medication. Thus, the use of these medications should be continued in patients with cardiac arrest. The AHA recommends that vasopressin (40 units IV) can be used as an alternate vasopressor therapy for cardiac arrest, indicated in the treatment of adult shock-refractory VF or pulseless VT as a 1-time alternative to epinephrine.[4]

PARASYMPATHOLYTIC MEDICATION (ATROPINE)

During cardiac arrest, parasympathetic tone is increased as a result of vagal stimulation, which leads to decreases in heart rate, systemic vascular resistance, and blood pressure. Atropine is a parasympatholytic drug that enhances both sinoatrial node automaticity and atrioventricular conduction via direct vagolytic action and competitive antagonism of acetylcholine at the sinoatrial and atrioventricular nodes. Because asystole can be precipitated or exacerbated by excess vagal tone, atropine provides a theoretic physiologic advantage. However, the literature on the use of atropine in cardiac arrest is limited. There are no prospective, randomized, controlled trials that support the use of atropine in asystole or PEA arrest, nor is there literature to suggest its harmful effects or dispute its use in cardiac arrest.

Brown and colleagues[14] examined the notion that atropine can aid in cardiac arrest via its parasympathetic blockade. They published a case series of 8 patients who had return of a regular rhythm after administration of atropine, 3 of whom ultimately survived to hospital discharge. The investigators' results suggest the value of atropine in the treatment of asystole. Stueven[15] published a retrospective review of 170 patients with asystole, of whom 43 patients received atropine for refractory asystole after the administration of epinephrine and sodium bicarbonate, whereas 41 patients did not. The investigator found 14% survival to hospital admission in the atropine group, with 0% in the nonatropine group, although there were no survivors to hospital discharge in either group. Coon and colleagues[16] evaluated the efficacy of atropine for treating asystolic prehospital cardiac arrests in a controlled prospective study. Twenty-one patients were divided into atropine-treated and nonatropine-treated (control) groups. The atropine-treated patients received 1 mg of atropine IV with a repeat dose at 1 minute if no rhythm change occurred, as well as the same additional medication therapy as the control group. Only 2 patients in each group were successfully resuscitated in the emergency department, and only 1 patient in the control group was discharged alive. The investigators therefore question the usefulness of atropine for brady-asystolic arrests.

Because no prospective clinical trials have examined the use of atropine in asystole or bradycardic PEA arrest combined with lower-level clinical studies providing conflicting evidence, in G2010 the AHA commented that atropine is unlikely to have a therapeutic benefit in cardiac arrest and was therefore removed from the ACLS algorithm.[4] This action is the first time that a major medication has been removed from the AHA ACLS guidelines. However, there is neither demonstrated benefit nor harm in such settings. On the contrary, the aggressive and early use of atropine in the prearrest setting (ie, patients with intact although compromised perfusion) has demonstrated benefit.[17,18]

ANTIARRHYTHMIC MEDICATIONS (LIDOCAINE AND AMIODARONE)

Lidocaine and amiodarone are the 2 most commonly used antiarrhythmic medications in cardiac arrest, although their benefit has not been clearly established in clinical trials. Lidocaine, well known and widely used as both an amide local anesthetic and an antiarrhythmic agent, increases the electrical stimulation threshold of the ventricle during diastole, thereby decreasing ectopic electrical myocardial activity. Paradoxically, this action has the unfortunate consequence of also serving to increase the defibrillation threshold. Amiodarone is the other primary antiarrhythmic agent that is indicated in VF and pulseless VT. The drug's primary effects are via sodium and calcium channel blockade, potassium efflux antagonism, and adrenergic blocking effects; thus, amiodarone acts via a multitude of mechanisms.

The use of lidocaine for ventricular arrhythmias was initially supported by animal studies, and 1 prehospital study reported that lidocaine usage improved short-term survival.[19] However, 3 additional randomized trials examined the effects of lidocaine during cardiac arrest and reported less-than-impressive end results. Weaver and colleagues[20] randomized 199 patients who suffered an out-of-hospital cardiac arrest to receive either epinephrine or lidocaine. The investigators determined that the rates of asystole were higher in patients who received lidocaine. Two additional studies directly compared the outcomes of patients who received lidocaine with those receiving amiodarone. Dorian and colleagues[21] demonstrated that the use of amiodarone leads to substantially higher rates of survival to hospital admission in patients with shock-resistant VF compared with lidocaine. A German study by Kentsch[22] also concluded that the use of lidocaine led to lower rates of ROSC compared with amiodarone. Thus, the evidence does not support the use of lidocaine in the management of shock-resistant VF or pulseless VT.

Although there are data to advocate the use of amiodarone rather than lidocaine for antiarrhythmic therapy in cardiac arrest, there are still questions on whether the administration of amiodarone improves long-term outcomes. In a study that enrolled 347 patients, Dorian and colleagues[21] concluded that the use of amiodarone leads to substantially higher rates of survival to hospital admission in patients with shock-resistant VF compared with lidocaine, but final outcomes were not different. Kudenchuck and colleagues[23] published a study comparing amiodarone with placebo for out-of-hospital cardiac arrest in patients with pulseless VT and VF. The investigators examined 504 patients and concluded that patients who received amiodarone had higher rates of survival to hospital admission, with an adjusted odds ratio of 1.6. The study, however, was not sufficiently powered to determine a difference to hospital discharge; no difference in ultimate outcome was found.

As a result of these studies, the AHA recommends the use of amiodarone for VF or pulseless VT that is unresponsive to CPR, shock, and a vasopressor (class IIb recommendation). Amiodarone is first given as a dose of 300 mg IV, which can be followed with a second dose of 150 mg IV after 5 minutes.[4] Furthermore, the AHA concludes that lidocaine has no proven short-term or long-term efficacy in cardiac arrest. However, given its widespread familiarity and few immediate side effects, lidocaine may still be considered an alternative to amiodarone for VF and pulseless VT, with a class indeterminate; the drug should be given at an initial dose of 1 to 1.5 mg/kg IV, followed by 0.5- to 0.75-mg/kg IV push at 5- to 10-minute intervals (maximum dose, 3 mg/kg) if VF or pulseless VT persists.[4]

OTHER MEDICATIONS

In addition to the vasopressor and antiarrhythmic medications, several other adjunctive therapies have been examined for use in cardiac arrest, including sodium bicarbonate, magnesium, calcium, and fibrinolytic agents. The common theme among these 4 general classes of medication is summarized by the following statement: the use of these agents in cardiac arrest management does not demonstrate benefit in all such patients; these agents, however, do potentially benefit specific patients in cardiac arrest, introducing the concept of niche application of these drugs in certain cardiac arrest scenarios. Examples of these situations include the patient with severe hyperkalemia, profound hypocalcemia, and diagnosed or highly suspected pulmonary embolism.

Sodium Bicarbonate

Sodium bicarbonate is a potent alkaline agent and an essential component in the maintenance of acid-base homeostasis in the human body. Because of its role as a potent buffer and presence in the AHA algorithms, sodium bicarbonate is frequently used in cardiac arrest; Bar-Joseph and colleagues[24] noted that bicarbonate is used in 54.5% of all cardiac arrests. They reviewed the use of bicarbonate in cardiac arrest therapy.[24] The BRCT III database comprises 2915 patients who experienced an out-of-hospital cardiac arrest. Although the initial objective of the study was to compare high-dose with standard-dose epinephrine during resuscitation, the investigators also examined sodium bicarbonate usage and determined that pre–basic life support or pre-ACLS intervals did not influence the decision to use sodium bicarbonate or when to administer it. They suggest that future guidelines for sodium bicarbonate use during resuscitation should emphasize the importance of pre-ACLS hypoxia time in contributing to acidosis and define more specifically the interval in which bicarbonate administration may be helpful. The investigators noted that both early and aggressive buffer use were associated with improved, although still poor, outcome in cardiac arrest resuscitation.[24]

There is, however, limited evidence to support its widespread use in cardiac arrest because it can adversely affect perfusion in certain vascular beds, thereby unfavorably altering acid-base status at the tissue and cell levels and promoting hyperosmolarity and hypernatremia. As a result of this information, the AHA currently gives sodium bicarbonate a level III recommendation for use in all patients in cardiac arrest.[4] There are several niche applications for sodium bicarbonate use, including severe acidosis, sodium channel blocking agent overdose, and significant hyperkalemia.

Magnesium

Magnesium is an electrolyte whose ions are essential to many enzymatic processes, most importantly, serving as a cofactor in the formation and use of the energy substrate adenosine triphosphate. Hypomagnesemia, an electrolyte disturbance in which there is an abnormally low level of magnesium in the blood, can precipitate sudden cardiac death. It has therefore been hypothesized that the use of magnesium may be beneficial in cardiac arrest.

Two case reports were published in the early 1990s that led to further investigation of the role of magnesium in cardiac arrest. Tobey and colleagues[25] reported the case of a 46-year-old man who suffered a VF arrest, received 62 minutes of ACLS care, and was successfully resuscitated on arrival in the emergency department when he received 4 g of IV magnesium sulfate ($MgSO_4$). Craddock[26] reports a similar case in which a 41-year-old woman experienced an asystolic cardiac arrest postoperatively and subsequent ROSC, which was temporally related to the administration of 8 g of IV $MgSO_4$.

Because of these 2 dramatic case reports, Fatovich and colleagues[27] conducted the MAGIC (Magnesium in Cardiac Arrest) trial to determine if high-dose magnesium was associated with increased survival from out-of-hospital cardiac arrest. A total of 67 patients were randomized to receive either 5 g $MgSO_4$ or placebo as first-line antiarrhythmic drug therapy, with the remainder of their management dictated by standard ACLS. In this small study, the investigators concluded that the use of magnesium as first-line drug therapy for out-of-hospital cardiac arrest was not associated with significantly improved survival. Thel and colleagues[28] examined the use of magnesium during in-hospital cardiac arrest, finding results similar to those of the Fatovich study,[27] and concluding that empiric magnesium supplementation did not improve the rate of successful resuscitation, survival to 24 hours, or survival to hospital discharge.[2]

There are 2 specific instances where its utility has been demonstrated: long QT-related polymorphic VT (torsades de pointes) and toxemia of pregnancy. Long QT-related polymorphic VT, or torsades de pointes, is a less common variety of VT that demonstrates the characteristic electrocardiographic findings of a twisting-about-the-points morphology of sequential QRS complexes around an isoelectric baseline. In this situation, magnesium is a negative inotrope and works by slowing electrical signals in the atrioventricular node. Magnesium is also useful in toxemia of pregnancy or eclampsia. Eclampsia affects the vasculature and leads to vasospasm and convulsions, which may become fatal. The vasodilatory properties of magnesium can modify these effects, and its administration is considered the standard of care in these cases.

The AHA does not recommend the routine use of magnesium for cardiac arrest, although it receives a level IIb recommendation for torsades de pointes and is considered standard of care for the treatment of toxemia.

Calcium

Calcium is essential for living organisms, particularly as related to cellular physiology, when the movement of calcium ions into and out of the cytoplasm functions as a signal for cellular processes. However, calcium abnormality as a cause of cardiac arrest is very rare. Because cardiac muscle depends on extracellular calcium ions for contraction and calcium exerts a stabilizing effect on myocardial cells, researchers have attempted to determine if the routine use of calcium during cardiac arrest alters survival. Like the other agents discussed in this article, conclusive evidence of a beneficial effect of calcium in cardiac arrest management is lacking.

One study by Stueven and colleagues[29] examined 179 patients who presented in asystole and 116 patients with electromechanical dissociation (ie, PEA). Calcium use was not significantly found in patients who were resuscitated; for both rhythms, patients who did not receive calcium were more likely to undergo successful resuscitation than those who received calcium. Harrison and Amey[30] examined 480 patients who suffered an out-of-hospital cardiac arrest and received calcium chloride during the course of the arrest. They determined that there was no positive effect on patient outcomes in cardiac arrest. Furthermore, Donovan and Propp[31] argue that the routine administration of calcium during cardiac arrest may even be deleterious because natural cellular accumulation of calcium within the myocardium occurs during cardiac arrest. Therefore, the AHA does not recommend the routine use of calcium during cardiac arrest.[4] There are, however, several potential niche applications for its use, including hyperkalemia, severe hypocalcemia, and calcium channel blocker overdose.[4,32]

Fibrinolytic Agents

Because coronary thrombosis and pulmonary thromboembolism are common precipitants of cardiac arrest, one final adjunctive medication that has been suggested in patients with persistent PEA arrest is the fibrinolytic agents. Fibrinolysis is the process by which a fibrin clot, the product of coagulation, is degraded. Fibrinolytic agents, such as tissue plasminogen activator (t-PA), convert plasminogen to active plasmin, which works to break down the fibrin mesh. Adults have been successfully resuscitated after the administration of t-PA when the condition leading to the arrest was acute pulmonary embolism or myocardial infarction.[33]

In one large clinical trial, Abu-Laban and colleagues[34] assessed whether the administration of t-PA during resuscitation would benefit patients with PEA of unknown cause. A total of 233 patients with cardiac arrest were enrolled and randomly assigned to receive 100 mg of t-PA or placebo IV along with standard resuscitation measures. One patient in the t-PA group survived to hospital discharge, compared with none in the placebo group, although more patients in the placebo group achieved ROSC. Neither of these outcomes reached statistical significance, and the investigators concluded that they found no evidence of a beneficial effect of fibrinolysis in patients with undifferentiated cardiac arrest and PEA. A second prospective, randomized, double-blind, placebo-controlled, multicenter trial was conducted by Bottiger and colleagues[35] to determine whether fibrinolysis with tenecteplase improves survival in adults with witnessed out-of-hospital arrest of presumed cardiac origin. After the enrollment of the first 443 patients, patients who presented in asystole were no longer enrolled because of low survival, and the trial was ultimately terminated by the Human Safety Committee of the sponsoring institution after the enrollment of 1050 patients for futility because there were no significant differences in 30-day survival, hospital admission, ROSC, 24-hour survival, survival to hospital discharge, or neurologic outcome. Furthermore, there were more intracranial hemorrhages in the tenecteplase group. The investigators therefore concluded that there was no improvement in outcome when tenecteplase was used for out-of-hospital cardiac arrest compared with placebo.

The AHA states that there is insufficient evidence to advocate for the routine use of fibrinolytic agents during cardiac arrest but that their use should be considered on a case-by-case basis; they receive a level IIb recommendation for cardiac arrest secondary to pulmonary embolism.[4]

SUMMARY

The goal of treating patients who present with cardiac arrest is to intervene as quickly as possible to affect the best possible outcome. The mainstays of these interventions, including early activation of the emergency response team, early initiation of CPR, and early defibrillation, are essential components with demonstrated positive impact on resuscitation outcomes. Conversely, the use of the code drugs as a component of advanced life support has not benefited patients with cardiac arrest in general. Although short-term outcomes are improved as a function of these medications, the ultimate outcome has not been altered, whether one considers survival to hospital discharge or neurologic status at discharge. Direct harm has not been conclusively demonstrated as a result of the use of these drugs. Furthermore, it is conceivable that selected individuals do benefit from such interventions. At present, no data exist that allow for the rapid identification of such patients who will derive benefit. Thus, the authors agree with the AHA's recommendations in the G2010 regarding the code drugs. Clinicians must be aware of this modest, at best, impact on cardiac arrest outcome of these agents and not allow their use to hinder, interrupt, or otherwise adversely affect management, namely, the timely performance of high-quality chest compressions and early electrical defibrillation.

REFERENCES

1. Out of hospital cardiac arrest: statistical guidelines. American Heart Association; 2007.
2. Stiell IG, Wells GA, Field B, et al. Advanced cardiac life support in out-of-hospital cardiac arrest. N Engl J Med 2004;351:647–56.
3. Stiell IG, Wells GA, DeMaio VJ, et al. Modifiable factors associated with improved cardiac arrest survival in a multicenter basic life support/defibrillation system: OPALS Study Phase I results. Ann Emerg Med 1999;33:44–50.
4. Neumar RW, Otto CW, Link MS, et al. 2010 American Heart Association guidelines for cardiopulmonary resuscitation and emergency cardiovascular care science. Part 8: adult advanced cardiovascular life support. Circulation 2010;122: S729–67.
5. Herlitz J, Ekstrom L, Wennerblom B, et al. Adrenaline in out-of-hospital ventricular fibrillation. Does it make any difference? Resuscitation 1995;29:195–201.

6. Callaham M, Madsen CD, Barton CW, et al. A randomized clinical trial of high-dose epinephrine and norepinephrine vs standard-dose epinephrine in prehospital cardiac arrest. JAMA 1992;268:2667–72.
7. Gueugniaud PY, Mols P, Goldstein P, et al. A comparison of repeated high doses and repeated standard doses of epinephrine for cardiac arrest outside the hospital. European Epinephrine Study Group. N Engl J Med 1998;339:1595–601.
8. Brown CG, Martin DR, Pepe PE, et al. A comparison of standard-dose and high-dose epinephrine in cardiac arrest outside the hospital. The Multicenter High-Dose Epinephrine Study Group. N Engl J Med 1992;327:1051–5.
9. Lindner KH, Brinkmann A, Pfehninger EG, et al. Effect of vasopressin on hemodynamic variables, organ blood flow, and acid-base status in a pig model of cardiopulmonary resuscitation. Anesth Analg 1993;77:427–35.
10. Stiell IG, Hebert PC, Wells GA, et al. Vasopressin versus epinephrine for inhospital cardiac arrest: a randomized controlled trial. Lancet 2001;358:105–9.
11. Guyette FX, Guimond GE, Hostler D, et al. Vasopressin administered with epinephrine is associated with a return of a pulse in out-of-hospital cardiac arrest. Resuscitation 2004;63:277–82.
12. Wenzel V, Krismer AC, Arntz HR, et al. A comparison of vasopressin and epinephrine for out-of-hospital cardiopulmonary resuscitation. N Engl J Med 2004;350: 105–13.
13. Gueugniaud PY, David JS, Canzy E, et al. Vasopressin and epinephrine vs epinephrine alone in cardiopulmonary resuscitation. N Engl J Med 2008;359: 21–30.
14. Brown DC, Lewis AJ, Criley JM. Asystole and its treatment: the possible role of the parasympathetic nervous system in cardiac arrest. JACEP 1979;8:448–52.
15. Stueven HA, Tonsfeldt DJ, Thompson BM, et al. Atropine in asystole: human studies. Ann Emerg Med 1984;13:815–7.
16. Coon GA, Clinton JE, Ruiz E. Use of atropine for bradyasystolic prehospital cardiac arrest. Ann Emerg Med 1981;10:462–7.
17. Brady WJ, Swart G, DeBehnke DJ, et al. The efficacy of atropine in the treatment of hemodynamically unstable bradycardia and atrioventricular block: prehospital and emergency department considerations. Resuscitation 1999;41:47–55.
18. Swart G, Brady WJ, DeBehnke DJ, et al. Acute myocardial infarction complicated by hemodynamically unstable bradyarrhythmia: prehospital and emergency department treatment with atropine. Am J Emerg Med 1999;17:647–52.
19. Herlitz J, Bang A, Holmberg M, et al. Rhythm changes during resuscitation from ventricular fibrillation in relation to delay until defibrillation, number of shocks delivered, and survival. Resuscitation 1997;34:17–22.
20. Weaver WD, Fahrenbruch CD, Johnson DD, et al. Effect of epinephrine and lidocaine therapy on outcome after cardiac arrest due to ventricular fibrillation. Circulation 1990;82:2027–34.
21. Dorian P, Cass D, Schwartz B, et al. Amiodarone as compared with lidocaine for shock-resistant ventricular fibrillation. N Engl J Med 2002;346:884–90.
22. Kentsch M, Berkel H, Bleifeld W. Intravenose amiodaron—applikation bei therapierefraktarem kammerflimmern. Intesivmedizin 1998;25:70–4 [in German].
23. Kudenchuck PJ, Cobb LA, Copass MK, et al. Amiodarone for resuscitation after out-of-hospital cardiac arrest due to ventricular fibrillation. N Engl J Med 1999; 341:871–8.
24. Bar-Joseph G, Abramson NS, Jansen-McWilliams L, et al. Clinical use of sodium bicarbonate during cardiopulmonary resuscitation—is it used sensibly? Resuscitation 2002;54:47–55.

25. Tobey RC, Birnbaum GA, Allegra JR, et al. Successful resuscitation and neurologic recovery from refractory ventricular fibrillation after magnesium sulfate administration. Ann Emerg Med 1992;21:92–6.
26. Craddock L, Miller B, Clifton G, et al. Resuscitation from prolonged cardiac arrest with high-dose intravenous magnesium sulfate. J Emerg Med 1991;9:469–76.
27. Fatovich DM, Prentice DA, Dobb GJ. Magnesium in cardiac arrest (the magic trial). Resuscitation 1997;35:237–41.
28. Thel MC, Armstrong AL, McNulty SE, et al. Randomised trial of magnesium in in-hospital cardiac arrest. Lancet 1997;350:1272–6.
29. Stueven H, Thompson BM, Aprahamian C, et al. Use of calcium in prehospital cardiac arrest. Ann Emerg Med 1983;12:136–9.
30. Harrison EE, Amey ED. The use of calcium in cardiac resuscitation. Am J Emerg Med 1983;1:267–73.
31. Donovan PJ, Propp DA. Calcium and its role in cardiac arrest: understanding the controversy. J Emerg Med 1985;3:105–16.
32. Parham WA, Mehdirad AA, Biermann KM, et al. Hyperkalemia revisited. Tex Heart Inst J 2006;33:40–7.
33. Bottiger BW, Arntz HR, Chamberlain DA, et al. Thrombolysis during resuscitation for out-of-hospital cardiac arrest. N Engl J Med 2008;359:2651–62.
34. Abu-Laban RB, Christenson JM, Innes GD, et al. Tissue plasminogen activator in cardiac arrest with pulseless electrical activity. N Engl J Med 2002;346:1522–8.
35. Bottiger BW, Bode C, Kern S, et al. Efficacy and safety of thrombolytic therapy after initially unsuccessful cardiopulmonary resuscitation: a prospective clinical trial. Lancet 2001;357:1583–5.

Airway Management in Cardiac Arrest

Jose V. Nable, MD, NREMT-P[a],*, Benjamin J. Lawner, DO, EMT-P[b,c],
Christopher T. Stephens, MD, EMT-P[d]

KEYWORDS

- Cardiac arrest • Airway management
- Cardiopulmonary resuscitation • Assisted ventilation
- Intubation • Ventilator

The mantra of airway, breathing, circulation (ABC) is well known to practitioners of emergency medicine. It positions airway management as a preeminent feature of any resuscitation and engenders memories of Dr Peter Safar and his groundbreaking work on artificial respiration. Recent discoveries surrounding the physiology of cardiac arrest have turned the ABC mnemonic around. Although effective exchange of oxygen is important to survival, it seems that maintenance of coronary and cerebral perfusion eclipses airway management as an overriding goal of any cardiac arrest situation. The last iteration of the American Heart Association (AHA) guidelines deemphasizes endotracheal intubation as the penultimate goal of airway intervention in cardiac arrest. Instead, emergency practitioners should focus on the rapid delivery of uninterrupted compressions and other basic life support interventions that have proved to increase both survival and neurologic recovery. Important questions about airway management persist. It is no longer a question of when a patient in cardiac arrest must be intubated. The decision to perform endotracheal intubation results from a complex synthesis of environmental and clinical factors. It may not be feasible for a system that lacks veteran paramedics to mandate securing the airway with an endotracheal tube. Recent advances in the understanding of cardiac arrest physiology suggest that airway management, in the immediate phase following cardiac arrest, is subordinate to interventions such as defibrillation and quality cardiac compressions. When intubation is performed, it should not interfere with the ongoing resuscitation and thereby

The authors have nothing to disclose.
[a] Department of Emergency Medicine, University of Maryland Medical Center, 110 South Paca Street, 6th Floor, Suite 200, Baltimore, MD 21201, USA
[b] Department of Emergency Medicine, University of Maryland School of Medicine, 110 South Paca Street, 6th Floor, Suite 200, Baltimore, MD 21201, USA
[c] Baltimore City Fire Department, Baltimore, MD, USA
[d] Division of Trauma Anesthesiology, Department of Anesthesiology, R Adams Cowley Shock Trauma Center, University of Maryland School of Medicine, 22 South Greene Street, Room S11C00, Baltimore, MD 21201, USA
* Corresponding author.
E-mail address: JVNABLE@gmail.com

Emerg Med Clin N Am 30 (2012) 77–90
doi:10.1016/j.emc.2011.09.009
0733-8627/12/$ – see front matter © 2012 Elsevier Inc. All rights reserved.

emed.theclinics.com

decrease the coronary perfusion that is so vital to survival. This article reviews the state of the art as it applies to airway management in the patient with cardiac arrest. Like any other medical intervention, the plan for airway management should proceed from a thorough understanding of current evidence, provider capability, and emergency medical services (EMS) system resources.

PARADIGM SHIFTS IN AIRWAY MANAGEMENT
Physiology of Cardiac Arrest Ventilation

Ventilation is the exchange of gas that occurs as a result of air movement caused by changes in pressure. During spontaneous respirations, contractions of respiratory muscles cause an expansion of the chest cavity. A negative intrathoracic pressure (ITP) is generated, resulting in air moving into the lungs.[1] This negative-pressure ventilation is replaced with positive pressures when medical personnel attempt resuscitation of a patient during cardiac arrest. Although positive-pressure ventilation (PPV) has been an essential component of resuscitating critically ill patients, understanding the physiology of PPV and how it relates to patients in cardiac arrest is crucial to optimizing conditions favoring successful resuscitations.

The physiologic effect of PPV reducing coronary perfusion has long been studied.[2] PPV forces air into the respiratory system, increasing ITP. This increased ITP impedes blood flow returning to the heart and causes a marked decrease in left and right ventricular end-diastolic volumes, thereby reducing preload.[3] The Starling law reveals that this reduction in preload results in a direct decrease in cardiac output during chest compressions, thus reducing coronary perfusion. Therefore, PPV has the paradoxic and potentially harmful effect of reducing cardiac output during the resuscitation of a patient during cardiac arrest.

In addition to reducing coronary perfusion, PPV reduces the effectiveness of chest compressions by preventing negative ITP from being generated during recoil of the chest wall.[4] This negative ITP during the recoil phase of chest compressions assists with blood return to the chest cavity.[5] Drawing blood back to the heart increases preload, which in turn increases cardiac output with the next chest compression. However, while performing PPV, the generation of a negative ITP during chest wall recoil is hindered. PPV can consequently make chest compressions less effective at generating sufficient cardiac output.

Furthermore, PPV causes an increase in intracranial pressure.[6] The excess intrathoracic pressure generated during PPV is transmitted to the intracranial space via the venous vasculature. This process can result in a reduction in cerebral blood flow. Even if the patient were to be successfully resuscitated, the potential for anoxic brain injury or other profound complications from reduced cerebral blood flow is a possible drawback of PPV. The reductions in coronary and cerebral perfusion during PPV have profound implications for the management of patients in cardiac arrest.

De-emphasizing PPV

The deleterious effects of PPV mandate that it must be avoided, or at least reduced. Despite AHA guidelines addressing concerns for hyperventilation, providers often ventilate at rates exceeding 30 breaths per minute.[7] So even when providers are specifically trained not to overventilate, they often continue to do so. A de-emphasis of PPV during training of providers, along with constant instruction by EMS medical directors and other continuing medical educators must highlight the potential harmfulness of PPV. Given the negative effects associated with ventilation, as discussed earlier, it is imperative to reduce PPV during cardiac arrest. The ABC mantra of resuscitation has been the standard teaching since at least the early 1960s,[8] so the reduction of PPV represents a major paradigm shift in the management of patients in cardiac arrest, for which the emphasis on early airway management including intubation has long been emphasized.

Shifting the focus of resuscitations away from ventilations may improve other aspects that have proved to be more beneficial, such as increasing the amount of time compressing the chest. The cardiocerebral resuscitation (CCR) algorithm reduces interruptions to compressions by specifically concentrating on continuous chest compressions.[9] CCR is composed of cycles of 200 continuous compressions, each followed by defibrillation, if indicated. No PPV is given until at least the third cycle, when intubation may be considered. Instead, rescuers use passive insufflations with nonrebreather masks. Kellum and colleagues[10] found that CCR greatly improved outcomes, with 48% of patients being discharged from hospital with good neurologic functions, versus 15% using standard cardiopulmonary resuscitation (CPR). CCR represents a major shift in the standard resuscitative techniques because it inverts ABC to CAB (circulation, airway, breathing).

The need to not interrupt chest compressions, at least during initial phases of resuscitation, cannot be overemphasized. Despite compression/ventilation ratios that underscore the need for more time compressing the chest, less than half the time spent resuscitating a patient by rescuers, particular EMS providers, includes performing chest compressions.[11] Chest compressions are vital to achieving needed coronary perfusion pressures (CPP). A study by Reynolds and colleagues[12] found that higher CPPs than previously thought were associated with return of spontaneous circulation (ROSC) after cardiac arrest. Interrupting compressions to ventilate results in lower CPP, thereby reducing ROSC. Continuous chest compression has been shown to improve neurologic outcome following cardiac arrest.[13] Given the importance of perfusion during resuscitation, good chest compressions while minimizing PPV should be emphasized. Resuscitation methods that reduce any interruptions to chest compressions are highly desirable.

The concept of uninterrupted compressions is further supported by data from compression-only resuscitation by bystanders. A large study in Japan convincingly found that compression-only resuscitation resulted in more favorable neurologic outcomes compared with traditional CPR in patients who were apneic, had a shockable rhythm, or whose resuscitations were begun within 4 minutes of cardiac arrest.[14] Moreover, chest compressions may also provide some ventilation in the form of passive chest recoil.[15] In this respect, chest compressions may be a form of ventilation management. As such, uninterrupted chest compressions should be stressed and prioritized rather than mechanical ventilation.

EMERGENCY MEDICINE AIRWAY MANAGEMENT: FROM PREHOSPITAL TO THE EMERGENCY DEPARTMENT

Recent studies and the latest iteration of the AHA guidelines have challenged the idea of endotracheal intubation as the gold standard for airway control in the arrested patient.[16] Prehospital providers, although capable of performing endotracheal intubation, are implementing less invasive strategies such as passive ventilation and supraglottic airways. The direct impact of endotracheal intubation to patient survival is a matter of debate. The focus of cardiac arrest management has shifted toward the delivery of excellent basic life support, uninterrupted compressions, and prompt defibrillation. Prehospital providers, emergency clinicians, and other critical care providers must have a thorough appreciation of the evidence base surrounding airway management of the patient in cardiac arrest. Definitive airway control in the form of endotracheal intubation should not be achieved at the expense of other interventions linked to increased survival and improved neurologic outcome.

Passive Airway Management

PPV, although long considered a staple of CPR, is being reevaluated. A retrospective study by Bobrow and colleagues[17] examined patients with out-of-hospital cardiac arrest who underwent airway management via passive insufflation or bag-valve-mask (BVM) ventilation. Responding paramedics were permitted, at their discretion, to deliver oxygen via BVM or nonrebreather facemask. In the subset of patients with witnessed arrest, passive ventilation was associated with increased neurologically intact survival to discharge. Despite study limitations that included a retrospective design and a lack of control for postarrest care, the association between neurologic recovery and passive oxygenation deserves consideration. Oxygen delivery via face mask does not require additional skills or equipment. It avoids the complications of hyperventilation and may minimize gastric distention. Although 1 retrospective study does not constitute a robust evidence base, it nevertheless reminds rescuers that a single strategy of airway control has potential complications. However, the AHA guidelines do not recommend removal of ventilation from CPR performed by advanced cardiac life support providers.[16]

Noninvasive Airway Management

BVM ventilation is a cornerstone of emergency airway management. BVM strategies are taught to all levels of EMS personnel, from basic to paramedic. AHA guidelines affirm that all health care providers should be familiar with BVM techniques.[16] Airway management of the patient in cardiac arrest requires considerable attention to detail. First, rescuers must ensure avoidance of hyperventilation. Overzealous inflation of the BVM is associated with negative patient outcomes and complications such as hypotension.[18] As previously discussed, hyperventilation increases intrathoracic pressure, diminishes venous return, and decreases coronary perfusion.[7,19] Current AHA guidelines recommend low-volume (600 mL) ventilations for patients in cardiac arrest. Rescuers should deliver 2 breaths during the brief pause that follows every 30 chest compressions. When an advanced airway is not deployed, rescuers should not synchronize ventilations with compressions. Other airway adjuncts, such as nasopharyngeal airway (NPA) and oropharyngeal airway (OPA), may assist with maintenance of a tight facemask seal. Use of the OPA and NPA may also decrease airway resistance through displacement of the tongue. Cricoid pressure is also addressed in the 2010 guidelines. Although long considered customary in nearly all airway management scenarios, the application of cricoid pressure is not grounded in evidence-based practice. Recent studies associate cricoid pressure with impaired glottic visualization, airway obstruction, and even esophageal perforation.[20,21] The potential for complications and the lack of proven patient benefit resulted in a recommendation to avoid the routine use of cricoid pressure.[16] Like any other skill, BVM ventilation requires ongoing training and skills maintenance. It may be technically difficult for one rescuer to achieve an adequate face mask seal and provide ventilation sufficient to achieve chest rise. AHA guidelines corroborate that the presence of 2 rescuers is key to the execution of excellent BVM technique.[16] Guiding principles of effective BVM ventilation include avoidance of hyperventilation, the delivery of low volumes, and the maintenance of an adequate mouth-to-mask seal.

Supraglottic Airway Device: Selection and Use

Providers are faced with many choices with respect to available airway management devices. Although BVM ventilation is often sufficient for the first few minutes of CPR, there is a perceived need to secure the patient's airway. Endotracheal intubation, long considered the optimum means of airway management for patients in arrest, has been supplanted by simpler and more rapid techniques that may have less potential for complication. Maintaining proficiency in endotracheal intubation is a significant barrier for many prehospital providers, and the link between prehospital intubation and survival in out-of-hospital cardiac arrest is not well established. Supraglottic airway devices mitigate some of the concerns and difficulties surrounding endotracheal intubation. In general, less training is required to achieve a baseline level of proficiency. Studies with supraglottic devices, including laryngeal mask airways (LMA) and laryngeal tube airways, indicate that basic-level emergency medical technicians (EMT) can successfully use these devices. Furthermore, time to ventilation is reliably shorter when a supraglottic device is chosen as the initial method for airway management. In the first few minutes of resuscitation, the importance of minimizing interruptions in CPR cannot be overstated. Even when performed by experienced providers, endotracheal intubation may result in unacceptable pauses in chest compressions.[22] Wang and colleagues[22] reported an alarmingly high rate of intubation-associated pauses. The investigators found that "the median total duration (sum) of endotracheal intubation-associated CPR interruptions was 109.5 seconds per patient." The AHA guidelines therefore endorse the use of supraglottic airways as a "reasonable alternative to bag-valve-mask ventilation and endotracheal intubation" in the management of cardiac arrest.[16] A supraglottic airway may confer additional advantages in the more austere out-of-hospital setting. Placement of these devices does not generally require visualization of the glottic opening. Blind insertion methods, such as those used for LMA insertion, obviate neck extension and airway manipulation.

The 2010 guidelines review 2 common types of supraglottic airway: the laryngeal mask and the laryngeal tube.[16] Insufficient exists to recommend one device rather than another. Providers deciding to implement a supraglottic strategy for airway control should be mindful of device-specific considerations. First, insertion of these airways necessitates that the patient have sufficient mouth opening. Trismus, trauma, or supraglottic obstruction interferes with proper device placement. Supraglottic airways are less effective in the ventilation of patients with a fixed decrease in airway compliance. Severe underlying airway obstruction and high airway resistance found in conditions such as cystic fibrosis and severe chronic obstructive pulmonary disease (COPD) may impair ventilation.[23] Gravid patients have decreased lower esophageal sphincter tone and may be at increased risk for aspiration. These considerations should be weighed against the ease of insertion when using a supraglottic device for a patient in cardiac arrest. The relative contraindications for a laryngeal mask airway may not be relevant for failed endotracheal intubation. The supraglottic airways feature prominently in existing algorithms for difficult airway management.[23,24] LMA use should complement other method for airway control. Certain patients may not be ventilated sufficiently with a supraglottic device. Providers directly responsible for airway management should therefore receive training in BVM ventilation and other strategies for airway control such as endotracheal intubation or esophageal tracheal combitube insertion.

Tracheal Intubation: Revisiting the Gold Standard (Polishing the Touchstone?)

Endotracheal intubation is the gold standard in advanced airway management. Benefits traditionally associated with endotracheal intubation include effective ventilation and protection from aspiration. Despite its long-standing place in emergency airway management, there is a paucity of data that link endotracheal intubation to improved survival and neurologic recovery from cardiac arrest. Clinically significant patient outcomes are consistently matched with the delivery of excellent basic life support to include uninterrupted and effective compressions. The performance of endotracheal intubation requires a considerable amount of initial provider training in addition to ongoing skills maintenance. The challenge of visualizing a glottic opening and placing a tube through the cords has been shown to interrupt the delivery of potentially life-saving cardiac compressions. As previously noted, these pauses are detrimental to achieving needed CPP associated with successful ROSC. Current AHA guidelines caution against interruption of CPR, and providers are encouraged to synchronize their intubation efforts with ongoing resuscitation. Further complicating the performance of endotracheal intubation is its unacceptably high complication rate. Hypoxemia, oropharyngeal trauma, and misplacement can result from failed or prolonged intubation attempts. The decision to tracheally intubate a patient in cardiac arrest is therefore contingent on several factors including level of provider training and experience. Frequent experience or frequent retraining is recommended for health care professionals authorized and trained to perform endotracheal intubation.[16]

Endotracheal intubation is also seldom performed compared with other procedures undertaken by prehospital providers. In a large study involving more than 40 EMS agencies, more than 30% of patients intubated in the prehospital setting required more than 1 attempt.[25] Multiple attempts at endotracheal intubation can be associated with airway trauma, aspiration, hypoxemia, and other serious complications.[26,27] Endotracheal intubation is a difficult procedure that requires a significant amount of time, and it is potentially associated with major complications, so it should be deemphasized in the management of patients in cardiac arrest.

The timing of endotracheal intubation may be critically important to the question of survival. In the first few moments of cardiac arrest, patient survival is most clearly linked to the preservation of coronary perfusion and minimally interrupted CPR.[10] Endotracheal intubation cannot therefore supplant the delivery of excellent and effective basic life support. AHA guidelines do not articulate or recommend a specific time interval for endotracheal intubation. No studies exist to directly address the relationship of advanced airway timing to improved survival. Immediate tracheal intubation is deemphasized.[16] In some cases, ventilation with a BVM or supraglottic airway may function as definitive airway control. Certain clinical situations may mandate endotracheal intubation. When protective airway reflexes are absent and frequent suctioning is required to maintain patency, the introduction of an endotracheal tube is key to ongoing airway management. Some patients cannot be ventilated with a BVM or supraglottic airway; these individuals require tracheal intubation for definitive control. For cardiac arrest, the AHA guidelines remind providers to limit intubation attempts to less than 10 seconds.[16]

Providers should be meticulous in the confirmation and subsequent anchoring of the endotracheal tube. Patient movement and transfer from ambulance stretcher to emergency department bed carry a risk of dislodgement.[28] Confirmation of placement is at once clinical and objective. Providers ideally should visualize the tube through the glottic opening, auscultate lung sounds, and use end-tidal carbon dioxide. A multimodal approach is desirable because any single strategy fails to detect the potentially lethal complication of tube misplacement or dislodgement: "Improper placement of endotracheal tubes into the esophagus…can remain undetected despite physical examination, chest radiography, and pulse oximetry methods."[28] The setting of cardiac arrest is time dependent. The imperative to rapidly secure the airway, coupled with a patient presenting in extremis, poses many challenges to both prehospital and hospital-based providers. An ideal strategy for tube confirmation should therefore require little time, a minimum amount of training, and exhibit high reliability. Despite several readily available methods and devices to assist providers with confirmation of placement, the single most reliable indicator of successful tracheal intubation remains detection of exhaled carbon dioxide.[29,30] Colorimetric detectors are simple devices that are easy to deploy. The devices answer the question of correct placement within the space of several PPVs. When managing the airway of a patient in full arrest, providers must pay meticulous attention to tube confirmation because the decreased exchange of carbon dioxide may lead to false-negative readings.[28,29] Although the presence of end-tidal carbon dioxide is specific for successful tube placement, no single confirmation modality approaches perfect sensitivity or 100% reliability. Because resuscitation is a dynamic event, it is prudent to continuously monitor carbon dioxide throughout treatment and transport. Waveform capnometry might not be readily available in all settings of emergency health care. However, waveform capnometry permits real-time assessment of tube position and permits early detection of tube dislodgement or ineffective air exchange.[30] As stated in the 2010 AHA guidelines, "providers should always use both clinical assessment and devices to confirm endotracheal tube location immediately after placement and throughout the resuscitation."[16]

VENTILATORY MANAGEMENT STRATEGIES
Avoidance of Hyperoxia

Successful resuscitation of the victim of cardiac arrest must rely on a team approach to airway management, as well as meaningful and thoughtful goals of oxygenation and ventilation. Much of the research has been focused on adequate perfusion techniques, showing the negative aspects of airway control regarding outcome. Oxygenation strategies must be considered during airway and ventilation management throughout resuscitation and ROSC. Most, if not all, attempts at reviving victims of cardiac arrest involve the use of oxygen delivery systems by health care providers. Therefore, oxygen should be considered a resuscitation drug and used as such. Most medical providers consider oxygen an important but benign aspect of emergency care. So how much oxygen is too much? Many experts think that oxygenation strategies are less important during resuscitation attempts, but are they? Is too little oxygen or too much oxygen deleterious to patient outcomes? Historically, oxygen has been a mainstay of emergency skills teaching since the early studies of CPR. The recommendation now is to assist ventilations during cardiac arrest with 100% forced inspiratory oxygen (Fio_2), 5 times that of room air. Could this aggressive oxygenation with 100% Fio_2 be causing further harm in an already compromised circulation? This goal of treating patients using hyperoxia should be carefully examined. There has been extensive research into examining the effects of high levels of oxygen during prolonged ventilation of patients in the intensive care unit. The theory is that such supranormal levels of oxygen are likely resulting in the production of oxygen free radicals (OFR). These OFRs are capable of interrupting cellular signaling pathways in addition to causing direct damage to the cells. In a recent multicenter cohort study, hyperoxic patients admitted to the intensive care unit (ICU) after being successfully resuscitated from cardiac arrest showed increased in-hospital mortality.[31] In this study, patients who were deemed to have arterial hyperoxia (defined as partial arterial oxygen tension [Pao_2] ≥ 300 mm Hg) were associated with a higher mortality than hypoxic patients ($Pao_2 < 60$ mm Hg).[31] In support of these observations, studies of cardiac arrest using hyperoxia have shown a worsened oxidative stress and, hence, impaired neurologic outcomes.[32–34] In addition to OFR-mediated oxidative stress, studies suggest that hyperoxia may compromise coronary perfusion and cardiac output through coronary and peripheral vasoconstriction, thus leading to worsened ischemia-reperfusion injury as well as fueling the inflammatory response.[35–37] Based on these results, the idea of oxygenating and ventilating cardiac arrest patients with 100% Fio_2 should perhaps be revisited. However, this issue is complex. Many experts argue that there is a major difference between early resuscitation and late resuscitation and/or ROSC. So is it necessary to titrate oxygen therapy throughout the phases of resuscitation? A study of experimental cardiopulmonary arrest suggested salutary effects of titrating oxygen delivery to arterial oxygen saturation in the early postresuscitation period.[32] In addition to oxygenation issues, ventilation after ROSC involves a careful and thoughtful plan to optimize patient outcomes.

Ventilation During Induced Hypothermia

In the past decade, there has been a renewed interest in hypothermic treatment of patients suffering from traumatic brain injury, stroke, and cardiac arrest. However, there has been a paucity of evidence to support the use of routine hypothermia in patients suffering from head injury or stroke. In contrast, there has been a significant amount of data to suggest that routine use of induced hypothermia in patients who have been resuscitated from cardiac arrest may improve neurologic outcome. The protective effects of induced hypothermia are thought to be secondary to decreased cerebral carbon dioxide production, decreased oxygen consumption, immunomodulation, and overall diminished cerebral edema and epileptic foci.[38–40] Despite a renewed interest in hypothermic techniques for cardiac arrest resuscitation and recovery, little has been studied with respect to ventilator therapy and lung mechanics. Clinical scientists have had to rely on ventilator outcome data from similar populations such as critically ill septic patients, patients having cardiac bypass, and patients with neurotrauma. The literature is lacking with respect to changes in lung physiology and ventilator management when caring for the patient in the ICU after arrest.

During the initial moments after ROSC, many tasks must be completed with respect to airway management. A goal-directed strategy must be implemented to ensure optimal oxygenation and ventilation. If a supraglottic airway device has been used in the field, it must be replaced by an endotracheal tube so that mechanical ventilation can be commenced. The patient will likely be cooled in the first minutes to hours after ROSC. To achieve the goals of induced hypothermia and improved neurologic outcome, the patient should be sedated if the neurologic and hemodynamic states warrant this.

Before the induction of hypothermia, a baseline panel of respiratory blood gases should be examined. Evidence shows that the hypothermic state slows metabolism and therefore likely alters normal gas exchange and cellular use. Hence, goals for mechanical ventilation include optimizing blood gas levels, preventing hemodynamic instability, and resting the patient. It can be assumed that all patients that are resuscitated and in a reperfusion state are at risk for hemodynamic instability, acute lung injury, acute respiratory distress syndrome (ARDS), and other lung-related disorders such as pneumonia, atelectasis, and pulmonary edema. Patients after arrest are at particularly high risk for acute lung injury and ARDS, especially those transported from the field. Many of these patients have associated lung comorbidities such as COPD and history of smoking in addition to their coronary disease. Furthermore, a large percentage of patients managed in the field have aspirated various amounts of gastric contents before the placement of a definitive secured airway. In addition to these pulmonary embarrassments, all resuscitated patients have the secondary insult of ischemia-reperfusion injury to tissue beds including the lung. As a result, attention must be focused on preventing further lung injury in these cooled, mechanically ventilated patients.

There are data suggesting that mild hypothermia may alter lung mechanics as well as respiratory gas production and use. Hypothermic reduction in carbon dioxide production may be masked by simultaneous alterations in lung compliance, resistance, and gas exchange.[41,42] To test this notion of altered lung mechanics during induced hypothermia, Aslami and colleagues[43] studied the effects of mild induced hypothermia on lung parameters in patients admitted to the ICU after resuscitation from cardiac arrest. Parameters included tidal volume, positive end-expiratory pressure (PEEP), plateau pressure, respiratory rate, end-tidal CO_2 (ET_{CO_2}), and Fio_2. In addition, static compliance and dead-space ventilation were recorded. The study cohort was mechanically ventilated in a pressure-controlled mode with an inspiratory/expiratory time of 1:2. $Paco_2$ was decreased during the hypothermic period with unchanged minute ventilation, whereas Pao_2/Fio_2 ratio increased without altering PEEP levels. During rewarming, $Paco_2$ was unchanged; however, ET_{CO_2} increased with the same minute ventilation. Dead-space ventilation was unchanged and decreased during hypothermia and rewarming, respectively. Conversely, respiratory static compliance was unaltered throughout both hypothermic and rewarming phases. Based on the results of these studies, it is likely that hypothermia decreases carbon dioxide production in the mechanically ventilated postarrest population. Furthermore, lower tidal volume, as used in patients with acute lung injury (ALI), may prove to be beneficial in this patient population by resting the ischemia-reperfused lung tissue in hypocapnia. Results suggest that tidal volumes as low as 4 mL/kg may be beneficial in these hypocapneic, hypothermic patients to prevent further lung injury. Although lung compliance has been shown to be altered in most critically ill ventilator-dependent patients, this may not be the case during temporary induction of hypothermia in postarrest ICU management. In addition to the potential of unaltered lung compliance in most patients, the suspected decrease in oxygen demand and use during induced hypothermia may allow reduction in Fio_2 as well as PEEP levels throughout the postarrest recovery phase. Based on the limited literature and anecdotal experience, ventilator management in the postarrest hypothermic patient should be targeted to resting the lungs, which can be accomplished through either a volume or pressure mode of ventilation, targeting smaller tidal volumes and plateau pressures. In addition, it may be prudent to use minimal to moderate PEEP in this patient population depending on the individual's oxygenation status. All patients undergoing a hypothermic postarrest protocol should be mechanically ventilated, using sedation and muscle relaxation. Muscle relaxants allow for controlled respirations, maintaining a narrow window of targeted blood gas values, in addition to preventing the shivering response, which could potentially alter metabolic goals.

Optimal Ventilator Support

Ventilatory management in patients with ROSC is critical to ensure metabolic recovery. During the initial stages of ROSC, there is considerable damage to the internal milieu of tissue beds and cells. Reperfusion injury results in catastrophic alterations in cellular signaling cascades and metabolic machinery. OFRs, inflammatory cytokines, and acids are an integral part of this process and clinical scientists must do whatever is necessary to prevent further cellular injury. Goals are therefore directed at maintaining the organism's physiology in the most homeostatic state possible, to allow recovery of viable tissues and cells, although this is easier said than done.

Studies have shown that optimal ventilatory support in critically ill patients should target strategies that minimize ALI and the potential for ARDS, as stated earlier. Traditional approaches used tidal volumes of 10 to 12 mL/kg and excessively high PEEPs. To minimize risks of barotrauma and volutrauma (risks for ALI and ARDS), tidal volume (Vt) must be set to lower levels (6–8 mL/kg) and best PEEP must be targeted, which is defined as the lowest PEEP possible to ensure optimal oxygenation and hemodynamic stability. High levels of PEEP result in several undesirable effects. High intrinsic PEEP or auto-PEEP leads to increased intrathoracic pressures, interrupting venous return, diminishing cardiac output, and ultimately compromising both coronary and global perfusion. In addition, high intrathoracic pressures may cause an increase in intracranial pressure (ICP), which can be deleterious in an already compromised recovering cerebrum.

Once the patient is stabilized, mechanical ventilator settings optimized, and hypothermic targets reached, a chest radiograph should be ordered to determine correct endotracheal tube placement and whether any lung disorder is present. Blood gas measurements should be followed closely in the first few hours of mechanical ventilation to ensure optimal respiratory physiology. ALI is suggested if the Pao_2/Fio_2 is less than or equal to 300 mm Hg. If Pao_2/Fio_2 is less than 200, this indicates ARDS. Strategies to improve pulmonary derangements during hypothermic protocol include titrated Fio_2 and PEEP levels based on dynamic lung physiology. Recommended guidelines suggest titrating the minimum Fio_2 to maintain arterial oxygen saturations at greater than or equal to 94%, with the goal of ensuring adequate oxygen delivery while preventing hyperoxia.[44] Studies of animal models of ROSC have shown that ventilating with Fio_2 of 100% in the first 15 to 60 minutes after ROSC worsens brain lipid peroxidation, metabolic dysfunction, neuron degeneration, and short-term functional outcome compared with ventilation with room air or titrating Fio_2 to arterial saturations between 94% and 96%.[33,34,45–48]

Hyperventilation was once thought to be the best method to aid in reversing a combined respiratory and metabolic acidosis that ensued after cardiac arrest. Although theoretically beneficial, we have determined this practice to be detrimental. Hyperventilating the hypothermic patient after arrest can be problematic for several reasons. Increased minute ventilation (respiratory rate and Vt) decreases Pco_2, thus shifting the oxyhemoglobin dissociation curve to the left, altering the delivery of oxygen to the tissues. In addition, lowered Pco_2 alters cerebral circulation. Hypocapnia causes cerebral vasoconstriction, thus diminishing cerebral blood flow and oxygenation, exacerbating neurologic ischemic injury. Hence, it is recommended to use conventional ventilator modes, aiming for normocapnia, best PEEP, carefully titrated to lowest Fio_2 possible to maintain arterial saturations greater than or equal to 94%, and a relaxed sedated patient. There is no compelling evidence to show that any special ventilation method should be used other than those described earlier. Clinicians must be vigilant and prevent hyperventilation, hypoventilation, and associated hypoxemia and hypercarbia, as well as ALI and/or ARDS. In addition to these lung-sparing guidelines, several monitoring techniques are equally important to help guide the clinician caring for the hypothermic patient after arrest.

Once the patient with ROSC has been stabilized in the ICU and is on mechanical ventilation, an arterial catheter should be placed to monitor hemodynamics as well as intermittent arterial blood gas measurements to help guide ventilator management. In addition, continuous arterial pulse oximetry should be used and targeted to 94% to 96%, which should correspond to a Pao_2 of 80 to 100 mm Hg. Fio_2 should be titrated down to reach these oxygenation goals. Continuous waveform capnography is now considered the gold standard for monitoring integrity of the intubated patient as well as to measure ET_{CO_2} and maintain a normocapneic state of approximately 35 to 40 mm Hg and Pa_{CO_2} of 40–45 mm Hg. Again, chest radiographs should be used as needed to determine correct endotracheal tube positioning and to follow any developing lung disorders.

Ventilatory management of the patient being resuscitated from cardiac arrest is a delicate balance that must take into account the goals of needing to optimize blood gas levels while resting the patient, maintaining hemodynamic stability. Because such patients have lung mechanics that closely resemble ARDS, the lowest possible PEEP must be used. Hyperventilation must also be avoided. Furthermore, careful titration of Fio_2 to achieve goal arterial saturations greater than or equal to 94% is recommended.

SUMMARY

Airway management of the patient in cardiac arrest is of prime importance. Paradigm shifts in the understanding of cardiac arrest physiology have resulted in changes to overall management strategies. Historically, the tracheal intubation was considered central to any successful resuscitation. Tracheal intubation confers advantages compared with noninvasive ventilation, but it can no longer be recommended without reservation. Neurologic recovery and improved survival is closely associated with uninterrupted compressions, high-quality CPR, and basic life support interventions. As opposed to placement of a tube through the glottic opening, the initial goal of emergency airway management is the provision of effective ventilation. Chest rise, as produced with a BVM or supraglottic airway, may be sufficient in the first few minutes of resuscitation. AHA guidelines and current research support the idea that deployment of an advanced airway may be deferred until the completion of 2 compression cycles.[10,16] Although the optimum timing for endotracheal intubation remains unclear, there are no data to support the idea that it must be performed immediately. Providers should focus on minimizing interruptions in compressions and delivering high-quality basic life support. Emergency providers capable of performing endotracheal intubation must do so with the goal of integrating intubation attempts into the resuscitation as opposed to expecting a protracted pause. Endotracheal intubation has complications, and providers should be sufficiently trained and retrained to maintain proficiency. Ideally, advanced airway placement should be confirmed clinically and with the presence of end-tidal carbon dioxide. The addition of continuous waveform capnometry capability permits early recognition of unsuccessful tube placement or dislodgement. Further, the goals of ventilator support of the resuscitated patient include the need to use the lowest possible PEEP while carefully titrating Fio_2 to avoid hyperoxia.

REFERENCES

1. Zin WA. Elastic and resistive properties of the respiratory system. In: Lucangelo U, Pelosi P, Zin WA, et al, editors. Respiratory system and artificial ventilation. New York: Springer; 2008. p. 21.
2. Cournand A, Motley HL, Werko L, et al. Physiologic studies of the effects of intermittent positive pressure breathing on cardiac output in man. Am J Physiol 1947; 152:162–74.
3. Fewell JE, Abendschein DR, Carlson CJ, et al. Continuous positive-pressure ventilation decreases right and left ventricular end-diastolic volumes in the dog. Circ Res 1980;46:125–32.
4. Aufderheide TP, Sigurdsson G, Pirrallo RG, et al. Hyperventilation-induced hypotension during cardiopulmonary resuscitation. Circulation 2004;109:1960–5.

5. Lurie KG, Zielinski T, McNight S, et al. Use of an inspiratory impedance valve improves neurologically intact survival in a porcine model of ventricular fibrillation. Circulation 2002;105:124–9.

6. Guerci AD, Shi AY, Levin H, et al. Transmission of intrathoracic pressure to the intracranial space during cardiopulmonary resuscitation in dogs. Circ Res 1985;56(1):20–30.

7. Aufderheide TP, Lurie KG. Death by hyperventilation. Crit Care Med 2004;32(9): S345–51.

8. Safar P, Elam JO, Jude JR, et al. Resuscitative principles for sudden cardiopulmonary collapse. Dis Chest 1963;43:34–49.

9. Ewy GA. Cardiocerebral resuscitation: the new cardiopulmonary resuscitation. Circulation 2005;111:2134–42.

10. Kellum MJ, Kennedy KW, Ewy GA. Cardiocerebral resuscitation improves survival of patients with out-of-hospital cardiac arrest. Am J Med 2006;119:335–40.

11. Valenzuela TD, Kern KB, Clark LL, et al. Interruptions of chest compressions during emergency medical systems resuscitation. Circulation 2005;112:1259–65.

12. Reynolds JC, Salcido DD, Menegazzi JJ. Coronary perfusion pressure and return of spontaneous circulation after prolonged cardiac arrest. Prehosp Emerg Care 2010;14:78–84.

13. Kern KB, Hilwig RW, Berg RA, et al. Importance of continuous chest compressions during cardiopulmonary resuscitation: improved outcome during a simulated single lay rescuer scenario. Circulation 2002;105:645–9.

14. SOS-KANTO study group. Cardiopulmonary resuscitation by bystanders with chest compression only (SOS-KANTO): an observational study. Lancet 2007; 369:920–6.

15. Noc M, Weil HM, Tang W, et al. Mechanical ventilation may not be essential for initial cardiopulmonary resuscitation. Chest 1995;108:821–7.

16. Neumar RW, Otto CW, Link MS, et al. Part 8: Adult advanced cardiac life support: 2010 American Heart Association guidelines for cardiopulmonary resuscitation and emergency cardiac care. Circulation 2010;1222(183):S727–67.

17. Bobrow BJ, Ewy GA, Clark L, et al. Passive oxygen insufflation is superior to bag valve mask ventilation for witnessed fibrillation out of hospital cardiac arrest. Ann Emerg Med 2009;54(5):656–62.

18. Davis DP. The impact of hypoxia and hyperventilation on outcome after paramedic rapid sequence intubation of severely head-injured patients. J Trauma 2004;57(1):1–8.

19. Wang HE, Yealy DM. Out of hospital endotracheal intubation: where are we. Ann Emerg Med 2006;47(6):532–41.

20. Hocking G, Roberts FL, Thew ME. Airway obstruction with cricoid pressure and lateral tilt. Anaesthesia 2001;56:825–8.

21. Hartsilver EL, Vanner RG. Airway obstruction with cricoid pressure. Anaesthesia 2000;55:208–11.

22. Wang HE, Simeone SJ, Weaver MD, et al. Interruptions in cardiopulmonary resuscitation from paramedic endotracheal intubation. Ann Emerg Med 2009;54: 645–52.

23. Barata I. The laryngeal mask airway: prehospital and emergency department use. Emerg Med Clin North Am 2008;26:1069–83.

24. Lavery GG, McCloskey BV. The difficult airway in adult critical care. Crit Care Med 2008;36(7):2163–73.

25. Wang HE, Yealy DM. How many attempts are required to accomplish out-of-hospital endotracheal intubation? Acad Emerg Med 2006;13:372–7.

26. Jaeger K, Ruschulte H, Osthaus A, et al. Tracheal injury as a sequence of multiple attempts of endotracheal intubation in the course of a preclinical cardiopulmonary resuscitation. Resuscitation 2000;43:147–50.

27. Mort TC. Emergency tracheal intubation: complications associated with repeated laryngoscopic attempts. Anesth Analg 2004;99:607–13.

28. Burton JH, Huff JS, Lavonas EJ. Verification of endotracheal tube placement. Dallas (TX): American College of Emergency Physicians; 2009.

29. Grmec S. Comparison of three different methods to confirm tracheal tube placement in emergency intubation. Intensive Care Med 2002;28:701–4.

30. Silvestri S, Ralls GA, Krauss B, et al. The effectiveness of out of hospital use of continuous end tidal carbon dioxide monitoring on the rate of unrecognized misplaced intubation within a regional emergency medical services system. Ann Emerg Med 2005;45:497–503.

31. Kilgannon JH, Jones AE, Shapiro NI, et al. Association between arterial hyperoxia following resuscitation from cardiac arrest and in-hospital mortality. JAMA 2010; 303:2165–71.

32. Balan IS, Fiskum G, Hazelton J, et al. Oximetry-guided reoxygenation improves neurological outcome after experimental cardiac arrest. Stroke 2006;37:3008–13.

33. Liu Y, Rosenthal RE, Haywood Y, et al. Normoxic ventilation after cardiac arrest reduces oxidation of brain lipids and improves neurological outcome. Stroke 1998;29:1679–86.

34. Zwemer CF, Whitesall SE, D'Alecy LG, et al. Cardiopulmonary-cerebral resuscitation with 100% oxygen exacerbates neurological dysfunction following nine minutes of normothermic cardiac arrest in dogs. Resuscitation 1994;27:159–70.

35. McNulty PH, Robertson BJ, Tulli MA, et al. Effect of hyperoxia and vitamin C on coronary blood flow in patients with ischemic heart disease. J Appl Physiol 2007;102:2040–5.

36. Lu J, Dai G, Egi Y, et al. Characterization of cerebrovascular responses to hyperoxia and hypercapnia using MRI in rat. Neuroimage 2009;45:1126–34.

37. Dyson A, Stidwill R, Taylor V, et al. The impact of inspired oxygen concentration on tissue oxygenation during progressive haemorrhage. Intensive Care Med 2009;35:1783–91.

38. Bernard SA, Gray TW, Buist MD, et al. Treatment of comatose survivors of out-of-hospital cardiac arrest with induced hypothermia. N Engl J Med 2002;346:557–63.

39. Polderman KH. Mechanisms of action, physiological effects, and complications of hypothermia. Crit Care Med 2009;37:S186–202.

40. Nordmark J, Enblad P, Rubertsson S. Cerebral energy failure following experimental cardiac arrest hypothermia treatment reduces secondary lactate/pyruvate-ratio increase. Resuscitation 2009;80:573–9.

41. Sitzwohl C, Kettner SC, Reinprecht A, et al. The arterial to end-tidal carbon dioxide gradient increases with uncorrected but not with temperature-corrected $PaCO_2$ determination during mild to moderate hypothermia. Anesth Analg 1998;86:1131–6.

42. Deal CW, Warden JC, Monk I. Effect of hypothermia on lung compliance. Thorax 1970;25:105–9.

43. Aslami H, Binnekade JM, Horn J, et al. The effect of induced hypothermia on respiratory parameters in mechanically ventilated patients. Resuscitation 2010; 81:1723–5.

44. Peberdy MA, Clifton W, Callaway RW, et al. Part 9: Post-cardiac arrest care: 2010 American Heart Association guidelines for cardiopulmonary resuscitation and emergency cardiovascular care. Circulation 2010;122:S768–86.

45. Marsala J, Marsala M, Vanicky I, et al. Post cardiac arrest hyperoxic resuscitation enhances neuronal vulnerability of the respiratory rhythm generator and some brainstem and spinal cord neuronal pools in the dog. Neurosci Lett 1992;146: 121–4.
46. Vereczki V, Martin E, Rosenthal RE, et al. Normoxic resuscitation after cardiac arrest protects against hippocampal oxidative stress, metabolic dysfunction, and neuronal death. J Cereb Blood Flow Metab 2006;26:821–35.
47. Richards EM, Fiskum G, Rosenthal RE, et al. Hyperoxic reperfusion after global ischemia decreases hippocampal energy metabolism. Stroke 2007;38:1578–84.
48. Richards EM, Rosenthal RE, Kristian T, et al. Postischemic hyperoxia reduces hippocampal pyruvate dehydrogenase activity. Free Radic Biol Med 2006;40: 1960–70.

Prognosis in Cardiac Arrest

Joseph P. Martinez, MD

KEYWORDS

• Cardiac arrest • Prognosis • Cardiopulmonary resuscitation
• Neurologic outcome

Cardiac arrest (CA) remains a worldwide challenge. Nearly 450,000 Americans suffer from CA annually, with another 350,000 to 700,000 Europeans involved.[1,2] Out-of-hospital CA is the third leading cause of death in the United States.[3] Survival rates remain low, averaging 2% to 5% in most studies, occasionally as high as 10%. In-hospital arrests fare slightly better, with survival rates still a dismal 15%.[4] Several prognostic factors have been identified. These factors may be broadly divided into prearrest factors, intra-arrest factors, and postarrest factors. Of note, the great majority of the research on this topic was conducted before the development of protocols for therapeutic hypothermia (TH) for comatose survivors of CA. It is unclear whether widespread adoption of TH will alter the prognostic capabilities of some of these factors.

PREARREST FACTORS

Several factors alter the prognosis of CA even before the initiation of advanced life support (ALS) measures. Some of these factors are specific to out-of-hospital CA (OHCA) whereas others relate to in-hospital CA (IHCA). Well-established factors in OHCA that influence the survival from CA include initial rhythm, location, age, witnessed arrest or not, bystander cardiopulmonary resuscitation (CPR), mode of arrest (respiratory vs cardiac), and delay to arrival of rescue team (**Table 1**). Other factors include time of day, day of week, and gasping or other abnormal respiratory efforts. Some factors more specific to IHCA include ward experience (more than 5 resuscitations per year), hospital location, use of automated external defibrillator (AED), and again, time of day/day of week (**Table 2**).

OUT-OF-HOSPITAL CARDIAC ARREST

It is clear that victims of OHCA have better outcomes if they present to emergency medical services (EMS) providers in a shockable rhythm such as ventricular fibrillation

Disclosures: None.
Department of Emergency Medicine, University of Maryland School of Medicine, 110 South Paca Street, Sixth Floor, Suite 200, Baltimore, MD 21201, USA
E-mail address: jmartinez@som.umaryland.edu

Emerg Med Clin N Am 30 (2012) 91–103
doi:10.1016/j.emc.2011.09.010
0733-8627/12/$ – see front matter © 2012 Elsevier Inc. All rights reserved.

emed.theclinics.com

Table 1
Prognostic factors in out-of-hospital cardiac arrest

Factor	Association
Initial rhythm	VF/VT survival 6 times as high
Location	Public arrest: survival 3–4 times more likely Workplace arrest: survival 6 times more likely
Age	Older age associated with worsened survival Young adults (18–35) with marginally better outcomes
CPR	Any form of bystander CPR greatly increases chance of survival
Time to defibrillation	AED use before EMS arrival 1.75-fold more likely to survive
Time of day	Peak incidence 8–10 AM; lowest survival midnight to 6 AM
Gasping	Survival 28% vs 8%; with bystander CPR survival 39% vs 9.4% if not gasping

Abbreviations: AED, automated external defibrillator; CPR, cardiopulmonary resuscitation; EMS, emergency medical services; VF/VT, ventricular fibrillation/ventricular tachycardia.

(VF) or pulseless ventricular tachycardia (VT). Survival when a patient presents in a shockable rhythm is up to 6 times as high as when they have a nonshockable rhythm.[5] These rhythms occur early in the course of an arrest and deteriorate to rhythms less amenable to intervention. Time to defibrillation is important. The use of an AED prior to EMS arrival is associated with a 1.75-fold increase in survival to hospital discharge.[6] People that have witnessed arrests in public places have a better outcome. Survival is 3 to 4 times more likely if a patient arrests in a public place and 6 times more likely if they arrest in the workplace.[7] In general, arrests in public or in the workplace tend to be younger, to be men, and to be in VF. Those that arrest at home are more likely to be elderly, female, unwitnessed, and not VF.[7] If the event is witnessed and a bystander performs CPR, outcomes from CA are improved. Delays to arrival of the rescue team and advanced age lead to worse outcomes.[5] It is interesting that although advanced age portends a poor prognosis, young adults (age 18–35) do not always fare better. In one study, their 1-month survival was only 6.3%. This group tended to suffer from "noncardiac" arrests (the majority were drug overdoses), were

Table 2
Prognostic factors in in-hospital cardiac arrest

Factor	Association
Rhythm	VF/VT still has a better outcome but occurs much less frequently than in OHCA (fewer than 20% of all IHCAs)
Time to CPR and defibrillation	Survival 33% if CPR started in less than 1 min (vs 14% if >1 min) Survival 38% if VF/VT defibrillated in <3 min (vs 21% if >3 min)
Hospital location	ICUs have better survival rates Wards with >5 arrests per year have better survival rates Hemodialysis units have better survival rates
Time of day	Night shift arrests have half the survival of daytime arrests
AED use	Worse survival (10.4% vs 15.4%) when used for nonshockable arrests No survival benefit in shockable arrests

Abbreviations: ICU, intensive care unit; IHCA, in-hospital cardiac arrest; OHCA, out-of-hospital cardiac arrest.

less likely to be witnessed, and were less likely to be in VF. Of those young adults who did present in VF, survival was nearly 21%.[8]

Several clinical prediction rules for the termination of resuscitation have been developed and validated. Separate criteria were developed for basic and ALS teams. The ALS rule stated that termination of resuscitation could be considered in the prehospital setting if there was no return of spontaneous circulation (ROSC) at any point during the resuscitation, no shock was given, the arrest was not witnessed by EMS personnel or bystanders, and no bystander CPR was delivered.[9] The basic life support rule recommended termination of resuscitation of patients treated by defibrillation-only emergency medical technicians if the following criteria were met: no ROSC before transport, no shock given, and the arrest not witnessed by EMS personnel.[10] In an effort to optimize consistency among EMS providers, the investigators performed a secondary cohort analysis and determined that using the basic life support criteria as a "universal" rule would result in a lower overall transport rate without missing any potential survivors.[11]

Recent study of the chronobiology of OHCA has elucidated several interesting principles. A study of nearly 10,000 patients in the United States and Canada showed that the frequency of OHCA varied significantly across time of day, day of week, and month of year. Even more interesting was that survival to hospital discharge also varied according to time of day and day of week. Dividing the day into 4 6-hour time blocks, it was shown that there is a daytime excess to CA with a peak between 8 AM and 10 AM. Significant variation across day of week was seen with the maximal number of CAs occurring on Saturdays. Contrary to other studies, there was no excess of CA on Mondays or workdays. The maximum number of CAs occurred in December without evidence of seasonal variability across these geographically distinct study centers. In terms of prognosis, survival to discharge was lowest in the midnight to 6 AM time block, likely due to these events occurring in private residences and being unwitnessed. Survival was highest for arrests occurring on Mondays, but overall survival was not different between weekdays and weekends.[12] Further research into this topic may assist hospitals with determining staffing patterns and resource allocation.

In a study using TH, the most important prognostic factor was time to ROSC, even in those patients with non-VF arrests. When time to ROSC was 25 minutes or less, survival to hospital discharge was 65.7% with nearly 58% of these patients having predominantly good neurologic outcome. Outcomes were dismal in the group where ROSC took longer than 25 minutes, with no survivors with good neurologic outcome.[13]

Gasping or abnormal breathing after CA has been recognized as an important prognostic factor; it is common but decreases rapidly with time. Gasping was seen in 33% of those patients who arrested after EMS arrival but only 7% of those in whom EMS arrival took longer than 9 minutes. Those who gasped were significantly more likely to survive (28% vs 8% in the nongasper group, $P<.0001$).[14] Gaspers who received bystander CPR had a survival of 39% whereas nongaspers who received CPR had a survival of only 9.4%. Gasping appears to indicate marginally adequate cerebral perfusion. In animal studies, gasping increased ventilation and cardiac output, decreased intracranial pressure, and increased cerebral perfusion pressure.[15,16] There are concerns that laypersons and even some health care professionals delay performing CPR when the victim is gasping, mistakenly believing that they are not in arrest. In an effort to ensure that the presence of gasping does not delay the institution of CPR, the 2010 American Heart Association Guidelines for Cardiopulmonary Resuscitation and Emergency Cardiovascular Care (AHA Guidelines for CPR and ECC) prompts lay rescuers to provide CPR if the victim is "not breathing or only gasping."[17]

IN-HOSPITAL CARDIAC ARREST

Survival from IHCA has not significantly changed in the last 30 years and hovers around 15% to 20%. Similar to OHCA, VF arrests have better outcomes. Such arrests can be treated promptly and seem to signify recent onset of CA. However, there is a lower prevalence of VF arrests in IHCA than in OHCA. VF/pulseless VT arrests occur in fewer than 20% of IHCA versus rates as high as 45% to 71% in some OHCA studies conducted in public locations.[18] In-hospital CA is more often caused by hypoxia or hypotension, which may contribute to lower survival rates. Time to CPR or defibrillation is one of the more important prognostic factors in IHCA. When CPR is started within 1 minute of arrest, survival is 33% versus 14%. In VF/VT arrests, defibrillation within 3 minutes yields survival rates of 38% versus 21% if the time interval is greater than 3 minutes.[19]

Hospital location changes prognosis in IHCA. CAs in intensive care units (ICUs) fare better, despite these units housing sicker patients. In ICUs all arrests are witnessed and monitored; there is immediate ALS availability, and often younger median age populations. In addition, patients selected for resuscitation may be more appropriate, due to better use of "Do Not Attempt Resuscitation" orders. Relative frequency of resuscitation events may contribute to survival rates. Wards that have more than 5 CAs per year have better survival rates, even if all ward personnel receive basic life support and advanced cardiac life support training.[20] Prognosis of arrest on hemodialysis units is better than on general wards, again more likely due to environmental factors (all witnessed arrests, vascular access in place, CPR equipment readily available) than underlying patient characteristics. Hemodialysis unit arrests are more common on Mondays and Tuesdays than on other days, presumably because of the longer hemodialysis-free interval of the weekend.[21] Time of day affects survival as well. Arrests occurring at night on general hospital wards have one-half the likelihood of survival.

A recent and disconcerting finding was that AED use during IHCA did not improve survival. The use of AEDs was actually associated with lower survival rates (16.3% vs 19.3% if AED not used, $P<.001$). This finding was primarily due to significantly worse survival in patients with nonshockable rhythms (10.4% vs 15.4%, $P<.001$). There was no offsetting survival benefit in patients with shockable rhythms (38.4% vs 39.8%, $P = .99$). These results were consistent across hospital wards and from monitored to unmonitored units.[22] As mentioned previously, the prevalence of VF arrests in OHCA is much higher than that of IHCA, which may partially account for the improved survival in OHCA after implementation of public AED programs. The investigators hypothesize that the lower survival in nonshockable rhythms may be a result of the time required for AEDs to assess these rhythms, thus leading to longer "hands-off" intervals during CPR. It is increasingly clear that high-quality CPR is the most effective intervention in resuscitations of nonshockable rhythms, and the use of an AED may hinder compression delivery.

INTRA-ARREST FACTORS

Several prognostic factors have been identified during the provision of active resuscitation (**Table 3**). These factors include partial pressure of end-tidal CO_2 (PETCO$_2$) and the use of cardiac sonography. The utility of ultrasound during resuscitation includes both detection of cardiac standstill and exclusion of reversible causes.

END-TIDAL CO$_2$ MONITORING

Circulating blood delivers the CO_2 that is produced in the body to the lungs. In CA, CO_2 is produced but not delivered to the lungs. Thus, PETCO$_2$ approaches zero. Initial

Table 3
Prognostic factors intra-arrest

Factor	Association
PETCO$_2$	Values less than 10 mm Hg at 20 min are not compatible with survival
	Abrupt and sustained increase indicates ROSC
Ultrasonography	Cardiac standstill on ultrasound is predictive of failed resuscitation
	regardless of rhythm on monitor

Abbreviations: PETCO$_2$, partial pressure of end-tidal CO$_2$; ROSC, return of spontaneous circulation.

PETCO$_2$ may be high in cases of respiratory arrest as the heart continues to deliver CO$_2$ to the lungs during the period of asphyxia (as opposed to the abrupt cessation of cardiac output in an arrest due to VF). With high-quality CPR, the main determinant of CO$_2$ delivery to the lungs is cardiac output. PETCO$_2$ therefore correlates with cardiac output. Kalenda[23] was the first to report a decrease in PETCO$_2$ in patients who could not be resuscitated and a significant increase in those in whom ROSC could be accomplished. In 1989, Sanders and colleagues[24] published data in the *Journal of the American Medical Association* showing that ETCO$_2$ levels were predictive of successful resuscitation in both IHCA and OHCA. A landmark study[25] published in the *New England Journal of Medicine* in 1997 showed that a 20-minute PETCO$_2$ level was able to predict mortality and was more reliable than the initial PETCO$_2$ level. Values less than 10 mm Hg after 20 minutes of CPR were not compatible with survival and were felt to be helpful with decisions about the termination of resuscitation.[25] More recently, it was found that a PETCO$_2$ of 1.9 kPa (14.3 mm Hg) at 20 minutes was predictive of death with a sensitivity, specificity, positive predictive value, and negative predictive value of 100%.[26] In the same study, no patient with an initial, average, maximum, or final PETCO$_2$ of less than 1.33 kPa (10 mm Hg) was successfully resuscitated.

The partial pressure of end-tidal CO$_2$ can be useful as a guide to optimize compression depth and rate and to predict fatigue in the provider performing compressions. Furthermore, an abrupt and sustained increase in PETCO$_2$ in an intubated patient indicates ROSC.[27–30] Pulse checks are often unreliable in arrest situations. Close monitoring of PETCO$_2$ trends may help to limit the amount of "hands-off" time during compressions for lengthy pulse checks. It should be noted that PETCO$_2$ may transiently increase after the administration of sodium bicarbonate (as the bicarbonate is converted to water and CO$_2$). This transient increase should not be confused with ROSC.

ULTRASONOGRAPHY

More emergency physicians are incorporating ultrasound into their daily practice. The indications for emergency ultrasonography are expanding greatly. Many emergency physicians are comfortable using ultrasound to evaluate for the presence or absence of pericardial effusions. Some emergency physicians possess sufficient expertise to estimate ejection fraction, assess for right ventricular enlargement, and examine the valves. Emergency ultrasound examination assesses for cardiac standstill and reversible causes such as cardiac tamponade. Clinicians who are more adept at ultrasound use are also using it to guide therapy in some cases. For example, a patient in pulseless electrical activity (PEA) with a dilated right ventricle and septal bowing into the left ventricle may receive thrombolytics to treat a presumed pulmonary embolism. A parasternal ultrasound view may reveal the presence of an acute thoracic aortic dissection and therefore alter the course of the resuscitation.

Several studies have been published on the use of ultrasonography during resuscitations. A 2005 study of 70 patients in CA found that of the 34 that were in PEA, only 23 of them truly had PEA; the other 11 had "pseudo-PEA" with detectable cardiac activity on ultrasound. All 36 patients in asystole and all 23 in true PEA had cardiac standstill on ultrasound and none had ROSC. Of the 11 in "pseudo-PEA" that had identifiable cardiac activity on ultrasound, 8 had ROSC.[31] Another study found survival to hospital admission was 27% in all patients with sonographic cardiac activity versus 3% in those without activity. The numbers were very similar in those thought to have PEA (26% vs 4%).[32] Clinicians who used ultrasonography thought that it provided clinically useful information in 97% of cases. A study that looked at 169 patients in CA found 136 had cardiac standstill on ultrasound despite the presence of a rhythm on cardiac monitoring in 71 cases. Of those with cardiac standstill, none survived to leave the emergency department regardless of initial rhythm.[33] The investigators hypothesized that cardiac standstill likely implies exhausted myocardial reserve that makes successful resuscitation impossible despite electrical activity on the monitor. On the other hand, if cardiac activity is visualized in a patient thought to have PEA, he or she may benefit from an infusion of volume or the initiation of inotropes. Of the 341 patients in these studies, 218 were found to have cardiac standstill on ultrasound. Only 2 of these had ROSC. Neither survival to hospital discharge nor favorable neurologic outcomes was reported.

A more recent study in *Resuscitation*[34] examined the use of transesophageal echocardiography (TEE) in CA. TEE is not part of the average emergency physician's arsenal. However, as more emergency physicians become adept at ultrasonography and the cost of these transducers becomes lower, it may become more commonplace. The advantages of TEE during resuscitation are that the images are not degraded by such factors as obesity or hyperinflated lungs, such as in a patient with chronic obstructive pulmonary disease. In addition, once the probe is in position it can be left there throughout the resuscitation, and the information is available to all members of the treatment team. This real-time monitoring provides information about the effectiveness of compressions, allows for identification of rhythms that may be amenable to shocking (such as fine VF), and shows ROSC without needing a lengthy pause for a pulse check.[34] Studies such as these led the American Heart Association to include the following statement in the 2010 AHA Guidelines for CPR and ECC: "Transthoracic or transesophageal echocardiography may be considered to diagnose treatable causes of CA and guide treatment decisions."[35] The use of ultrasound in resuscitation has the potential to dramatically alter its course.

POSTARREST FACTORS

The prognostic factors examined up to this point have all been prior to the point of ROSC. Once there has been ROSC, it is helpful to identify factors that predict survival to discharge. Even more important is the quality of survival, typically the patient's neurologic outcome. Some immediate predictors of survival after ROSC have included postarrest rhythm, heart rate variability, and lactate clearance. Prognosticating neurologic outcome requires a more complex algorithm that takes into account clinical factors, biochemical testing, and other complex neurologic testing.

IMMEDIATE POSTARREST FACTORS

One small study examined the immediate postarrest rhythms in patients after ROSC. Tsai and colleagues[36] found that in patients who had an accelerated idioventricular rhythm (AIVR) after arrest, 38% required repeated CPR (vs 4% in the non-AIVR group) and none survived at 7 days (vs 50% in the non-AIVR group). Typically regarded as a "benign" rhythm, AIVR is even considered to be a marker of reperfusion after thrombolysis. This study suggests that AIVR after CA may not be as benign. Another factor that has been studied to greater depth is that of heart rate variability (HRV). HRV refers to the beat-to-beat fluctuations in heart rate during sinus rhythm, and reflects the level of autonomic modulations to heart rhythm. After CA, patients with a more potent stress response have a better outcome.[37] This stress response may include immediate baroreceptor sensing, which initiates an autonomic nervous response. This response is assessed by HRV. A decrease in HRV is associated with an increase in mortality in patients with critical illness and in survivors of CA.[38–42] Typically a 24-hour measurement, more recently it was demonstrated that a mere 10-minute electrocardiography recording performed 30 to 60 minutes after a successful resuscitation could be analyzed and used to identify patients at risk of 24-hour mortality.[43] Another study of HRV in survivors treated with TH showed that patients treated with TH had higher HRVs and improved outcomes.[44]

Elevated lactate levels after CA imply tissue hypoperfusion. Lactate clearance has been shown to correlate with decreased mortality in patients with trauma, burns, and sepsis.[45–48] It has been shown that an elevated lactate level 48 hours after CA is an independent predictor of mortality and unfavorable neurologic outcome.[49] Early, effective lactate clearance is associated with decreased early mortality and decreased overall hospital mortality in survivors of CA.[50] High lactate clearance at 12 hours postarrest is predictive of 24-hour survival.

NEUROLOGIC PREDICTORS

The ultimate question faced by providers and asked by families regards the quality of life that survivors of CA will have. While many studies of resuscitation will use ROSC or survival to hospital discharge as end points, the true measure that should be reported are those survivors with favorable neurologic outcomes. This topic has been one of much research and is of renewed interest in this era of TH. Several different factors have been evaluated, from clinical parameters, to biomarkers, to electrophysiological signs and advanced neuroimaging (**Table 4**). This research has led the American Academy of Neurology (AAN) to publish an algorithm for use in predicting the outcome of comatose survivors of CA.[51] This algorithm uses these different factors in a stepwise

Table 4
Prognostic factors regarding neurologic outcome

Factor	Association	Caveats
Brainstem reflexes	Absence at day 3 predicts poor outcome	May be affected by clinical situation (sedatives/paralytics)
Myoclonic status epilepticus	Predictive of in-hospital death or poor outcome	Even if brainstem reflexes are intact
Somatosensory evoked potentials	Bilateral absence of N20 peak predicts poor outcome	May be present initially and lost later
Neuron-specific enolase	Value >33 µg/L on day 3 is universally associated with poor outcome	May be falsely elevated by hemolysis
S-100B	Elevated levels associated with poor prognosis	Peaks earlier than neuron-specific enolase

fashion over several days. Though regarded as a valuable tool, the algorithm has limited utility in the emergency department.

CLINICAL SIGNS

Studies of neurologic outcome frequently cite the false-positive rate (FPR) of the test. FPR refers to an outcome better than poor despite positive a test result. In other words, a high FPR means that despite the test predicting poor neurologic outcome, there are survivors with meaningful recovery. An FPR of zero means that the test correctly predicts absence of meaningful recovery. Absent pupillary reaction to light seems to portend a poor prognosis for meaningful recovery. However, the FPR at time of admission is unacceptably high. Of more utility is the absence of pupillary reaction to light at day 3 with an FPR of zero. Absence of other brainstem reflexes at 72 hours (corneal reflex, oculocephalic reflex) show similar FPRs.[52] Likewise, motor response to noxious stimuli that is no better than extensor posturing carries a poor prognosis. However, in a study involving TH, just under 15% of the very small sample developed recovery of awareness on day 6 after extensor posturing on day 3.[53] Thus, it is cautioned that in patients treated with TH, using the motor response alone should be avoided on day 3 and repeated on day 6.

Myoclonus status epilepticus is defined as spontaneous, repetitive, unrelenting, generalized multifocal myoclonus involving the face, limbs, and axial musculature in comatose patients. The presence of myoclonus status epilepticus was uniformly associated with in-hospital death or poor outcome.[54,55] This finding was true even in patients with intact brainstem reflexes or some motor activity. This presentation at 24 hours is ominous and accurately predicts poor outcome.

ELECTROPHYSIOLOGICAL TESTING

Another accurate predictor of poor outcome is the measurement of somatosensory evoked potentials (SSEPs). The principal measurement is the N20 response from the primary somatosensory cortex. N20 refers to a negative polarity peak measured by an electrode over this area of the cortex 20 milliseconds after electrical stimulation of the median nerve at the wrist. Bilateral absence of this peak on days 1 to 3 or later accurately predicts poor outcome. The N20 response may be preserved initially only to disappear later.[56] Also, the presence of the N20 response is not helpful in predicting outcome, as a normal N20 is associated with arousal from coma in only 60% of subjects.[57] Thus, only its absence bilaterally is of any utility.

BIOCHEMICAL TESTING

Although clinical parameters are easily evaluated, are readily available, and of virtually no cost, they are also often affected by the clinical situation, including the use of sedative agents or paralytics. Biochemical markers, especially the well-studied neuron-specific enolase (NSE) and S-100B, appear to have a predictive value superior to clinical signs, though they are not readily available in a timely fashion at many centers.

NSE is the neuronal form of the intracytoplasmic glycolytic enzyme enolase. It is found mainly in neurons and neuroendocrine cells. NSE peaks in the serum and cerebrospinal fluid at 72 hours after injury.[58] It has been demonstrated that an NSE value of greater than 33 µg/L at days 1 to 3 after CPR was universally associated with a poor outcome with an FPR of zero.[54] A caveat is that small amounts of NSE can be found in platelets and red cells, so hemolysis (or traumatic lumbar punctures, if measured in cerebrospinal fluid) can falsely elevate the levels. S-100B is a protein present in glial cells and Schwann cells. It is a sensitive marker for glial damage and peaks at 24 hours, declining then over the next 48 hours. Despite many studies of S-100B, this marker predicts poor outcome with lesser confidence than NSE.[54,59–62] Therefore, the AAN guidelines recommend using NSE preferentially. However, given the earlier peak of S-100B, it may be more clinically useful than NSE at predicting outcome when measured early in the course (such as in the emergency department).[63] Further studies will need to be undertaken to delineate the utility of measuring this biomarker in the emergency department.

NEUROIMAGING

Computed tomography (CT) is readily available in most emergency departments, and is often used as a screening tool in patients with neurologic dysfunction. Cerebral edema seen on a noncontrast head CT may be a sign of global brain ischemia. A study using CT Hounsfield units to quantify cerebral edema found that a difference in gray matter/white matter ratio of less than 1.18 at the basal ganglia level was 100% predictive of death.[64] Advances in magnetic resonance (MR) imaging techniques have dramatically altered the evaluation of acute ischemic strokes, and show promise as an adjunct to assessing neurologic outcome after CA. However, its advantages are offset by the inherent difficulties of obtaining an MR image of a critically ill patient.

Multivariate assessment of the post-CA patient is clearly of more utility than relying on one modality. The use of clinical signs in combination with biochemical markers, electrophysiological examinations, and even advanced neuroimaging is under investigation. The AAN guidelines use a combination of clinical signs including the absence of brainstem reflexes or presence of myoclonic status epilepticus, combined with SSEP testing and measurement of NSE, to develop an algorithm to help clinicians predict the outcome of comatose survivors of CA. This algorithm may require further validation or modification as more information is gained about neurologic outcomes in this era of TH.

SUMMARY

CA remains a tremendous problem throughout the world, with rates of successful resuscitation remaining low. The ability to predict outcome from resuscitation remains elusive although several variables that are of value prearrest, intra-arrest, and postarrest have been identified. In the prearrest phase, initial rhythm is the most valuable prognostic factor. Shockable rhythms show survival rates 5 to 10 times as high as nonshockable ones. Several other environmental and demographic factors have been described, although many of them relate to the likelihood of the arrest being discovered early while the patient remains in a shockable rhythm. Intra-arrest prognostic factors include the values of the PETCO$_2$, trends in PETCO$_2$, and the findings of cardiac standstill on ultrasound. After ROSC, some early outcome measures include lactate clearance and HRV. The ability to predict favorable or unfavorable neurologic outcome requires a multivariate approach, combining clinical examination, biochemical markers, electrophysiological testing, and advanced neuroimaging. The influence of TH in all of these prognostic factors has not been fully elucidated, and remains a subject of intense research interest.

REFERENCES

1. Callans DJ. Out-of-hospital cardiac arrest—the solution is shocking. N Engl J Med 2004;351:632–4.

2. Sans S, Kesteloot H, Kromhout D. The burden of cardiovascular diseases mortality in Europe. Task Force of the European Society of Cardiology on Cardiovascular Mortality and Morbidity Statistics in Europe. Eur Heart J 1997;18: 1231–48.
3. Nichol G, Aufderheide TP, Eigel B, et al. Regional systems of care for out- of-hospital cardiac arrest: a policy statement from the American Heart Association. Circulation 2010;121:709–29.
4. Schneider AP II, Nelson DJ, Brow DD. In-hospital cardiopulmonary resuscitation: a 30-year review. J Am Board Fam Pract 1993;6:91–101.
5. Herlitz J, Engdahl J, Svensson L, et al. Factors associated with an increased chance of survival among patients suffering from an out-of-hospital cardiac arrest in a national perspective in Sweden. Am Heart J 2005;149(1):61–6.
6. Weisfeldt ML, Sitlani CM, Ornato JP, et al, ROC Investigators. Survival after application of automatic external defibrillators before arrival of the emergency medical system: evaluation in the resuscitation outcomes consortium population of 21 million. J Am Coll Cardiol 2010;55(16):1713–20.
7. Iwami T, Hiraide A, Nakanishi N, et al. Outcome and characteristics of out-of-hospital cardiac arrest according to location of arrest: a report from a large-scale, population-based study in Osaka, Japan. Resuscitation 2006;69:221–8.
8. Herlitz J, Svensson L, Silfverstolpe J, et al. Characteristics and outcome amongst young adults suffering from out-of-hospital cardiac arrest in whom cardiopulmonary resuscitation is attempted. J Intern Med 2006;260:435–41.
9. Morrison LJ, Verbeek PR, Vermeulen MJ, et al. Derivation and evaluation of a termination of resuscitation clinical prediction rule for advanced life support providers. Resuscitation 2007;74(2):266–75.
10. Morrison LJ, Visentin LM, Kiss A, et al. Validation of a rule for termination of resuscitation in out-of-hospital cardiac arrest. N Engl J Med 2006;355:478–87.
11. Morrison LJ, Verbeek PR, Zhan C, et al. Validation of a universal prehospital termination of resuscitation clinical prediction rule for advanced and basic life support providers. Resuscitation 2009;80:324–8.
12. Brooks SC, Schmicker RH, Rea TD, et al. Out-of-hospital cardiac arrest frequency and survival: Evidence for temporal variability. Resuscitation 2010;81:175–81.
13. Oddo M, Ribordy V, Feihl F, et al. Early predictors of outcome in comatose survivors of ventricular fibrillation and non-ventricular fibrillation cardiac arrest treated with hypothermia: a prospective study. Crit Care Med 2008;36(8):2296–301.
14. Bobrow BJ, Zuercher M, Ewy GA, et al. Gasping during cardiac arrest in humans is frequent and associated with improved survival. Circulation 2008;118: 2550–4.
15. Xie J, Weil MH, Sun S, et al. Spontaneous gasping generates cardiac output during cardiac arrest. Crit Care Med 2004;32:238–40.
16. Srininvasan V, Nadkarnin VM, Yannopoulos D, et al. Spontaneous gasping decreases intracranial pressure and improves cerebral perfusion in a pig model of ventricular fibrillation. Resuscitation 2006;69:329–34.
17. Field JM, Hazinski MF, Sayre MR, et al. Part 1: executive summary: 2010 American Heart Association guidelines for cardiopulmonary resuscitation and emergency cardiovascular care. Circulation 2010;122(Suppl 3):S640–56.
18. Valenzuela TD, Roe DJ, Nichol G, et al. Outcomes of rapid defibrillation by security officers after cardiac arrest in casinos. N Engl J Med 2000;43(17):1206–9.
19. Sandroni C, Nolan J, Cavallaro F, et al. In-hospital cardiac arrest: incidence, prognosis and possible measures to improve survival. Intensive Care Med 2007;33: 237–45.

20. Hou S-K, Chern C-H, How C-K, et al. Is ward experience in resuscitation effort related to the prognosis of unexpected cardiac arrest? J Chin Med Assoc 2007;70(9):385–91.
21. Lafrance J-P, Nolin L, Senécal L, et al. Predictors and outcome of cardiopulmonary resuscitation (CPR) calls in a large haemodialysis unit over a seven-year period. Nephrol Dial Transplant 2006;21:1006–12.
22. Chan PS, Krumholz HM, Spertus JA, et al. Automated external defibrillators and survival after in-hospital arrest. JAMA 2010;304(19):2129–36.
23. Kalenda Z. The capnogram as a guide to the efficacy of cardiac massage. Resuscitation 1978;6:259–63.
24. Sanders AB, Kern KB, Otto CW, et al. End-tidal carbon dioxide monitoring during cardiopulmonary resuscitation: a prognostic indicator for survival. JAMA 1989; 262:1347–51.
25. Levine RL, Wayne MA, Miller CC. End-tidal carbon dioxide and outcome of out-of-hospital cardiac arrest. N Engl J Med 1997;337:301–6.
26. Kolar M, Krizmaric M, Klemen P, et al. Partial pressure of end-tidal carbon dioxide successfully predicts cardiopulmonary resuscitation in the field: a prospective observational study. Critical Care 2008;12:R115.
27. Garnett AR, Ornato JP, Gonzalez ER, et al. End-tidal carbon dioxide monitoring during cardiopulmonary resuscitation. JAMA 1987;257:512–5.
28. Bhende MS, Karasic DG, Karasic RB. End-tidal carbon dioxide changes during cardiopulmonary resuscitation after experimental asphyxial cardiac arrest. Am J Emerg Med 1996;14:349–50.
29. Falk JL, Rackow EC, Weil MH. End-tidal carbon dioxide concentration during cardiopulmonary resuscitation. N Engl J Med 1988;318:607–11.
30. Pokorna M, Necas E, Kratochvil J. A sudden increase in partial pressure end-tidal carbon dioxide ($PETCO_2$) at the moment of return of spontaneous circulation. J Emerg Med 2010;38(5):614–21.
31. Salen P, Melniker L, Chooljian C, et al. Does the presence or absence of sonographically identified cardiac activity predict resuscitation outcomes of cardiac arrest patients? Am J Emerg Med 2005;23:459–62.
32. Salen P, O'Connor R, Sierzenski P, et al. Can cardiac sonography and capnography be used independently and in combination to predict resuscitation outcomes? Acad Emerg Med 2001;8:610–5.
33. Blaivas M, Fox JC. Outcome in cardiac arrest patients found to have cardiac standstill on the bedside emergency department echocardiogram. Acad Emerg Med 2001;8:616–21.
34. Blaivas M. Transesophageal echocardiography during cardiopulmonary arrest in the emergency department. Resuscitation 2008;78:135–40.
35. Neumar RW, Otto CW, Link MS, et al. Part 8: adult advanced cardiovascular life support: 2010 American Heart Association guidelines for cardiopulmonary resuscitation and emergency cardiovascular care. Circulation 2010;122(18 Suppl 3): S768–86.
36. Tsai M-S, Huang C-H, Chen H-R, et al. Postresuscitation accelerated idioventricular rhythm: a potential prognostic factor for out-of-hospital cardiac arrest survivors. Intensive Care Med 2007;33:1628–32.
37. Ito T, Saitoh D, Takasu A, et al. Serum cortisol as a predictor marker of the outcome in patients resuscitated after cardiopulmonary arrest. Resuscitation 2004;62:55–60.
38. Goldstein B, Fiser DH, Kelly MM, et al. Decomplexification in critical illness and injury: relationship between heart rate variability, severity of illness, and outcome. Crit Care Med 1998;26:352–7.

39. Yien HW, Hseu SS, Lee LC, et al. Spectral analysis of systemic arterial pressure and heart rate signals as a prognostic tool for the prediction of patient outcome in the intensive care unit. Crit Care Med 1997;25:258–66.
40. Chen WL, Kuo CD. Characteristics of heart rate variability can predict impending septic shock in emergency department patients with sepsis. Acad Emerg Med 2007;14:392–7.
41. Huikuri HV, Linnaluoto MK, Seppanen T, et al. Circadian rhythm of heart rate variability in survivors of cardiac arrest. Am J Cardiol 1992;70:610–5.
42. Dougherty CM, Burr RL. Comparison of heart rate variability in survivors and non-survivors of sudden cardiac arrest. Am J Cardiol 1992;70:441–8.
43. Chen W-L, Tsai T-H, Huang C-C, et al. Heart rate variability predicts short-term outcome for successfully resuscitated patients with out-of-hospital cardiac arrest. Resuscitation 2009;80:1114–8.
44. Tiainen M, Parikka HJ, Makijarvi MA, et al. Arrhythmias and heart rate variability during and after therapeutic hypothermia for cardiac arrest. Crit Care Med 2009; 37:403–9.
45. Blow O, Magliore L, Claridge JA, et al. The golden hour and the silver day: detection and correction of occult hypoperfusion within 24 h improves outcome from major trauma. J Trauma 1999;47(5):964–9.
46. Levraut J, Ichai C, Petit I, et al. Low exogenous lactate clearance as an early predictor of mortality in normolactatemic critically ill septic patients. Crit Care Med 2003;31(3):705–10.
47. Nguyen HB, Rivers EP, Knoblich BP, et al. Early lactate clearance is associated with improved outcome in severe sepsis and septic shock. Crit Care Med 2004;32(8):1637–42.
48. Kamolz LP, Andel H, Schramm W, et al. Lactate: early predictor of morbidity and mortality in patients with severe burns. Burns 2005;31(8):986–90.
49. Kliegel A, Losert H, Sterz F, et al. Serial lactate determinations for prediction of outcome after cardiac arrest. Medicine 2004;83(5):274–9.
50. Donnino MW, Miller J, Goyal N, et al. Effective lactate clearance is associated with improved outcome in post-cardiac arrest patients. Resuscitation 2007;75:229–34.
51. Wijdicks EF, Hijdra A, Young GB, et al. Practice parameter: prediction of outcome in comatose survivors after cardiopulmonary resuscitation (an evidence-based review): report of the Quality Standards Subcommittee of the American Academy of Neurology. Neurology 2006;67:203–10.
52. Young GB. Neurologic prognosis after cardiac arrest. N Engl J Med 2009;361(6): 605–11.
53. Al Thenayan E, Savard M, Sharpe M, et al. Predictors of poor neurologic outcome after induced mild hypothermia following cardiac arrest. Neurology 2008;71: 1535–7.
54. Zandbergen EG, Hijdra A, Koelman JHTM, et al. For the PROPAC study group. Prediction of poor outcome within the first three days of postanoxic coma. Neurology 2006;66:62–8.
55. Wijdicks EF, Parisi JE, Sharbrough FW. Prognostic value of myoclonus status in comatose survivors of cardiac arrest. Ann Neurol 1994;35:239–43.
56. Zingler VC, Krumm B, Bertsch T, et al. Early prediction of neurological outcome after cardiopulmonary resuscitation: a multimodal approach combining neurobiochemical and electrophysiological investigations may provide high prognostic certainty in patients after cardiac arrest. Eur Neurol 2003;49:79–84.
57. Rothstein TL. The role of evoked potentials in anoxic-ischemic coma and severe brain trauma. J Clin Neurophysiol 2000;17:486–97.

58. Rosen H, Sunnerhagen KS, Herlitz J, et al. Serum levels of the brain-derived proteins S-100 and NSE predict long-term outcome after cardiac arrest. Resuscitation 2001;49:183–91.
59. Pfeifer R, Borner A, Figulla H. Outcome after cardiac arrest - predictive values and limitations of the neuroproteins neuron-specific enolase and protein S100 and the Glasgow Coma Scale. Resuscitation 2005;65:49–55.
60. Tiainen M, Roine RO, Pettila V, et al. Serum neuron-specific enolase and S-100B protein in cardiac arrest patients treated with hypothermia. Stroke 2003;34: 2881–6.
61. Martens P, Raabe A, Johnsson P. Serum S-100 and neuron-specific enolase for prediction of regaining consciousness after global cerebral ischemia. Stroke 1998;29:2363–6.
62. Rosen H, Rosengren L, Herlitz J, et al. Increased serum levels of the S-100 protein are associated with hypoxic brain damage after cardiac arrest. Stroke 1998;29:473–7.
63. Shinozaki K, Oda S, Sadahiro T, et al. S-100B and neuron-specific enolase as predictors of neurological outcome in patients after cardiac arrest and return of spontaneous circulation: a systematic review. Critical Care 2009;13:R121.
64. Torbey MT, Selim M, Knorr J, et al. Quantitative analysis of the loss of distinction between gray and white matter in comatose patients after cardiac arrest. Stroke 2000;31:2163–7.

"Putting It All Together" to Improve Resuscitation Quality

Robert M. Sutton, MD, MSCE[a],*, Vinay Nadkarni, MD, MS[a],
Benjamin S. Abella, MD, MPhil[b]

KEYWORDS

- Cardiopulmonary resuscitation • Cardiac arrest
- Feedback • Debriefing

Cardiac arrest is a major public health problem affecting thousands of individuals each year in both the before hospital and in-hospital settings. However, although the scope of the problem is large, the quality of care provided during resuscitation attempts frequently does not meet quality of care standards, despite evidence-based cardiopulmonary resuscitation (CPR) guidelines, extensive provider training, and provider credentialing in resuscitation medicine. Although this fact may be disappointing, it should not be surprising. Resuscitation of the cardiac arrest victim is a highly complex task requiring coordination between various levels and disciplines of care providers during a stressful and relatively infrequent clinical situation. Moreover, it requires a targeted, high-quality response to improve clinical outcomes of patients. Therefore, solutions to improve care provided during resuscitation attempts must be multifaceted and targeted to the diverse number of care providers to be successful.

In the "2010 American Heart Association Guidelines for Cardiopulmonary Resuscitation and Emergency Cardiovascular Care (AHA Guidelines),"[1,2] the focus of resuscitation priorities during cardiac arrest has shifted from early airway and breathing management toward providing high quality uninterrupted chest compressions and early defibrillation for shockable rhythms, which is exemplified in the acronym change

Financial Disclosures or Conflicts of Interest: Vinay Nadkarni receives unrestricted research grant support from the Laerdal Foundation for Acute Care Medicine. Robert Sutton is supported through a career development award from the Eunice Kennedy Shriver National Institute of Child Health & Human Development (K23HD062629). Benjamin Abella receives research funding from Philips Healthcare, the American Heart Association, and the Doris Duke Foundation, and has received speaking honoraria from Philips Healthcare.

[a] Department of Anesthesiology and Critical Care Medicine, University of Pennsylvania and the Children's Hospital of Philadelphia, 7th Floor Central Wing: 7C09, 34th Street and Civic Center Boulevard, Philadelphia, PA 19104, USA

[b] Department of Emergency Medicine, Center for Resuscitation Science, University of Pennsylvania, 3400 Spruce Street, Philadelphia, PA 19104, USA

* Corresponding author.

E-mail address: suttonr@email.chop.edu

from Airway-Breathing-Circulation, or ABC, to Circulation-Airway-Breathing, or CAB. There have been numerous studies supporting this simplified approach, including a recent clinical trial demonstrating that even administration of advanced cardiac life support (ACLS) medications may not provide a survival benefit to cardiac arrest patients.[3,4] Consequently, it seems that providing high quality CPR (summarized in the AHA Guidelines catchphrase "Push Hard, Push Fast") with minimal interruptions and prompt defibrillation may be the most important actions during cardiac arrest that will translate into a survival benefit.

Given the complexity of the care required during cardiac arrest resuscitation, it should not be surprising that, even though in many locales cardiac arrest survival rates have improved, overall, strategies to improve resuscitation quality and outcomes are not fully implemented. An adult in-hospital cardiac arrest (IHCA) registry study has documented a rate of survival to discharge for adult in-hospital arrest at 19%; pediatric rates of survival are slightly higher, exceeding 25%.[5–10] Out-of-hospital cardiac arrest (OHCA) survival rates are much lower for both groups at less than 10%, with survival depending on location of arrest, initial rhythm, as well as patient and rescuer factors.[11,12] The variability of survival rates among different locations given the same rhythm and same setting suggests that resuscitation performance may be a contributing factor.[11] This variability in performance can be explained by several factors. These events occur infrequently from the perspective of any given rescuer, most rescuers are uncomfortable in these highly stressful situations,[13] and this feeling of unease is only magnified by the existing training programs that follow a low-frequency paradigm (ie, certification every 2–4 years). Clearly, new approaches, both technological and educational, are needed. In this article, we review some of the new approaches to improving cardiac arrest resuscitation performance. The focus will be on a continuous quality improvement paradigm (ie, before, during, after): to improve resuscitation outcomes, we must improve training methods before actual cardiac arrest events, monitor quality during resuscitation attempts, and feedback care deficiencies to frontline care providers after the events using quantitative debriefing programs.

CURRENT STATE OF RESUSCITATION PERFORMANCE

Recent resuscitation literature, assisted by CPR-recording devices, large cardiac arrest event registries, and high-fidelity ACLS simulation studies, have focused on and provide a significant amount of objective data regarding rescuer performance during actual and simulated cardiac arrests. Unfortunately, a common theme from these studies was that resuscitation performance frequently does not meet established care guidelines during IHCA, OHCA, and simulated cardiac arrests. Even more troubling, these deficiencies in care spanned the literature on both pediatric and adult patients.[14–16] To illustrate, Wik and colleagues[15] reported that during adult OHCA resuscitations, 33% of chest compressions were too shallow and were being delivered only 48% of the time during the arrest (ie, nearly half the time when the heart had stopped and there was little or no cardiac output, no chest compressions were being performed). Although one might expect such care deficiencies during the sometimes chaotic resuscitation of OHCA victims, similar deficiencies (23% of chest compressions with incorrect rates; 36% of chest compressions too shallow) were also seen during adult in-hospital arrest care.[14] Sutton and colleagues,[16] in the only pediatric report of actual arrest resuscitation quality to date, demonstrated that even with the provision of defibrillator automated corrective feedback during the arrest, resuscitation efforts still did not consistently meet established care guidelines. However, this pediatric study did seem to demonstrate improved care compliance in comparison to previous adult investigations. The investigators hypothesized that their improved care was related to a bedside CPR training program instituted at their institution,[17] highlighting a possible target for improving resuscitation outcomes (see later discussion).

In addition to difficulties with chest compression delivery, ventilation rates exceeding AHA recommendations have also been problematic.[18,19] Why are incorrect ventilation rates troubling? During the low-flow state of CPR, cardiac output and pulmonary blood flow are approximately 25% to 50% of that during normal sinus rhythm. Therefore, much less ventilation is necessary for adequate gas exchange from the blood traversing the pulmonary circulation. Furthermore, both laboratory and clinical data indicate that a rapid rate of assisted ventilation ("over-ventilation" from aggressive rescue breathing) during CPR is common and can substantially compromise venous return and cardiac output by increasing intrathoracic pressure.[18,19] These detrimental hemodynamic effects are compounded when one considers the effect of interruptions in CPR to provide airway management and rescue breathing.[20-22] Several studies have supported these results during adult resuscitation attempts[23,24] and, as a result, the AHA now recommends the CAB approach, emphasizing that the rescuer should focus on providing high quality chest compressions with minimal interruptions. However, given that most pediatrics arrests are actually asphyxial in nature, controlled ventilation is still recommended. A recent large pediatric series from Japan supported the need for ventilation in pediatric arrest victims. In this study, favorable neurologic outcome 1 month after arrest was improved in patients who received conventional CPR compared with compression-only CPR for an arrest that was noncardiac in nature.[25] In short, the resuscitation technique should be titrated to the physiology of the patient to optimize patient outcome.

Performance of actual chest compressions and ventilations is only one aspect of resuscitation quality. In addition to deficiencies in these psychomotor skills, appropriate recognition and treatment of cardiac arrest rhythms has also been shown to be problematic in actual practice. The treatment of choice for short-duration ventricular fibrillation (VF) is prompt defibrillation. Nevertheless, a large recent registry study showed that defibrillation was delayed beyond 2 minutes in nearly one-third of in-hospital VF-ventricular tachycardia (VT) arrests. In general, as the mortality rate increases by 7% to 10% per minute of delay to defibrillation, such delays in treatment must be avoided.[26] Furthermore, the wrong treatment decisions are frequently made with respect to defibrillation. In a study involving emergency medical providers (EMS) providers and medical residents, although manual defibrillation decreased pauses in chest compressions compared with semiautomatic defibrillation, more inappropriate shocks were delivered (26%) with a manual approach. In this study, nearly 80% of these shocks were delivered for an organized cardiac rhythm.[27] Currently, the resuscitation literature is lacking a report of rhythm recognition and treatment during real pediatric cardiac arrest. However, during simulated resuscitations, pediatric residents at an academic teaching hospital delayed defibrillation by greater than 3 minutes after onset of pulseless VT over half of the time.[28] This is particularly troubling because recent studies indicate that VF and VT (ie, shockable rhythms) occur in 27% of in-hospital pediatric cardiac arrests at some time during the resuscitation,[7] with as many as 41% of pediatric cardiac intensive care arrests associated with VF or VT.[29] Programs to improve rhythm recognition and treatment are needed in both the adult and pediatric realm.

IMPROVING PERFORMANCE IMPROVES OUTCOMES

Although numerous studies have documented that resuscitation quality frequently does not meet established care guidelines, it also appears that this substandard care is adversely affecting hemodynamics during, and outcomes from, cardiac arrest resuscitation. For example, increasing chest compression depth to the AHA Guideline standard results in favorable hemodynamic changes, such as an increased arterial blood pressure, in adult humans[30] and an increase in coronary blood flow in mature pigs.[31] In addition, in both human and animal studies of adult subjects, the minimal interruption of chest compressions seems to be a critically important element of CPR quality because even short pauses in chest compressions (4–5 seconds) decreases coronary perfusion pressure, short-term clinical outcome (eg, defibrillation success), and survival.[23,32] Most importantly, studies in adults have established that aggressive implementation of the AHA Guidelines substantially improves adult cardiac arrest survival outcomes, including more favorable neurologic outcomes.[33,34] Thus, there seems to be evidence that improving resuscitation quality will translate to improved outcomes for patients.

BEFORE: RESUSCITATION TRAINING

Because the quality of CPR is directly related to survival outcomes,[23,35,36] several studies have implicated the existing educational programs for teaching CPR skills as a prime target for interventions to improve survival after cardiac arrest. Although most hospitals in the United States require either basic life support or ACLS certification for most care providers, this is often the only resuscitation training practitioners receive, and there is a growing body of literature supporting the notion that basic life support and ACLS certification may not necessarily even translate to adequate performance of these resuscitation skills during actual arrest events, especially given that most providers have poor retention of these skills 3 to 6 months after traditional training. Deficiencies with not only operational performance in simulated scenarios,[37–40] but also with self-perceived rescuer confidence,[13] are all too common. Better programs to improve training success are desirable with the expectation that this would translate into higher quality CPR performed during actual resuscitation attempts.

A multifaceted approach is needed to improve existing resuscitation training methods. Alternative training strategies in addition to the standard certification courses should be used to supplement existing resuscitation training. Techniques, such as higher fidelity simulation,[41–43] automated quantitative feedback during training,[44] post-event debriefing,[45] and regular refresher training[17,46,47] have shown promise. Individually or together, these techniques can be used to augment resuscitation performance (**Fig. 1**) and will be discussed in more detail.

Simulation has shown to be an effective tool to teach resuscitation skills.[41–43] Moreover, there is a growing body of literature supporting that higher fidelity training methods and scenarios achieve superior training targets (ie, the more realistic the manikin and scenario, the better the educational outcomes).[41] Importantly, the superiority of high fidelity training is not limited to simulated scenarios. For example, in the realm of critical care and/or emergency medicine, recent simulation science has demonstrated that training in central line insertion and daily maintenance not only improves patient outcomes (eg, decreased complications with insertion[48] and catheter-related infections[49]) but, also, the cost[50] associated with performance errors. Furthermore, one recent study confirmed that simulation-based education could, in fact, result in higher quality of care provided during an actual resuscitation events[43] (ie, these studies have demonstrated that improving operational performance on

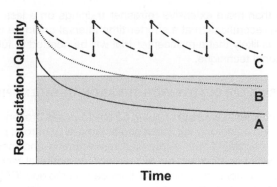

Fig. 1. Resuscitation quality after training. Curve A depicts quality decline after traditional instruction. Note fall into gray shaded zone of poor quality several months after initial training. Curve B represents the theoretical addition of high realism simulation and expert debriefing. Although there is no change in rate of psychomotor skill quality decrement over time, resuscitation quality is maintained longer owing to higher level of initial skill acquisition. Curve C represents addition of frequent refresher training in addition to simulation to prevent decrement to poor quality.

manikins can improve operational performance in real life). Why does simulation work? First, it provides the benefit of enhancing team work and increasing familiarity with resuscitation equipment, thereby avoiding more frequent errors. As previously mentioned, cardiac arrest resuscitations are relatively uncommon events for a given care provider. Simulation provides the opportunity to make these stressful clinical situations more "common," in a protected educational environment. Although the literature regarding simulation and improving team work is still evolving, it is likely that simulation is among the best-suited instruments to observe and improve on team dynamics and other human factors during rare-occurring, stressful situations, such as cardiac arrests.[51]

In a study by Verplancke and colleagues,[52] noncritical-care nurses reported an average of 59 months since their last actual delivery of CPR and 18 months since their last CPR training. It is likely that this gap in CPR training and experience is present in other hospitals and care settings, which ultimately leads to a decline in resuscitation performance. As a result, brief, but more frequent training "refreshers" may offer one solution to this problem. Three pediatric studies, all evaluating health care providers in both ICUs and general inpatient floors, have established that brief, intermittent "refresher" CPR training can improve both CPR skill acquisition as well as skill retention in a simulated cardiac arrest scenario.[17,46,47] The idea that a brief, relatively infrequent training can improve CPR performance may seem illogical considering that the high-intensity, standard, AHA programs demonstrate poor retention rates. The success of these refresher training programs is grounded in educational precepts and it takes into account the principles of adult learning. Adult learning theory states that there are certain characteristics common to successful adult educational programs: they must be focused, practical, and the need for obtaining the information must be apparent.[53–55] Because the education can be concentrated in refresher trainings (<2 minutes in these pediatric investigations), participants do not have to attend formal classroom instruction, making the program both practical and relevant. However, although refreshers may improve CPR skill acquisition and CPR performance, the optimal frequency of these refreshers, length of refresher training modules, and content of training still remains undetermined. Short and frequent refreshers may be more effective than more extensive refresher trainings on a less frequent basis. However, requiring recertification at a shorter time interval could be time consuming and impractical. It is likely that a multicenter trial will be needed to fully evaluate this promising educational technique.

DURING: MONITORING CPR QUALITY WITH TITRATION TO PATIENT PHYSIOLOGY

The evaluation of the effectiveness of ongoing CPR efforts has proven difficult. Several methods that are used commonly (eg, presence of femoral or carotid pulsations, pulse oximetry) have not correlated with successful resuscitation and may even mislead rescuers. The following is a discussion of real-time audiovisual feedback systems, arterial blood pressure monitoring, and end-tidal carbon dioxide (CO_2) capnography as methods to guide resuscitation quality.

Real-time Audiovisual Feedback

Interest in improving CPR quality through real-time feedback devices has been evolving since the early 1990s. Human,[56,57] animal,[58] and manikin studies[59–62] have shown improvement in quantitative measures of CPR quality and surrogates of survival outcomes (eg, end-tidal CO_2) when CPR feedback devices were used. Given the improvements seen in previous investigations, these technologies offer promise as we look for ways to strengthen our training methods, particularly in light of the fact that one of the problems highlighted concerning existing educational programs has been the poor ability of instructors to actually perceive CPR error in class participants.[63] As a result, the AHA now suggests that training programs consider use of automated real-time feedback devices to improve overall training efficacy by providing a quantitative assessment of the CPR performed by trainees.[64]

During the past decade, innovative technologies have extended the ability to monitor real-time CPR process from manikins used for training purposes to use in actual cardiac arrest victims. Using force transducer and/or accelerometer technology through pads placed between the rescuer's hands and the patient's chest, quantitative CPR quality information can be recorded, analyzed, and fed back to the rescuer in an effort to correct CPR deficiencies. Feedback can be given on chest compressions rate, depth, ventilation rate, pauses, and incomplete chest wall recoil (leaning). Feedback-enabled defibrillators, in before-and-after design trials (ie, studies with retrospective controls) have shown to improve CPR quality delivered by EMS providers and in-hospital care providers.[36,65] In one study of adult OHCA, feedback increased the mean compression depth from 34 mm to 38 mm and increased the percentage of compressions within AHA Guidelines recommendations for depth from 24% to 53%.[36] In similar fashion, another clinical study demonstrated that feedback improved in-hospital CPR quality by reducing the variability of CPR, conforming more to the AHA Guidelines recommendations.[65] In the pediatric environment, two studies from a single institution have further confirmed the positive effect of feedback in improving CPR quality. In the study by Sutton and colleagues,[16] compliance rates for chest compression depth and rate approached 70%. Unfortunately, this study was observational and lacked a before-period control group to fully evaluate the effect of feedback technology. However, the compliance rates far exceed those published in the adult-care and pediatric-care literature to date. Furthermore, in a small subset of patients from this same cohort, the investigators demonstrated a marked reduction in leaning because of feedback.[66] In accordance with the 2010 International Liaison Committee on Resuscitation recommendations, feedback technologies can improve quantitative measure of CPR quality, in training and real cardiac arrest situations.

However, although automated feedback devices can support improvements in CPR quality, questions have been raised regarding whether these devices actually improve patient outcomes.[44] None of the studies mentioned so far showed a significant improvement in any type of survival, but they were also not powered to do so. So, although it is clear that feedback technologies can coach providers to achieve quantitative feedback targets, whether achieving these targets through automated feedback technologies improves outcomes remains in question. A recent British Medical Journal publication by Hostler and colleagues,[67] using a cluster randomized design from three sites within the Resuscitation Outcomes Consortium in the United States and Canada, although demonstrating improvement in CPR quality, did not show a difference in survival outcomes. Does this mean that CPR quality is not related to clinical outcome? Unfortunately, the feedback targets used in this study were based on 2005 guidelines and, as a result, even with feedback, the average chest compression depth reached only 40 mm. Currently the AHA Guidelines recommend a depth of at least 50 mm to improve outcomes from adult cardiac arrest. In short, it seems that feedback technologies are effective at getting providers to achieve the programmed quality targets. It is the responsibility of resuscitation scientists to determine the best targets for CPR quality that will translate into improved clinical outcomes.

A particularly helpful technology used in feedback enabled defibrillators is the ability to display a signal that filters CPR artifact from the ECG tracing so that rhythm analysis can occur during chest compressions. The obvious benefit is that a rescuer would no longer have to pause chest compressions every 2 minutes to analyze cardiac rhythms. As a result, with fewer interruptions, there would be improved coronary and cerebral perfusion and likelihood of return of spontaneous circulation (ROSC). To date, there is no published literature regarding the clinical use of this feature incorporated into defibrillators. There is a modicum of literature regarding the accuracy of similar technology.[68] If this approach is shown to be reliable and not lead to incorrect rhythm interpretations, it has the potential to enhance CPR performance by decreasing interruptions in chest compressions.

Arterial Blood Pressure and End-tidal CO$_2$

Although CPR quality monitoring defibrillators have been highlighted in recent literature, older technology, such as monitoring of arterial blood pressure and end-tidal CO$_2$, during resuscitation can provide the rescuer with CPR quality information. Why monitor arterial blood pressure? Diastolic blood pressure is a major determinant of myocardial perfusion pressure (MPP), the driving force for myocardial blood flow during CPR.[69–72] Aortic diastolic pressure (AoDP) is related to MPP by the following equation: MPP = AoDP – right atrial diastolic pressure (RADP). Because the right atrial diastolic pressure does not change substantially during CPR,[73,74] arterial diastolic blood pressure is the most important variable affecting MPP and myocardial blood flow. Because adequate myocardial blood flow is necessary for successful resuscitation from cardiac arrests,[75–77] it follows that increasing arterial diastolic pressure will improve resuscitation outcomes. Evidence supporting diastolic blood pressure augmentation to improve the chance of resuscitation comes from numerous studies demonstrating that provision of vasoactive agents, such as epinephrine or vasopressin, or the application of abdominal binders, by raising AoDP, improve MPP and resuscitation success.[78–83] These laboratory investigations show that arterial diastolic pressures of at least 30 mmHg during CPR are typically necessary for adequate myocardial blood flow and successful resuscitation. Animals with arterial diastolic pressures less than 25 mmHg rarely survived. There is also supporting evidence from clinical adult arrest studies that diastolic pressures greater than 30 mmHg are associated with return of spontaneous circulation.[84] Therefore, an approach of "goal-directed" CPR, where a provider monitors arterial blood pressure and titrates chest compression force and vasoactive agents to achieve hemodynamic goals, seems reasonable.

Given the unexpected nature of many cardiac arrests and the sometimes chaotic nature of resuscitation, particularly during OHCA, placement of invasive arterial monitoring is not always feasible. In these situations, continuous end-tidal monitoring CO_2 (ie, capnography) can be used as an alternative to monitor CPR quality. In numerous experimental models, noninvasive end-tidal CO_2 correlates well with cardiac output, MPP, and resuscitation success.[85–89] Furthermore, the utility of end-tidal CO_2 monitoring during clinical investigations is not a new discovery and has been described since the 1970s when Kalenda[90] described three patients who were monitored for expired CO_2 during cardiac arrest. He described using CO_2 levels to monitor for rescuer fatigue and saw improvement in end-tidal CO_2 levels when a new rescuer started (presumably because the new provider was performing better CPR). He was also the first to show that ROSC could be recognized by a sudden rise in expired CO_2. By recognizing ROSC without having to interrupt chest compressions to check for a pulse or arterial blood pressure, one can anticipate that interruptions in chest compressions can be minimized (**Fig. 2**). Finally, building on this work, other studies have documented differences in end-tidal CO_2 levels between survivors and nonsurvivors after adult cardiac arrest, suggesting that end-tidal CO_2 can also be used as a prognostic tool during cardiac arrest.[86] As a result, continuous end-tidal CO_2 monitoring is now recommended during cardiac arrest resuscitation when available.

In conclusion, several technologies, some old and some rather new, are available to providers in both OHCA and IHCA settings. Although there can be arguments made about the superiority of a given technology, the first step in developing plans to improve resuscitation quality is to monitor the care provided during the arrest so that targeted treatment plans can be developed.

Matching Cardiac Arrest Physiology to Resuscitation

Beginning in 2005, the AHA and European Resuscitation Council guidelines for CPR were adjusted to better match the physiologic needs of the cardiac arrest

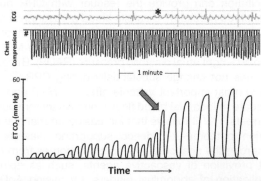

Fig. 2. Using end-tidal (ET) CO_2 to detect ROSC. From onset of arrest (#), note slow increase in end-tidal CO_2 as compressions are delivered. With ROSC (*arrow*), organized ECG rhythm begins to appear under chest compression artifact (*asterisk*) and end-tidal CO_2 rises suddenly to greater than 50 mmHg. Providers could have used the rapid rise in end-tidal CO_2 as a clinical guide that there was a return of spontaneous circulation, without having to pause chest compressions and risk interruption of CPR for a rhythm check.

victim, focusing on the delivery of high quality chest compressions with provision of "adequate" ventilation. What defines adequate ventilation? Once cardiac arrest has ensued and the heart has stopped beating, there is little to no blood flow throughout the body. At that point, during the low-flow state of CPR, cardiac output and blood flow are approximately 25% to 50% of that during normal sinus rhythm. As a result, less ventilation is needed for adequate gas exchange. In addition, there is the concern that excessive ventilation from rescuers may have detrimental effects on hemodynamics during resuscitation and survival outcomes.[18,19] These detrimental hemodynamic effects are compounded when one considers the effect of interruptions in CPR to provide airway management and rescue breathing. As a result, the chest compression to ventilation ratio was increased from 15:2 to 30:2 in 2005 to ensure chest compressions were being delivered for a greater proportion of the time during CPR. In 2009, a large prospective observational study corroborated the association between increased chest compression fraction (the proportion of resuscitation time without spontaneous circulation during which chest compressions are administered) and improved outcome, with two highest groups of chest compression fraction more than twice as likely to survive.[91]

The next obvious question raised by the developing body of literature supporting increased chest compression fraction was whether ventilation was needed at all (ie, compression-only resuscitation). Between 2005 and 2010, several studies were focused on investigating an alternative resuscitation strategy, known as cardiocerebral resuscitation (CCR).[92–95] CCR entails providing more uninterrupted chest compressions to ensure optimal cerebral and cardiac perfusion. In Arizona, Bobrow and colleagues[94] described a variant of CCR termed minimally interrupted cardiac resuscitation, which minimizes interruptions in chest compressions by delaying endotracheal intubation and positive pressure ventilations, instead initially providing passive oxygen insufflation via an oral pharyngeal airway and non-rebreather face mask. The study demonstrated a significant improvement in survival to discharge for OHCA. Since then, several other EMS systems have demonstrated comparable improvements in survival by implementing similar protocols that emphasized uninterrupted chest compressions and delayed intubation.[93,95]

During the same period that CCR was being investigated for OHCA by EMS providers, resuscitation scientists began to establish whether compression-only CPR was preferable to standard CPR for bystanders. Because bystander CPR is one of the most important determinants of resuscitation outcome,[96] the hope was by removing the need for ventilation delivery, more bystander CPR would be provided and outcomes from OHCA would be improved. After several studies demonstrated the efficacy of bystander-initiated compression-only CPR, this technique was endorsed in the 2010 AHA and European Resuscitation Council guidelines for CPR as a reasonable alternative to conventional CPR for adult OHCA.[97,98] Most recently, using survival to hospital discharge as the primary outcome, a meta-analysis was recently published in Lancet and concluded that compression-only CPR is preferably to conventional CPR with rescue breathing for adult OHCA.[99] However, in pediatrics, given that most arrests are actually asphyxial in nature, controlled ventilation is still recommended. A recent large pediatric series from Japan supported this approach and found that favorable neurologic outcome 1 month after arrest was improved in patients who received conventional CPR compared with compression-only CPR for arrest that was noncardiac in nature.[25] In short, this is one of the take-home points of this article: resuscitation technique and quality should be monitored and titrated to the physiology of the patient to optimize outcome.

Mechanical CPR Devices

As high-quality chest compressions with minimal interruptions seem to be a determinant of IHCA and OHCA survival, it follows that mechanical compression devices may be useful during resuscitation attempts. Piston-type devices and circumferential constriction band devices have been evaluated during cardiac arrest resuscitation and they have shown promise in improving hemodynamic and short-term clinical outcomes.[100–102] Although these devices can easily deliver high-quality chest compressions, rescuers must be cautious to limit interruptions in the deployment of said devices.[103] See discussion of these devices elsewhere in this issue.

AFTER: PERFORMANCE DEBRIEFING

Health care debriefing is defined as a facilitator-led participant discussion of events with reflection and assimilation of learning into practice. Structured debriefing can trace its origins back to the military in World War II. General George Marshall ordered soldiers under his command to give an account of their experience on return home from a mission. Although the initial intent was to gather tactical information or strategize for future battles, he noticed that debriefings were also spiritually healing and morale building for his soldiers. The technique was further refined in the military and aviation industries, and although initially used as a means to minimize the stress response and improve psychological outcomes from traumatic and infrequent situations,[104–108] currently debriefing is conceptualized as a method to improve care during rare and stressful events.

The value of debriefing starts with resuscitation training. Structured debriefing has been established as a useful tool to improve compliance of in-hospital adult care providers during simulated cardiac arrest. Although debriefing or automated feedback alone improved CPR quality modestly in a study from the University of Pennsylvania, the combination led to a more considerable improvement in quality.[109] Similarly, debriefing with pediatric in-hospital care providers has also shown the positive effects of debriefing during resuscitation training. In a study from the Children's Hospital of Philadelphia, the combination of instructor-led training and debriefing with automated defibrillator feedback improved CPR quality compared with either the training or debriefing method alone.[46] Therefore, in addition to quantitative monitoring of trainee performance, it seems prudent to ensure that performance is fed back to trainees in an attempt to achieve the best educational outcomes.

The first study published demonstrating efficacy of debriefing to improve outcomes from cardiac arrest came from the University of Chicago where the combination of resuscitation debriefing interventions and audiovisual feedback via defibrillators produced a marked improvement in resuscitation performance and a 33% increase in ROSC.[45] This particular debriefing program consisted of weekly sessions that reviewed transcripts of quantitative data downloaded from defibrillators, including CPR-quality ECG data (**Fig. 3**). Although this study was a designed before-after study using historical controls, the benefit of structured debriefing was apparent with improved CPR quality target compliance and ROSC.

Although these investigations reported positive findings with the addition of debriefing, a European study in the pre-hospital setting failed to show any benefit after incorporating performance evaluation.[110] However, this study should not deter resuscitation scientists from recommending performance debriefing. Instead, this study highlighted an important aspect of successful debriefing: the process must be completed with front-line care providers. In the European study, CPR performance data were presented to EMS leadership or local CPR instructors, not to front-line

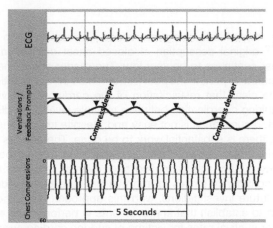

Fig. 3. Representative CPR quantitative recording. Provides ability to review ECG, ventilation, and chest compression data after events to improve future resuscitation quality. Note prompts given to rescuers to "compress deeper" when the chest compressions are too shallow. The arrow heads indicate ventilations, in this recording provided at a rate of approximately 60 per minute (too fast!). These recordings can be used to provide a structured quantitative postevent review for rescuers who participated in the resuscitation.

care providers. This prohibited the "self-reflection" and "assimilation" that is of paramount importance to debriefing success. Therefore, this study highlights the importance of having a highly structured debriefing process performed with front-line providers.

EVIDENCE THAT PUTTING IT ALL TOGETHER IMPROVES OUTCOMES

Although this article is focused on techniques to improve resuscitation performance (eg, innovative training methods, monitors to enable providers to titrate the resuscitation to arrest physiology, real-time feedback-enabled CPR monitoring defibrillators, and a systematic post-cardiac arrest debriefing process), it is likely that a bundled approach incorporating two to several of these techniques will be necessary to improve long-term patient outcomes. As a promising recent example, the "Take Heart America" program was a comprehensive, community-wide, systems-based approach to the treatment of cardiac arrest.[111] This program consisted of widespread cardiopulmonary resuscitation skills training in schools and businesses, retraining of all EMS personnel in methods to deliver high quality CPR, deploying additional automated external defibrillators in schools and public places (ie, enabling prompt defibrillation when needed), and establishing treatment protocols regarding transport to and treatment by cardiac arrest centers. As a result of this intensive program, bystander CPR rates increased from 20% to 29% ($P = .086$, odds ratio 1.7, 95% confidence interval 0.96–2.89), hypothermia therapy for admitted out-of-hospital cardiac arrest victims increased from 0% to 45%, and, most importantly, survival to hospital discharge for all patients after out-of-hospital cardiac arrest in these two sites improved from 8.5% to 19% ($P = .011$, odds ratio 2.60, confidence interval 1.19–6.26). Although this study used historical controls, the magnitude of improvement in survival outcomes provides strong evidence that initiation of a resuscitation care bundle or system will be effective to improve outcomes from cardiac arrest.

SUMMARY

In spite of the remarkable progress made in resuscitation science since Kouwenhoven's[112] original description of closed chest cardiac massage, survival from cardiac arrest continues to be very low. The reader should be convinced that this could be attributed, in part, to the poor performance of resuscitation care. Furthermore, it should be clear that resuscitation of the cardiac arrest victim is a highly complex task requiring coordination between multiple levels and disciplines of care providers. In short, resuscitation is not easy and, despite improvements in care over the past 50 years, there is substantial work to be done. The authors argue that using a continuous quality improvement bundle (ie, improving training before, monitoring and titrating quality during, and debriefing after events) seems to hold promise as the resuscitation community strives to improve the care that we deliver to cardiac arrest victims. In future investigations, with this approach, we expect resuscitation scientists to begin to establish that improvements in performance will subsequently translate into better survival rates for victims of sudden cardiac arrest.

ACKNOWLEDGMENTS

The authors would like to thank Dr Robert A. Berg and Dana Niles for their help in preparation of this article. We would also like to acknowledge Marion Leary, Lori Boyle, and Jessica Leffelman, who have supported resuscitation science at the University of Pennsylvania and Children's Hospital of Philadelphia.

REFERENCES

1. Berg RA, Hemphill R, Abella BS, et al. Part 5: adult basic life support: 2010 American Heart Association guidelines for cardiopulmonary resuscitation and emergency cardiovascular care. Circulation 2010;122(18 Suppl 3):S685–705.
2. Berg MD, Schexnayder SM, Chameides L, et al. Part 13: pediatric basic life support: 2010 American Heart Association guidelines for cardiopulmonary resuscitation and emergency cardiovascular care. Circulation 2010;122(18 Suppl 3):S862–75.
3. Olasveengen TM, Sunde K, Brunborg C, et al. Intravenous drug administration during out-of-hospital cardiac arrest: a randomized trial. JAMA 2009;302(20): 2222–9.
4. van Walraven C, Stiell IG, Wells GA, et al. Do advanced cardiac life support drugs increase resuscitation rates from in-hospital cardiac arrest? The OTAC study group. Ann Emerg Med 1998;32(5):544–53.
5. Lloyd-Jones D, Adams R, Carnethon M, et al. Heart disease and stroke statistics—2009 update: a report from the American Heart Association Statistics Committee and Stroke Statistics Subcommittee. Circulation 2009;119(3):480–6.
6. Tibballs J, Kinney S. A prospective study of outcome of in-patient paediatric cardiopulmonary arrest. Resuscitation 2006;71(3):310–8.
7. Samson RA, Nadkarni VM, Meaney PA, et al. Outcomes of in-hospital ventricular fibrillation in children. N Engl J Med 2006;354(22):2328–39.
8. Nadkarni VM, Larkin GL, Peberdy MA, et al. First documented rhythm and clinical outcome from in-hospital cardiac arrest among children and adults. JAMA 2006;295(1):50–7.
9. Meaney PA, Nadkarni VM, Cook EF, et al. Higher survival rates among younger patients after pediatric intensive care unit cardiac arrests. Pediatrics 2006; 118(6):2424–33.

10. de Mos N, van Litsenburg RR, McCrindle B, et al. Pediatric in-intensive-care-unit cardiac arrest: incidence, survival, and predictive factors. Crit Care Med 2006; 34(4):1209–15.
11. Nichol G, Thomas E, Callaway CW, et al. Regional variation in out-of-hospital cardiac arrest incidence and outcome. JAMA 2008;300(12):1423–31.
12. Donoghue AJ, Nadkarni V, Berg RA, et al. Out-of-hospital pediatric cardiac arrest: an epidemiologic review and assessment of current knowledge. Ann Emerg Med 2005;46(6):512 22.
13. Hayes CW, Rhee A, Detsky ME, et al. Residents feel unprepared and unsupervised as leaders of cardiac arrest teams in teaching hospitals: a survey of internal medicine residents. Crit Care Med 2007;35(7):1668–72.
14. Abella BS, Alvarado JP, Myklebust H, et al. Quality of cardiopulmonary resuscitation during in-hospital cardiac arrest. JAMA 2005;293(3):305–10.
15. Wik L, Kramer-Johansen J, Myklebust H, et al. Quality of cardiopulmonary resuscitation during out-of-hospital cardiac arrest. JAMA 2005;293(3):299–304.
16. Sutton RM, Niles D, Nysaether J, et al. Quantitative analysis of CPR quality during in-hospital resuscitation of older children and adolescents. Pediatrics 2009;124(2):494–9.
17. Niles D, Sutton RM, Donoghue A, et al. "Rolling refreshers": a novel approach to maintain CPR psychomotor skill competence. Resuscitation 2009;80(8):909–12.
18. Aufderheide TP, Lurie KG. Death by hyperventilation: a common and life-threatening problem during cardiopulmonary resuscitation. Crit Care Med 2004; 32(Suppl 9):S345–51.
19. Aufderheide TP, Sigurdsson G, Pirrallo RG, et al. Hyperventilation-induced hypotension during cardiopulmonary resuscitation. Circulation 2004;109(16): 1960–5.
20. Yannopoulos D, Aufderheide TP, Gabrielli A, et al. Clinical and hemodynamic comparison of 15:2 and 30:2 compression-to-ventilation ratios for cardiopulmonary resuscitation. Crit Care Med 2006;34(5):1444–9.
21. Ewy GA. Continuous-chest-compression cardiopulmonary resuscitation for cardiac arrest. Circulation 2007;116(25):2894–6.
22. Ewy GA, Zuercher M, Hilwig RW, et al. Improved neurological outcome with continuous chest compressions compared with 30:2 compressions-to-ventilations cardiopulmonary resuscitation in a realistic swine model of out-of-hospital cardiac arrest. Circulation 2007;116(22):2525–30.
23. Edelson DP, Abella BS, Kramer-Johansen J, et al. Effects of compression depth and pre-shock pauses predict defibrillation failure during cardiac arrest. Resuscitation 2006;71(2):137–45.
24. Valenzuela TD, Kern KB, Clark LL, et al. Interruptions of chest compressions during emergency medical systems resuscitation. Circulation 2005;112(9): 1259–65.
25. Kitamura T, Iwami T, Kawamura T, et al. Conventional and chest-compression-only cardiopulmonary resuscitation by bystanders for children who have out-of-hospital cardiac arrests: a prospective, nationwide, population-based cohort study. Lancet 2010;375(9723):1347–54.
26. Chan PS, Krumholz HM, Nichol G, et al. American Heart Association National Registry of Cardiopulmonary Resuscitation Investigators. Delayed time to defibrillation after in-hospital cardiac arrest. N Engl J Med 2008;358(1):9–17.
27. Kramer-Johansen J, Edelson DP, Abella BS, et al. Pauses in chest compression and inappropriate shocks: a comparison of manual and semi-automatic defibrillation attempts. Resuscitation 2007;73(2):212–20.

28. Hunt EA, Vera K, Diener-West M, et al. Delays and errors in cardiopulmonary resuscitation and defibrillation by pediatric residents during simulated cardiopulmonary arrests. Resuscitation 2009;80(7):819–25.
29. Rhodes JF, Blaufox AD, Seiden HS, et al. Cardiac arrest in infants after congenital heart surgery. Circulation 1999;100(19 Suppl):194–9.
30. Ornato JP, Levine RL, Young DS, et al. The effect of applied chest compression force on systemic arterial pressure and end-tidal carbon dioxide concentration during CPR in human beings. Ann Emerg Med 1989;18(7):732–7.
31. Bellamy RF, DeGuzman LR, Pedersen DC. Coronary blood flow during cardiopulmonary resuscitation in swine. Circulation 1984;69(1):174–80.
32. Berg RA, Sanders AB, Kern KB, et al. Adverse hemodynamic effects of interrupting chest compressions for rescue breathing during cardiopulmonary resuscitation for ventricular fibrillation cardiac arrest. Circulation 2001;104(20): 2465–70.
33. Aufderheide TP, Yannopoulos D, Lick CJ, et al. Implementing the 2005 American Heart Association guidelines improves outcomes after out-of-hospital cardiac arrest. Heart Rhythm 2010;7(10):1357–62.
34. Thigpen K, Davis SP, Basol R, et al. Implementing the 2005 American Heart Association guidelines, including use of the impedance threshold device, improves hospital discharge rate after in-hospital cardiac arrest. Respir Care 2010;55(8): 1014–9.
35. Abella BS, Sandbo N, Vassilatos P, et al. Chest compression rates during cardiopulmonary resuscitation are suboptimal: a prospective study during in-hospital cardiac arrest. Circulation 2005;111(4):428–34.
36. Kramer-Johansen J, Myklebust H, Wik L, et al. Quality of out-of-hospital cardiopulmonary resuscitation with real time automated feedback: a prospective interventional study. Resuscitation 2006;71(3):283–92.
37. Arshid M, Lo TY, Reynolds F. Quality of cardio-pulmonary resuscitation (CPR) during paediatric resuscitation training: time to stop the blind leading the blind. Resuscitation 2009;80(5):558–60.
38. Perkins GD, Boyle W, Bridgestock H, et al. Quality of CPR during advanced resuscitation training. Resuscitation 2008;77(1):69–74.
39. DeVita MA, Schaefer J, Lutz J, et al. Improving medical crisis team performance. Crit Care Med 2004;32(Suppl 2):S61–5.
40. Smith KK, Gilcreast D, Pierce K. Evaluation of staff's retention of ACLS and BLS skills. Resuscitation 2008;78(1):59–65.
41. Donoghue AJ, Durbin D, Nadel F, et al. Effect of high-fidelity simulation on pediatric advanced life support training in pediatric housestaff: a randomized trial. Pediatr Emerg Care 2009;25(3):139–44.
42. Wayne DB, Butter J, Siddall VJ, et al. Simulation-based training of internal medicine residents in advanced cardiac life support protocols: a randomized trial. Teach Learn Med 2005;17(3):210–6.
43. Wayne DB, Didwania A, Feinglass J, et al. Simulation-based education improves quality of care during cardiac arrest team responses at an academic teaching hospital: a case-control study. Chest 2008;133(1):56–61.
44. Yeung J, Meeks R, Edelson D, et al. The use of CPR feedback/prompt devices during training and CPR performance: a systematic review. Resuscitation 2009; 80(7):743–51.
45. Edelson DP, Litzinger B, Arora V, et al. Improving in-hospital cardiac arrest process and outcomes with performance debriefing. Arch Intern Med 2008; 168(10):1063–9.

46. Sutton RM, Niles D, Meaney PM, et al. "Booster" training; evaluation of instructor-led bedside cardiopulmonary resuscitation skill training and automated corrective feedback to improve cardiopulmonary resuscitation compliance of pediatric basic life support providers during simulated cardiac arrest. Pediatr Crit Care Med 2011;12(3):e116–21.

47. Sutton RM, Niles D, Meaney PA, et al. Low-dose, high-frequency CPR training improves skill retention of in-hospital pediatric providers. Pediatrics 2011; 128(1):e145–51.

48. Barsuk JH, McGaghie WC, Cohen ER, et al. Simulation-based mastery learning reduces complications during central venous catheter insertion in a medical intensive care unit. Crit Care Med 2009;37(10):2697–701.

49. Barsuk JH, Cohen ER, Feinglass J, et al. Use of simulation-based education to reduce catheter-related bloodstream infections. Arch Intern Med 2009;169(15): 1420–3.

50. Cohen ER, Feinglass J, Barsuk JH, et al. Cost savings from reduced catheter-related bloodstream infection after simulation-based education for residents in a medical intensive care unit. Simul Healthc 2010;5(2):98–102.

51. Hunt EA, Shilkofski NA, Stavroudis TA, et al. Simulation: translation to improved team performance. Anesthesiol Clin 2007;25(2):301–19.

52. Verplancke T, De Paepe P, Calle PA, et al. Determinants of the quality of basic life support by hospital nurses. Resuscitation 2008;77(1):75–80.

53. Knowles M. The adult learner: a neglected species. 4th edition. Houston (TX): Gulf Publishing Company; 1990.

54. Kaufman DM. Applying educational theory in practice. BMJ 2003;326(7382): 213–6.

55. DeWitt TG. The application of social and adult learning theory to training in community pediatrics, social justice, and child advocacy. Pediatrics 2003; 112(3 Part 2):755–7.

56. Berg RA, Sanders AB, Milander M, et al. Efficacy of audio-prompted rate guidance in improving resuscitator performance of cardiopulmonary resuscitation on children. Acad Emerg Med 1994;1(1):35–40.

57. Kern KB, Sanders AB, Raife J, et al. A study of chest compression rates during cardiopulmonary resuscitation in humans. The importance of rate-directed chest compressions. Arch Intern Med 1992;152(1):145–9.

58. Milander MM, Hiscok PS, Sanders AB, et al. Chest compression and ventilation rates during cardiopulmonary resuscitation: the effects of audible tone guidance. Acad Emerg Med 1995;2(8):708–13.

59. Sutton RM, Donoghue AJ, Myklebust H, et al. The voice advisory manikin (VAM): an innovative approach to pediatric lay provider basic life support skill education. Resuscitation 2007;75(1):161–8.

60. Wik L, Thowsen J, Steen PA. An automated voice advisory manikin system for training in basic life support without an instructor. A novel approach to CPR training. Resuscitation 2001;50(2):167–72.

61. Wik L, Myklebust H, Auestad BH, et al. Retention of basic life support skills 6 months after training with an automated voice advisory manikin system without instructor involvement. Resuscitation 2002;52(3):273–9.

62. Wik L, Myklebust H, Auestad BH, et al. Twelve-month retention of CPR skills with automatic correcting verbal feedback. Resuscitation 2005;66(1):27–30.

63. Kaye W, Rallis SF, Mancini ME, et al. The problem of poor retention of cardiopulmonary resuscitation skills may lie with the instructor, not the learner or the curriculum. Resuscitation 1991;21(1):67–87.

64. Mancini ME, Soar J, Bhanji F, et al, Education, Implementation, Teams Chapter Collaborators. Part 12: education, implementation, and teams: 2010 international consensus on cardiopulmonary resuscitation and emergency cardiovascular care science with treatment recommendations. Circulation 2010; 122(16 Suppl 2):S539–81.

65. Abella BS, Edelson DP, Kim S, et al. CPR quality improvement during in-hospital cardiac arrest using a real-time audiovisual feedback system. Resuscitation 2007;73(1):54–61.

66. Niles D, Nysaether J, Sutton R, et al. Leaning is common during in-hospital pediatric CPR, and decreased with automated corrective feedback. Resuscitation 2009;80(5):553–7.

67. Hostler D, Everson-Stewart S, Rea TD, et al. Effect of real-time feedback during cardiopulmonary resuscitation outside hospital: prospective, cluster-randomised trial. BMJ 2011;342:512.

68. Berger RD, Palazzolo J, Halperin H. Rhythm discrimination during uninterrupted CPR using motion artifact reduction system. Resuscitation 2007;75(1):145–52.

69. Voorhees WD, Babbs CF, Tacker WA Jr. Regional blood flow during cardiopulmonary resuscitation in dogs. Crit Care Med 1980;8(3):134–6.

70. Michael JR, Guerci AD, Koehler RC, et al. Mechanisms by which epinephrine augments cerebral and myocardial perfusion during cardiopulmonary resuscitation in dogs. Circulation 1984;69(4):822–35.

71. Halperin HR, Tsitlik JE, Guerci AD, et al. Determinants of blood flow to vital organs during cardiopulmonary resuscitation in dogs. Circulation 1986;73(3):539–50.

72. Schleien CL, Dean JM, Koehler RC, et al. Effect of epinephrine on cerebral and myocardial perfusion in an infant animal preparation of cardiopulmonary resuscitation. Circulation 1986;73(4):809–17.

73. Dean JM, Koehler RC, Schleien CL, et al. Improved blood flow during prolonged cardiopulmonary resuscitation with 30% duty cycle in infant pigs. Circulation 1991;84(2):896–904.

74. Berkowitz ID, Gervais H, Schleien CL, et al. Epinephrine dosage effects on cerebral and myocardial blood flow in an infant swine model of cardiopulmonary resuscitation. Anesthesiology 1991;75(6):1041–50.

75. Ralston SH, Voorhees WD, Babbs CF. Intrapulmonary epinephrine during prolonged cardiopulmonary resuscitation: improved regional blood flow and resuscitation in dogs. Ann Emerg Med 1984;13(2):79–86.

76. Ditchey RV, Lindenfeld J. Failure of epinephrine to improve the balance between myocardial oxygen supply and demand during closed-chest resuscitation in dogs. Circulation 1988;78(2):382–9.

77. Pellis T, Weil MH, Tang W, et al. Evidence favoring the use of an alpha2-selective vasopressor agent for cardiopulmonary resuscitation. Circulation 2003;108(21): 2716–21.

78. Redding JS, Pearson JW. Resuscitation from ventricular fibrillation. Drug therapy. JAMA 1968;203(4):255–60.

79. Redding JS, Pearson JW. Evaluation of drugs for cardiac resuscitation. Anesthesiology 1963;24:203–7.

80. Redding JS. Abdominal compression in cardiopulmonary resuscitation. Anesth Analg 1971;50(4):668–75.

81. Yakaitis RW, Otto CW, Blitt CD. Relative importance of alpha and beta adrenergic receptors during resuscitation. Crit Care Med 1979;7(7):293–6.

82. Pearson JW, Redding JS. The role of epinephrine in cardiac resuscitation. Anesth Analg 1963;42:599–606.

83. Pearson JW, Redding JS. Peripheral vascular tone on cardiac resuscitation. Anesth Analg 1965;44(6):746–52.
84. Paradis NA, Martin GB, Rivers EP, et al. Coronary perfusion pressure and the return of spontaneous circulation in human cardiopulmonary resuscitation. JAMA 1990;263(8):1106–13.
85. Weil MH, Bisera J, Trevino RP, et al. Cardiac output and end-tidal carbon dioxide. Crit Care Med 1985;13(11):907–9.
86. Sanders AB, Kern KB, Otto CW, et al. End-tidal carbon dioxide monitoring during cardiopulmonary resuscitation. A prognostic indicator for survival. JAMA 1989;262(10):1347–51.
87. Sanders AB, Ewy GA, Bragg S, et al. Expired PCO2 as a prognostic indicator of successful resuscitation from cardiac arrest. Ann Emerg Med 1985;14(10): 948–52.
88. Sanders AB, Atlas M, Ewy GA, et al. Expired PCO2 as an index of coronary perfusion pressure. Am J Emerg Med 1985;3(2):147–9.
89. Gudipati CV, Weil MH, Bisera J, et al. Expired carbon dioxide: a noninvasive monitor of cardiopulmonary resuscitation. Circulation 1988;77(1):234–9.
90. Kalenda Z. The capnogram as a guide to the efficacy of cardiac massage. Resuscitation 1978;6(4):259–63.
91. Christenson J, Andrusiek D, Everson-Stewart S, et al. Chest compression fraction determines survival in patients with out-of-hospital ventricular fibrillation. Circulation 2009;120(13):1241–7.
92. Kellum MJ, Kennedy KW, Ewy GA. Cardiocerebral resuscitation improves survival of patients with out-of-hospital cardiac arrest. Am J Med 2006;119(4): 335–40.
93. Kellum MJ, Kennedy KW, Barney R, et al. Cardiocerebral resuscitation improves neurologically intact survival of patients with out-of-hospital cardiac arrest. Ann Emerg Med 2008;52(3):244–52.
94. Bobrow BJ, Clark L, Ewy GA, et al. Minimally interrupted cardiac resuscitation by emergency medical services for out-of-hospital cardiac arrest. JAMA 2008; 299(10):1158–65.
95. Garza AG, Gratton MC, Salomone JA, et al. Improved patient survival using a modified resuscitation protocol for out-of-hospital cardiac arrest. Circulation 2009;119(19):2597–605.
96. Gilmore CM, Rea TD, Becker LJ, et al. Three-phase model of cardiac arrest: time-dependent benefit of bystander cardiopulmonary resuscitation. Am J Cardiol 2006;98(4):497–9.
97. Bohm K, Rosenqvist M, Herlitz J, et al. Survival is similar after standard treatment and chest compression only in out-of-hospital bystander cardiopulmonary resuscitation. Circulation 2007;116(25):2908–12.
98. SOS-KANTO study group. Cardiopulmonary resuscitation by bystanders with chest compression only (SOS-KANTO): an observational study. Lancet 2007; 369(9565):920–6.
99. Hupfl M, Selig HF, Nagele P. Chest-compression-only versus standard cardiopulmonary resuscitation: a meta-analysis. Lancet 2010;376(9752):1552–7.
100. Dickinson ET, Verdile VP, Schneider RM, et al. Effectiveness of mechanical versus manual chest compressions in out-of-hospital cardiac arrest resuscitation: a pilot study. Am J Emerg Med 1998;16(3):289–92.
101. Ward KR, Menegazzi JJ, Zelenak RR, et al. A comparison of chest compressions between mechanical and manual CPR by monitoring end-tidal PCO2 during human cardiac arrest. Ann Emerg Med 1993;22(4):669–74.

102. Casner M, Andersen D, Isaacs SM. The impact of a new CPR assist device on rate of return of spontaneous circulation in out-of-hospital cardiac arrest. Prehosp Emerg Care 2005;9(1):61–7.
103. Wang HC, Chiang WC, Chen SY, et al. Video-recording and time-motion analyses of manual versus mechanical cardiopulmonary resuscitation during ambulance transport. Resuscitation 2007;74(3):453–60.
104. Troiani TA, Boland RT. Critical incident stress debriefing: keeping your flight crew healthy. J Air Med Transp 1992;11(10):21–4.
105. FitzGerald ML, Braudaway CA, Leeks D, et al. Debriefing: a therapeutic intervention. Mil Med 1993;158(8):542–5.
106. Samter J, Fitzgerald ML, Braudaway CA, et al. Debriefing: from military origin to therapeutic application. J Psychosoc Nurs Ment Health Serv 1993;31(2):23–7.
107. Mitchell AM, Sakraida TJ, Kameg K. Critical incident stress debriefing: implications for best practice. Disaster Manag Response 2003;1(2):46–51.
108. Ireland S, Gilchrist J, Maconochie I. Debriefing after failed paediatric resuscitation: a survey of current UK practice. Emerg Med J 2008;25(6):328–30.
109. Dine CJ, Gersh RE, Leary M, et al. Improving cardiopulmonary resuscitation quality and resuscitation training by combining audiovisual feedback and debriefing. Crit Care Med 2008;36(10):2817–22.
110. Olasveengen TM, Tomlinson AE, Wik L, et al. A failed attempt to improve quality of out-of-hospital CPR through performance evaluation. Prehosp Emerg Care 2007;11(4):427–33.
111. Lick CJ, Aufderheide TP, Niskanen RA, et al. Take Heart America: a comprehensive, community-wide, systems-based approach to the treatment of cardiac arrest. Crit Care Med 2011;39(1):26–33.
112. Kouwenhoven WB, Jude JR, Knickerbocker GG. Closed-chest cardiac massage. JAMA 1960;173:1064–7.

Postresuscitation Care

Daniel Boutsikaris, MD, Michael E. Winters, MD*

KEYWORDS

- Post–cardiac arrest • Post–cardiac arrest syndrome
- Therapeutic hypothermia • Cardiac arrest
- Return of spontaneous circulation (ROSC)
- Cardiac catheterization

Cardiac arrest accounts for approximately 350,000 resuscitations per year in North America.[1–3] The incidence of cardiac arrest requiring interventions by emergency medical services (EMS) personnel is 50 to 55 per 100,000 population each year in the United States and Canada.[2] The primary goals of resuscitation are the return of spontaneous circulation (ROSC) and meaningful neurologic recovery. Care of the patient with ROSC after cardiac arrest is complex and challenging; it has a strong impact on patient morbidity and mortality.[1,3–5] Important components of post–cardiac arrest care are appropriate ventilation and oxygenation, hemodynamic optimization, induction of therapeutic hypothermia, early cardiac catheterization, and correction of metabolic derangements. It is imperative that the emergency physician (EP) be knowledgeable of the systematic and multisystem approach to the patient with ROSC following cardiac arrest. Given the urgency of treatment along with the increasing emergency department (ED) lengths of stay for many critically ill patients, it is the EP, rather than the intensivist, who can have the most significant impact on morbidity and mortality in this select population of critically ill patients in the ED.[6] This article focuses on the ED management of the patient with ROSC following cardiac arrest. The information complies with the recently updated guidelines for post–cardiac arrest care, published by the American Heart Association (AHA).[7]

POST–CARDIAC ARREST SYNDROME

Following ROSC, a complex array of pathophysiologic processes begins to occur. These processes, which constitute the post–cardiac arrest syndrome (PCAS), are grouped into 4 categories: systemic ischemia/reperfusion response, brain injury,

Funding support/financial disclosures/conflicts of interest: None.
Combined Emergency Medicine/Internal Medicine/Critical Care Program, University of Maryland School of Medicine, 110 South Paca Street, 6th Floor, Suite 200, Baltimore, MD 21201, USA
* Corresponding author.
E-mail address: mwint001@umaryland.edu

Emerg Med Clin N Am 30 (2012) 123–140
doi:10.1016/j.emc.2011.09.011
0733-8627/12/$ – see front matter © 2012 Elsevier Inc. All rights reserved.

myocardial dysfunction, and persistence of the precipitating cause of the arrest (**Table 1**).[3]

Systemic Ischemia-Reperfusion Response

With ROSC, ischemic tissue is reperfused, sending toxic substrates to the central circulation and potentially perpetuating organ dysfunction. The systemic ischemia/reperfusion response is thought to be mediated by increased cytokine production, alterations in coagulation, oxygen free-radical formation, adrenal dysfunction, and disruption of the blood-brain barrier.[3,8,9] The extent of injury caused by reperfusion depends on the duration of ischemia, existing comorbidities, and the cause of the

Table 1
Components of the post–cardiac arrest syndrome

	Pathophysiology	Clinical Manifestation	Potential Treatments

Brain injury	Reactive oxygen species
	Protein oxidation
	Lipid peroxidation
	Impaired
	  cerebrovascular
	  autoregulation
	Cerebral edema
		Coma
		Seizures
		Myoclonus
		Persistent
		  vegetative state
		Stroke
		Brain death
			Therapeutic
			  hypothermia
			Hemodynamic
			  optimization
			Seizure control
			Controlled
			  reoxygenation

Myocardial
  dysfunction
	Direct injury from CPR
	  and defibrillation
	Catecholamine surge
	Oxygen free radicals
	Acute coronary
	  syndrome
		Hypotension
		Dysrhythmias
		Global hypokinesis
		Circulatory collapse
			Early revascularization
			Hemodynamic
			  optimization
			Mechanical support
			  with IABP, LVAD,
			  ECMO

Systemic ischemia/
  reperfusion
  response
	Mediated by cytokines
	Impaired coagulation
	Oxygen free-radical
	  formation
	Adrenal dysfunction
	Increased susceptibility
	  to infection
		Hypovolemia
		Hypotension
		Circulatory collapse
		Multiorgan failure
			Hemodynamic
			  optimization
			Temperature control

Persistent
  precipitating
  cause
	ACS
	COPD, asthma
	CVA
	PE
	Overdose
	Sepsis
	Hypovolemia
	Hemorrhage
		Specific to cause	Disease-specific
			  interventions

Abbreviations: ACS, acute coronary syndrome; COPD, chronic obstructive pulmonary disease; CPR, cardiopulmonary resuscitation; CVA, cerebrovascular accident; ECMO, extracorporeal membrane oxygenation; IABP, intra-aortic balloon pump; LVAD, left ventricular assist device; PE, pulmonary embolism.

Data from Neumar RW, Nolan JP, Adrie C, et al. Post-cardiac arrest syndrome: epidemiology, pathophysiology, treatment, and prognostication. A consensus statement from the International Liaison Committee on Resuscitation (American Heart Association, Australian and New Zealand Council on Resuscitation, European Resuscitation Council, Heart and Stroke Foundation of Canada, InterAmerican Heart Foundation, Resuscitation Council of Asia, and the Resuscitation Council of Southern Africa); the American Heart Association Emergency Cardiovascular Care Committee; the Council on Cardiovascular Surgery and Anesthesia; the Council on Cardiopulmonary, Perioperative, and Critical Care; the Council on Clinical Cardiology; and the Stroke Council. Circulation 2008;118:2452–83.

arrest.[3] If ROSC can be achieved quickly, the systemic ischemia/reperfusion response can be limited.[3]

The PCAS can be considered similar to sepsis.[8,10] Like patients with sepsis, patients with PCAS have a significant increase in the production of cytokines and inflammatory mediators. This results in increased activation of neutrophils and the vascular endothelium leading to a potent pro-inflammatory response.[10] More recently studies have indicated that ischemia may also stimulate such mediators as vascular endothelial growth factor (VEGF), which was noted for its potential effects on vascular permeability.[9] Overall, the increased presence of cytokines, activation of endothelium, and upregulation of mediators such as VEGF is believed to lead to increased vascular permeability with resultant volume loss, as well as vascular dysregulation.[8–10] In addition, ischemia disrupts coagulation, generally favoring an overall pro-coagulant state.[3,10–12] Finally, increased cytokine production results in an entity called "endotoxin tolerance," which may initially be helpful against an overwhelming inflammatory response, but ultimately leads to immune dysfunction and a heightened risk of infection.[3,10]

In addition to this proinflammatory, procoagulant state, adrenal dysfunction can also develop in patients with reperfusion injury. The initial response to stress (eg, cardiac arrest) is an increased secretion of cortisol from the adrenal glands. Following ROSC after cardiac arrest, a relative adrenal insufficiency can emerge. This relative insufficiency is common in patients after cardiac arrest and can contribute to circulatory collapse.[13,14]

Overall, the systemic ischemia/reperfusion response is characterized by intravascular volume depletion from increased vascular permeability, impaired vasoregulation, prothrombotic state, and increased susceptibility to infection.[3] An early, goal-directed approach to resuscitation and management seems to limit the progression of the systemic ischemia/reperfusion response.[3,5,15,16]

Brain Injury

Most deaths in patients with ROSC from out-of-hospital cardiac arrest occur from neurologic injury.[17] Although a detailed discussion of neuronal cell death is beyond the scope of this article, it is important to briefly review the mechanisms that lead to it.

With ROSC, reactive oxygen species are generated by mitochondria in ischemic neuronal tissues. These reactive oxygen species trigger a cascade of cellular and molecular events, including protein oxidation, lipid peroxidation, and DNA damage, all of which can induce neuronal cell death.[18,19] Recent evidence suggests that sustained increases in arterial oxygen content (hyperoxia) may further increase the quantity of reactive oxygen species and increase the mortality.[20] In addition to creating reactive oxygen species, ischemia induces activation of transcription factors, resulting in apoptosis, inflammation, and sustained oxidative stress.[21] Many of these pathologic processes occur hours to days following ROSC.[3]

The brain can also be injured following ROSC after cardiac arrest by impaired autoregulation of the cerebral vasculature and cerebral edema. Although data are limited, vascular autoregulatory mechanisms may be either impaired or absent.[22] As a result, patients after cardiac arrest may need a higher mean arterial pressure (MAP) to sustain cerebral perfusion pressure and oxygen delivery.[22] Some degree of cerebral edema is typically seen on imaging studies of comatose survivors of cardiac arrest. The clinical significance of cerebral edema following ROSC remains controversial.[23–25] Torbey and colleagues[23] investigated the impact of cerebral edema by calculating the ratio (in Hounsfield units) between the cerebral gray matter (GM) and white matter (WM). They found that a GM/WM ratio of less than 1.18 at the level of the basal ganglia was 100% predictive of death. The cause of cardiac arrest may contribute to the degree of cerebral edema. Morimoto and colleagues[25] determined that cerebral edema was more common when the arrest had respiratory causes. Based on the available literature, the clinical relevance of impaired autoregulation and cerebral edema cannot be determined. Consensus opinion suggests that transient cerebral edema during the early post–cardiac arrest period is rarely associated with clinically relevant increases in intracranial pressure (ICP) or outcome.[3]

Myocardial Dysfunction

Although neurologic injury is the leading cause of death in patients after cardiac arrest, myocardial dysfunction is common and may contribute to increased morbidity and mortality.[3,17,26–29] Laurent and colleagues[26] showed that 50% to 70% of patients after cardiac arrest without evidence of coronary occlusion on angiography develop myocardial dysfunction.[30] Typically, myocardial dysfunction occurs within 8 hours following ROSC and is manifested by increased cardiac filling pressures, decreased cardiac index, and a decrease in both systolic and diastolic function.[26,27] In most patients, the cardiac index returns to baseline within 24 to 48 hours; however, supportive treatment with vasoactive agents may be necessary for up to 72 hours following ROSC. In rare cases, myocardial dysfunction persists for weeks or months before returning to the patient's prearrest cardiac function.[30]

Myocardial dysfunction is thought to occur from several factors. First, the myocardium may be injured directly from closed chest compressions or defibrillation. In addition, the surge in catecholamines that occurs following ROSC, or the use of epinephrine during resuscitation, has been associated with myocardial dysfunction in the post–cardiac arrest period.[30,31] At the cellular level, it is hypothesized that depletion of adenosine triphosphate stores diminishes myocardial performance, and several days may be needed to restore it. Additional theories on myocardial dysfunction in the post–cardiac arrest period include the generation of oxygen free radicals, alterations in sarcoplasmic calcium metabolism, and upregulation of heat shock proteins.[27]

Persistent Precipitating Cause

Following ROSC, the EP is challenged with identifying and treating the cause of the cardiac arrest. Cardiac causes are most common for out-of-hospital arrests, accounting for approximately 50% of cases.[32] Importantly, ST-segment abnormalities and complaints of chest pain are poor predictors of acute coronary occlusion in the patient after cardiac arrest.[32] It is estimated that 70% of deaths from acute myocardial infarction occur as out-of-hospital cardiac arrests.[33] Pulmonary embolism (PE) is another common cause of cardiac arrest, accounting for 5% to 10% of cases.[34,35] Although pulseless electrical activity is commonly associated with PE, asystole and ventricular fibrillation can occur.[34] Hess and colleagues[35] found that respiratory failure was the most common noncardiac cause of out-of-hospital cardiac arrest, accounting for approximately 35% of cases. In their study, PE accounted for 13.3% of arrests. Less common causes include drug overdose, electrolyte abnormalities, sepsis, near drowning, hypothermia, environmental exposures, and intracranial catastrophes.[3,35]

ED MANAGEMENT OF THE PATIENT AFTER CARDIAC ARREST

To improve morbidity and mortality, ED management of the patient after cardiac arrest should consist of a multisystem approach, with emphasis on appropriate oxygenation and ventilation, hemodynamic optimization, institution of therapeutic hypothermia for appropriate candidates, early cardiac catheterization when indicated, and management of metabolic derangements.

Oxygenation

Following ROSC, it is common practice to place all patients on 100% forced inspiratory oxygen (F_iO_2) regardless of intubation status. As previously discussed, there is mounting evidence to suggest that high partial pressures of arterial oxygen (P_aO_2) may be deleterious.[36–38] Kilgannon and colleagues[20] evaluated more than 6000 adult patients with ROSC after cardiac arrest and found that hyperoxia, defined in the study as a P_aO_2 greater than 300 mm Hg, was associated with worsened outcome compared with patients whose P_aO_2 ranged between 60 and 300 mm Hg. The optimal oxygen saturation (S_pO_2) and P_aO_2 remain unknown. The most recent guidelines from the AHA recommend titrating supplemental oxygen therapy to maintain an S_pO_2 greater than 94% and a P_aO_2 around 100 mm Hg.[7] For intubated patients, positive end-expiratory pressure (PEEP) can be titrated to maintain target oxygen saturation levels while minimizing exposure to high levels of inspired oxygen.

Ventilation

Following cardiac arrest, patients are at risk of developing acute respiratory distress syndrome.[7] Although optimal settings for mechanical ventilation of the patient after cardiac arrest have not yet been determined, current guidelines recommend implementing a low–tidal volume ventilatory strategy with the selection of initial tidal volumes between 6 and 8 mL/kg of ideal body weight.[7,39–41] A respiratory rate that avoids hyperventilation should be chosen. Hyperventilation increases intrathoracic pressures, potentially worsening hemodynamic instability, and induces hypocapnia.[7,42] Conversely, hypercapnia can increase ICP and exacerbate any preexisting acidosis.[3,41] An initial respiratory rate between 16 and 18 breaths per minute is suggested but must be followed with serial arterial blood gas measurements to determine the partial pressure of carbon dioxide (P_aCO_2). Similar to P_aO_2, minute ventilation should be adjusted to maintain normal levels of P_aCO_2 (40–45 mm Hg).[7] In recent years, evidence has mounted in support of the efficacy of monitoring end-tidal carbon dioxide concentration ($P_{et}CO_2$). The EP can use $P_{et}CO_2$, if it is available, as a method to monitor ventilation, with the target being 35 to 40 mm Hg. To minimize ventilator-induced lung injury, serial measurements of the plateau pressure should be obtained, with the goal plateau pressure being less than or equal to 30 cm H_2O.[7,39,40] Tidal volume may be decreased to as little as 4 mL/kg ideal body weight if the plateau pressure remains greater than 30 cm H_2O.

Hemodynamic Optimization

Hemodynamic optimization of the patient after cardiac arrest focuses on restoring intravascular volume, maintaining adequate perfusion pressure, monitoring oxygen delivery, identifying and correcting precipitating causes, and providing supportive care during the period of myocardial dysfunction.[3] Early hemodynamic optimization is essential to improving outcomes.[5,43] In many ways, the approach to the patient after cardiac arrest parallels that for other disease states, such as sepsis, with an early, goal-directed approach to hemodynamic resuscitation.[15,16] Therefore, many of the recommended resuscitation end points for patients after arrest are extrapolated from guidelines for the management of septic or critically ill postoperative patients.[15,16]

Restoring intravascular volume is an integral component of hemodynamic optimization. As discussed earlier, patients with PCAS are generally volume depleted as a result of increased vascular permeability. Isotonic crystalloid fluids should be administered to restore volume status and optimize right heart filling pressures.[3,5,7,15,16] Between 3 and 5 L of crystalloid fluid may be required to maintain these filling pressures during the first 24 hours following ROSC.[26] However, the best means of accurately assessing volume status remains controversial. Previous guidelines recommended the use of central venous pressure (CVP) to assess volume status, with a resuscitation end point for CVP of 8 to 12 mm Hg.[15,16] However, evidence for CVP as a reliable estimate of intravascular volume status is lacking. Numerous conditions, such as tricuspid valve abnormalities, PE, cardiac tamponade, tension pneumothorax, and right-sided myocardial infarction, can increase CVP, thereby giving inaccurate information on volume status.[3] Current methods for assessing intravascular volume status include respirophasic changes in the inferior vena cava, as measured with ultrasonography; pulse pressure variation; and systolic pressure variation. These dynamic indices of volume responsiveness provide a better estimate of volume status than CVP. In addition, urine output can be followed as an indirect marker of volume status and renal perfusion. Current guidelines recommend targeting a urine output of greater than or equal to 0.5 mL/kg/h.[3]

Maintaining adequate perfusion pressure is as important as restoring intravascular volume. MAP, rather than systolic blood pressure, is a better physiologic surrogate for organ perfusion pressure and should be followed. No prospective study designed to identify the optimal MAP in these patients has been reported.[3,7] Nevertheless, current guidelines recommend a MAP greater than 65 mm Hg for patients after cardiac arrest.[7] Recognizing the limitations of the literature, the EP must determine the optimal MAP for each patient. Some patients may require a higher MAP to maintain adequate cerebral perfusion and oxygen delivery. Several studies have found that MAPs between 90 and100 mm Hg give good outcomes.[5,44,45] MAPs greater than 100 mm Hg are unlikely to provide additional therapeutic benefit and may be detrimental.[3,44] Given the importance of maintaining an adequate perfusion pressure, patients after cardiac arrest should have an arterial line placed for continuous measurement of MAP.

If the MAP remains less than 65 mm Hg despite restoration of intravascular volume, a vasopressor should be administered. To date, no vasopressor agent has been shown to be superior. Current guidelines recommend the use of dopamine, norepinephrine, or epinephrine to maintain MAP greater than 65 mm Hg in the patient after cardiac arrest.[7] DeBacker and colleagues[46] evaluated the use of norepinephrine and dopamine in more than 1600 patients with undifferentiated shock. Although no survival benefit was shown with either agent, dopamine was associated with an increased number of adverse events and a trend toward a higher mortality for patients with cardiogenic shock.

Titrating therapy to optimize hemodynamic parameters in the patient after cardiac arrest also depends on assessing the adequacy of oxygen delivery. Oxygen delivery is assessed via global markers of hypoperfusion, namely the serum lactate concentration and central venous oxygen saturation ($S_{cv}O_2$). $S_{cv}O_2$ is measured from a central line placed in the internal jugular or subclavian vein. Values less than 70% indicate inadequate oxygen delivery and indicate the need for continued aggressive resuscitation. Current guidelines recommend maintaining $S_{cv}O_2$ greater than or equal to 70%.[3,7,15,16] Clinically, the interpretation of $S_{cv}O_2$ in the setting of cardiac arrest can be difficult because of venous hyperoxia, which tends to occur in patients who have received high doses of epinephrine (eg, during cardiopulmonary resuscitation [CPR]).[47] Recent evidence suggests that measuring serial lactate values and determining the lactate clearance rate is adequate for assessment of oxygen delivery.[48,49] In a recent noninferiority trial, Jones and colleagues[50] showed that titrating therapy in accordance with the lactate clearance rate was comparable with therapy based on $S_{cv}O_2$ values in patients with sepsis. However, lactate clearance can be impaired in hepatic dysfunction, convulsive seizures, and hypothermia. Regardless of whether

$S_{cv}O_2$ or lactate clearance is used, the adequacy of oxygen delivery should be assessed. For patients who have poor oxygen delivery, as shown by a lactate clearance rate of less than 10% for serial measurements or an $S_{cv}O_2$ of less than 70% despite adequate intravascular volume and MAP, administration of an inotropic agent should be considered. Dobutamine, the inotropic agent of choice, has been shown to be effective in the reversal of systolic and diastolic dysfunction following cardiac arrest.[51–53]

If restoration of intravascular volume and the addition of vasopressor and inotropic agents fail to maintain an adequate perfusion pressure or oxygen delivery, mechanical assistance may be considered.[3] In these circumstances, emergent cardiac catheterization is indicated to allow the placement of an intra-aortic balloon pump (IABP) or left ventricular assist device (LVAD). However, the routine use of mechanical support is not recommended, because studies have not shown a consistent survival benefit.[7,54,55] A summary of oxygenation, initial settings for the mechanical ventilator, and hemodynamic goals are listed in **Box 1**.

Therapeutic Hypothermia

Although case reports on the potential benefits of therapeutic hypothermia date back to the 1950s, it was not until after 2002, when 2 landmark studies were published in The New England Journal of Medicine, that the AHA incorporated therapeutic hypothermia into its recommendations for postresuscitation care.[7,56–58] Current AHA guidelines recommend the use of therapeutic hypothermia in all comatose survivors of cardiac arrest.[7] Comatose is defined by the AHA as a lack of meaningful response to verbal commands.[7]

At present, knowledge gaps exist regarding patient selection, method of induction, goal temperature, duration of the maintenance phase, and the rate of rewarming with therapeutic hypothermia.[3,7] Despite the recommendations to cool all comatose survivors of cardiac arrest, no prospective, randomized trials have evaluated the outcome of therapeutic hypothermia in patients who had an initial cardiac arrest rhythm other than pulseless ventricular tachycardia (VT) or ventricular fibrillation (VF). Literature on patients with non-VT/VF rhythms is limited to case reports, case series, and observation studies, which do seem to show a beneficial effect of therapeutic hypothermia.[5,59–63]

Patients receiving therapeutic hypothermia should be cooled as soon as possible. Data from the 2 largest, prospective trials suggest that the window for therapeutic hypothermia is between 2 and 8 hours following ROSC.[56,57] Patients should be cooled to a target temperature between 32 and 34°C.[3,7,56,57] Although the ideal temperature is not clear, a temperature less than 32°C may result in greater risk of complications without a clear morbidity or mortality benefit. Patients can be cooled easily and inexpensively with the infusion of crystalloid fluid at a temperature of 4°C. Lactated Ringer solution or 0.9% normal saline can be administered as a bolus between 500 mL and 30 mL/kg.[7,64] In addition to cold intravenous fluids, surface cooling techniques such as ice packs to the groin, axilla, head, and neck and cooling blankets can be used.[65–67] Iced saline gastric lavage through a Salem Sump (Covidien, Mansfield, Massachusetts) nasogastric tube is another strategy that can be used to achieve the target temperature. More recent methods explored the use of endovascular cooling devices with feedback technology to assist with maintenance therapy.[3,63] These devices have not been shown to be superior in achieving or maintaining the target temperature compared with cold intravenous fluids, ice packs, and cooling blankets.

Monitoring axillary, oral, or tympanic temperatures is not adequate in the patient in whom therapeutic hypothermia is being induced.[7] Instead, in nonanuric patients, core

Box 1

Oxygenation, initial mechanical ventilation settings, and hemodynamic goals

Oxygenation

- Titrate F_iO_2 to maintain S_pO_2 at greater than 94% and P_aO_2 around 100 mm Hg
- Titrate PEEP to maintain target S_pO_2

Initial mechanical ventilator settings

- Tidal volume: 6 to 8 mL/kg of ideal body weight
- Respiratory rate: 16 to 18 bpm
- PEEP: 5 cm H_2O
- Maintain
  - P_aCO_2: 40 to 45 mm Hg
  - $P_{et}CO_2$: 35 to 40 mm Hg
  - pH: 7.3 to 7.4
- Monitor and maintain plateau pressure less than or equal to 30 cm H_2O

Hemodynamic

- Maintain euvolemia
- Urine output: greater than or equal to 0.5 mL/kg/h
- MAP: greater than or equal to 65 mm Hg
- $S_{cv}O_2$: greater than or equal to 70%
- Lactate clearance of greater than 10% at 2-hour intervals until normal
- Vasopressors and inotropic agents as needed
- Consider mechanical assist device (eg, LVAD, IABP)

Data from Neumar RW, Nolan JP, Adrie C, et al. Post-cardiac arrest syndrome: epidemiology, pathophysiology, treatment, and prognostication. A consensus statement from the International Liaison Committee on Resuscitation (American Heart Association, Australian and New Zealand Council on Resuscitation, European Resuscitation Council, Heart and Stroke Foundation of Canada, InterAmerican Heart Foundation, Resuscitation Council of Asia, and the Resuscitation Council of Southern Africa); the American Heart Association Emergency Cardiovascular Care Committee; the Council on Cardiovascular Surgery and Anesthesia; the Council on Cardiopulmonary, Perioperative, and Critical Care; the Council on Clinical Cardiology; and the Stroke Council. Circulation 2008;118:2452–83; and Peberdy MA, Callaway CW, Neumar RW, et al. Part 9: post-cardiac arrest care: 2010 American Heart Association Guidelines for Cardiopulmonary Resuscitation and Emergency Cardiovascular Care. Circulation 2010; 22:S768–86.

temperature should be monitored with a temperature-sensing Foley catheter or an esophageal thermometer, provided that iced saline gastric lavage is not being used.[7] A pulmonary artery catheter can be used to monitor temperature if it has been placed for other reasons.[7,68] A rectal thermometer may be used if no other option for core temperature monitoring is available.

Patient shivering can be problematic when attempting to reach goal temperature and should be treated aggressively. Although there is sparse evidence to guide the selection of medications to prevent shivering, current recommendations suggest an opioid in combination with an anxiolytic. Additional medications used to treat shivering in the patient after cardiac arrest receiving therapeutic hypothermia include propofol, meperidine, fentanyl, and dexmedetomidine. If the patient continues to shiver despite aggressive sedation and analgesia, neuromuscular blockade may be necessary in intermittent bolus doses.[3,7] Hypothermia can reduce medication clearance, which is especially important when using neuromuscular agents and sedatives. Hypothermia can reduce the clearance of these agents by as much as 30%.[3,69] Shivering can also be reduced by warming the skin: for every 4°C increase in skin temperature, there is a 1°C decrease in the shivering threshold.[3,69] Typically, warming the skin to treat shivering is feasible only when using intravascular cooling devices.

Once patients achieve the target temperature of 32 to 34°C, the second phase, the maintenance phase, of hypothermic therapy begins. The goal of this phase is to maintain a steady core body temperature, which is best achieved by methods that use a closed-feedback temperature-sensing loop.[3,7,66] Cold intravenous fluids alone should not be used for the maintenance phase. Cooling blankets and ice packs, although not optimal, are feasible.[3,66] The optimal duration of the maintenance phase of therapeutic hypothermia is unknown. Based on expert opinion and studies to date, current guidelines recommend that the duration of therapy should be between 12 and 24 hours.[3,7,56,57] Durations of hypothermia longer than 24 hours have not been studied.

Following 12 to 24 hours of hypothermia, patients should be rewarmed. Similar to the induction and maintenance phases of therapeutic hypothermia, there is scant literature to guide the rewarming phase. Current guidelines, based primarily on consensus opinion, recommend rewarming patients at a rate of 0.25°C to 0.5°C per hour.[3] Transitioning from hypothermia to normothermia can result in significant effects on metabolism, electrolyte concentrations, medications levels, and hemodynamics.[3] If rewarming speeds are too high, the catabolic processes could be reinitiated, worsening patient outcome.[69]

Throughout the induction, maintenance, and rewarming phases of therapeutic hypothermia, it is important to continue to monitor oxygenation, ventilation, and hemodynamic optimization. All patients should remain on continuous cardiac monitoring, pulse oximetry, and end-tidal carbon dioxide, with the goals of maintaining S_{pO_2} greater than 94%, euvolemia, MABP greater than 65 mm Hg, and a P_{etCO_2} of 35 to 40 mm Hg.

The complications of therapeutic hypothermia include bradycardia, increased systemic vascular resistance, and decreased cardiac output.[69,70] Cooling also has significant effects on the kidneys and can induce diuresis, resulting in hypophosphatemia, hypokalemia, hypomagnesemia, hypocalcemia, and hypovolemia.[3,69,70] Electrolyte levels should be monitored frequently and replaced to high normal values.[69] Hypothermia can also induce insulin resistance and decreased insulin secretion. Significant hyperglycemia can be seen even in patients without a history of diabetes.[3,69] Coagulopathy is another common effect of hypothermia, mediated through platelet dysfunction and its effects on the clotting cascade.[69] In addition, hypothermia can suppress the immune system through inhibition of proinflammatory mediators. Literature to date suggests a trend toward increased infections; however, values have not reached statistical significance.[3,69] A summary of the 3 phases of therapeutic hypothermia is listed in **Box 2**.

Early Cardiac Catheterization

The rates of coronary artery disease in patients resuscitated from out-of-hospital cardiac arrest are as high as 71%; up to 50% have an acute coronary occlusion.[32,71] Cardiac catheterization provides definitive therapy for patients with an occlusion and has been independently associated with improved outcome.[3,7,32,71] Complaints of chest pain and ST-segment increase seen on an electrocardiogram (ECG) are poor predictors of acute arterial occlusion.[3,7,32,71] Therefore, all patients with a presumed cardiac cause of an arrest should be considered for emergent cardiac catheterization, despite the absence of ST-segment increase on ECG.[3,4,7,32,71] If PCI is not

> **Box 2**
> **Therapeutic hypothermia**
>
> *Induction phase*
>
> - Cool as early as possible, even if going for percutaneous coronary intervention (PCI)
> - Target temperature 32 to 34°C
> - Administer cold intravenous fluids (30 mL/kg bolus of isotonic crystalloid)
> - Use surface cooling methods
> - Place temperature-sensing Foley catheter, esophageal temperature probe, rectal probe, or intravascular device
> - Control shivering
>
> *Maintenance phase*
>
> - Maintain hypothermia at 32 to 34°C
> - Continue for 12 to 24 hours
> - Monitor electrolytes and replace to high normal values
>   - Magnesium
>   - Phosphate
>   - Potassium
>   - Calcium
> - Monitor glucose and treat hyperglycemia
> - Monitor coagulation parameters
>   - Prothrombin time
>   - Activated partial thromboplastin time
>   - Platelets
>
> *Rewarming phase*
>
> - Rewarm at a rate of 0.25 to 0.5°C/h
> - Monitor electrolytes and replace to high normal values
> - Rapid rewarming may reinitiate catabolic processes and worsening outcome

immediately available and ST-segment increase is present, or if there is strong suspicion for an ischemic cardiac event, thrombolytic therapy should be considered.[3]

PCI should not be delayed or withheld because of the use of therapeutic hypothermia. Rittenberger and colleagues[60] and Wolfrum and colleagues[72] showed that the 2 procedures can be done together safely. The theoretic risk of increased bleeding during hypothermia was not observed in either of these studies.[60,72] Early PCI in the setting of hypothermia is associated with improved survival and neurologic outcome.[32,60,71,73] Cardiac catheterization can also provide a means for advanced hemodynamic monitoring and support as well as placement of mechanical assist devices (ie, IABP or LVAD).

SUPPORTIVE CARE
Dysrhythmias

The treatment of dysrhythmias that occur during the post–cardiac arrest period do not differ from standard treatment of dysrhythmias in the patient who has not had a cardiac arrest.[7] These treatments can be electrical and medication therapies. Following ROSC, all patients should be placed on continuous cardiac monitoring and a 12-lead ECG should be obtained. Although patients may have received antidysrhythmic therapy during resuscitation, current guidelines recommend against the use of prophylactic antidysrhythmic medications.[7]

For stable patients with a normal QT interval who develop VT, procainamide or amiodarone may be administered.[3] Amiodarone has been shown to improve survival to hospital admission, but not overall survival or survival to discharge.[74,75] For patients who develop VT in the setting of a prolonged QT interval, amiodarone can be administered. Patients with a prolonged QT interval who develop polymorphic VT should receive magnesium sulfate.[74] Magnesium is unlikely to be effective in the setting of polymorphic VT with a normal QT interval.[74]

Because the underlying cause of a substantial number of out-of-hospital cardiac arrests is cardiac ischemia, the definitive dysrhythmic therapy is reperfusion with PCI or thrombolytics.[32]

Transfusions

Blood transfusion remains controversial outside the setting of hemorrhagic cardiac arrest and in the critically ill. In the initial study on early goal-directed treatment of sepsis, patients whose hemoglobin was less than 10 g/dL in the setting of an $S_{cv}O_2$ less than 70% received transfusions.[16] The transfusion threshold of a hemoglobin less than 10 g/dL in patients with potentially persistent hypoperfusion remains controversial. Currently, there are data to suggest that restrictive transfusion practices (transfusion hemoglobin trigger <7 g/dL) may be beneficial.[76] Blood transfusion should be strongly considered in the patient after cardiac arrest whose hemoglobin concentration is less than 6 g/dL. There is almost no indication to transfuse patients after cardiac arrest whose hemoglobin is greater than 10 g/dL.[77]

Seizure Management

Seizures are common in comatose survivors of cardiac arrest. It is estimated that the clinical course of 5% to 20% of patients after cardiac arrest is complicated by seizures.[5,7] Prolonged seizure activity can have detrimental neurologic effects in the patient after cardiac arrest and has been associated with increased mortality.[78] Current guidelines recommend continuous electroencephalographic monitoring in all comatose survivors of cardiac arrest.[3,7]

Patients who experience seizures during the postresuscitation period typically have a poor response to antiepileptic medications, especially if myoclonus is present.[79] If myoclonus is observed, clonazepam is considered the drug of choice. Sodium valproate and levetiracetam may also be effective.[80] Post–cardiac arrest seizures have also been treated with benzodiazepines, phenytoin, propofol, and barbiturates. Maintenance therapy with antiepileptic medications should be initiated once control of seizure activity is achieved.[3] For patients after cardiac arrest without seizure activity, there is no benefit to the routine administration of antiepileptic medications.[7,81,82]

Hyperglycemia

Hyperglycemia is common in patients after cardiac arrest and may be detrimental.[7,78] This topic has been investigated in critically ill patients and following cardiac arrest.[83–85] In both settings, research has shown that glycemic control is important.[83,84] However, the optimal glucose value remains controversial. In several studies, intensive insulin therapy to aggressively target a normal serum glucose (80–110 mg/dL) value did not affect the mortality rate and markedly increased the incidence of severe hypoglycemia.[83,85] Therefore, current guidelines recommend moderate glycemic control, with a goal serum glucose between 144 and 180 mg/dL.[7]

Hyperthermia

Hyperthermia (>37.6°C) increases the risk of poor neurologic outcome in patients after cardiac arrest.[86] If hyperthermia develops, it should be treated aggressively with antipyretic medications or active cooling therapies.[3,7] If hyperpyrexia develops during the rewarming phase of therapeutic hypothermia, the patient must be monitored closely and the temperature corrected as quickly as possible.[3,7]

A summary of supportive treatment is provided in **Box 3**.

REGIONALIZATION OF RESUSCITATION CENTERS

Out-of-hospital cardiac arrest (OOHCA) affects 236,000 to 325,000 people in the United States each year.[1] The national average survival rate to hospital discharge is only 8.4%.[1] This number does not describe neurologic status at discharge; many of these patients probably have severe and permanent neurologic injury.

Regarding survival to hospital discharge, there is great variation between regions and even among hospitals within the same region.[1–3] There is roughly a fivefold regional variation in outcome by EMS-treated patients of OOHCA.[1,2] Seattle and King County reached a 16.3% survival rate of EMS-treated patients with any initial rhythm, and a 39.9% survival rate when the initial rhythm was VF. Rochester, Minnesota, reported a similar survival rate of 49% after bystander-witnessed VF arrest.[1,2] Survival rates, as well as the likelihood of good neurologic recovery, are highly contingent on several interventions. Interventions such as bystander CPR and defibrillation are beyond the control of the EP, but EMS transport to an appropriate facility can be directed by the EP.[87] Interventions such as emergent PCI, induction of therapeutic hypothermia, and provider experience have all been shown to improve outcomes after OOHCA.[3,5,7,32,56,59,72]

Similar to the current designation of trauma centers, ST-segment elevation myocardial infarction (STEMI) centers, and stroke centers, cardiac arrest center designation is on the horizon.[1,3,88] Cardiac arrest centers must be staffed with experienced personnel who have access to the necessary resources to provide the efficient and definitive care these patients require.[1,3,32,59,71,72,89] The ability to perform emergent coronary angiography is an independent predictor of improved outcome and must be within the capabilities of a cardiac arrest center.[1,3,32,71,89] The availability of cardiac catheterization is also important, because some studies have shown rates of coronary artery disease as high as 71% in the postarrest population.[1]

There is increasing evidence that it is safe to transport patients with ROSC to a resuscitation center and bypass closer facilities.[88,90] However, the nearest facility should be bypassed only to provide primary transport to a cardiac arrest center. If CPR remains in progress, EMS personnel should transport the patient to the nearest facility for resuscitation. If the patient has ROSC during the prehospital phase of care, transport to a cardiac arrest center should be arranged.[90]

Regionalization and designation decisions regarding cardiac arrest centers are largely extrapolated from previous work done to establish designated trauma, stroke, and STEMI centers. Longer primary transport times to reach these designated centers has been shown to be safe for patients and to improve patient outcomes, and this is likely the case for future cardiac arrest centers, which will be able to provide definitive treatment under the direction of highly experienced care providers. However, many EMS systems lack standard protocols for patients after cardiac arrest, many of

---

Box 3
Supportive care

Dysrhythmia

- Obtain 12-lead electrocardiogram
- Continuous cardiac monitoring
- Standard medical and electrical therapies
- Normal QT with VT: amiodarone or procainamide
- Prolonged QT with VT: amiodarone
- Prolonged QT with polymorphic VT: magnesium sulfate
- Consider need for reperfusion therapy

Red blood cell transfusion

- Strongly consider if:
  - Hemoglobin less than 7.0 g/dL and
  - $S_{cv}O_2$ less than 70% or lactate clearance less than 10% following 2 hours of resuscitation
- Unlikely if hemoglobin greater than 10 g/dL

Seizure control

- Initiate electroencephalogram monitoring for all comatose survivors
- For myoclonic seizure activity:
  - Clonazepam drug of choice
  - Valproate and levetiracetam may also be used
- For general seizure activity, all of the following are acceptable:
  - Benzodiazepines
  - Phenytoin
  - Propofol
  - Barbiturates
- Initiate maintenance therapy once seizure controlled
- No indication for routine administration of antiepileptic therapies in absence of seizure activity

Hyperglycemia

- Monitor glucose every 1 to 2 hours
- Goal serum glucose 144 to 180 mg/dL
- Administer insulin if serum glucose outside goal range

Hyperthermia

- Aggressively control with antipyretics, surface cooling devices

---

whom are transported to the nearest facility, which may not have the resources needed to adequately care for these complex patients.

SUMMARY

Caring for the ED patient with ROSC after cardiac arrest is challenging. A coordinated and systematic approach to post–cardiac arrest care can improve the mortality rate and the chance of meaningful neurologic recovery. By achieving appropriate targets for oxygenation, ventilation, and hemodynamic parameters, along with initiating therapeutic hypothermia and arranging early PCI, the EP can have the most significant impact on patients who have just been revived from death.

ACKNOWLEDGMENTS

The authors would like to thank Linda J. Kesselring, MS, ELS, the technical editor for the Department of Emergency Medicine at the University of Maryland School of Medicine, for her assistance in the preparation of this article.

REFERENCES

1. Nichol G, Aufderheide TP, Eigel B, et al. Regional systems of care for out-of-hospital cardiac arrest: a policy statement from the American Heart Association. Circulation 2010;121:709–29.
2. Nichol G, Thomas E, Callaway CW, et al. Regional variation in out-of-hospital cardiac arrest incidence and outcome. JAMA 2008;300:423–31.
3. Neumar RW, Nolan JP, Adrie C, et al. Post-cardiac arrest syndrome: epidemiology, pathophysiology, treatment, and prognostication. A consensus statement from the International Liaison Committee on Resuscitation (American Heart Association, Australian and New Zealand Council on Resuscitation, European Resuscitation Council, Heart and Stroke Foundation of Canada, InterAmerican Heart Foundation, Resuscitation Council of Asia, and the Resuscitation Council of Southern Africa); the American Heart Association Emergency Cardiovascular Care Committee; the Council on Cardiovascular Surgery and Anesthesia; the Council on Cardiopulmonary, Perioperative, and Critical Care; the Council on Clinical Cardiology; and the Stroke Council. Circulation 2008;118:2452–83.
4. Nolan JP, Soar J. Postresuscitation care: entering a new era. Curr Opin Crit Care 2010;16:216–22.
5. Sunde K, Pytte M, Jacobsen D, et al. Implementation of a standardised treatment protocol for post resuscitation care after out-of-hospital cardiac arrest. Resuscitation 2007;73:29–39.
6. Bernstein SL, Asplin BR. Emergency department crowding: old problem, new solutions. Emerg Med Clin North Am 2006;24:821–37.
7. Peberdy MA, Callaway CW, Neumar RW, et al. Part 9: post-cardiac arrest care: 2010 American Heart Association Guidelines for Cardiopulmonary Resuscitation and Emergency Cardiovascular Care. Circulation 2010;22:S768–86.
8. Adrie C, Adib-Conquy M, Laurent I, et al. Successful cardiopulmonary resuscitation after cardiac arrest as a "sepsis-like" syndrome. Circulation 2002;106:562–8.
9. Karimova A, Pinsky DJ. The endothelial response to oxygen deprivation: biology and clinical implications. Intensive Care Med 2001;27:19–31.
10. Adrie C, Laurent I, Monchi M, et al. Postresuscitation disease after cardiac arrest: a sepsis-like syndrome? Curr Opin Crit Care 2004;10:208–12.
11. Adrie C, Monchi M, Laurent I, et al. Coagulopathy after successful cardiopulmonary resuscitation following cardiac arrest: implication of the protein C anticoagulant pathway. J Am Coll Cardiol 2005;46:21–8.
12. Shoemaker WC, Appel PL, Kram HB. Role of oxygen debt in the development of organ failure sepsis, and death in high-risk surgical patients. Chest 1992;02:208–15.
13. Miller JB, Donnino MW, Rogan M, et al. Relative adrenal insufficiency in post-cardiac arrest shock is under-recognized. Resuscitation 2008;76:221–5.

14. Hekimian G, Baugnon T, Thuong M, et al. Cortisol levels and adrenal reserve after successful cardiac arrest resuscitation. Shock 2004;22:116–9.
15. Pearse R, Dawson D, Fawcett J, et al. Early goal-directed therapy after major surgery reduces complications and duration of hospital stay: a randomised, controlled trial [ISRCTN38797445]. Crit Care 2005;9:R687–93.
16. Rivers E, Nguyen B, Havstad S, et al. Early goal-directed therapy in the treatment of severe sepsis and septic shock. N Engl J Med 2001;345:1368–77.
17. Laver S, Farrow C, Turner D, et al. Mode of death after admission to an intensive care unit following cardiac arrest. Intensive Care Med 2004;30:2126–8.
18. Jung JE, Kim GS, Chen H, et al. Reperfusion and neurovascular dysfunction in stroke: from basic mechanisms to potential strategies for neuroprotection. Mol Neurobiol 2010;41:172–9.
19. Chen H, Yoshioka H, Kim GS, et al. Oxidative stress in ischemic brain damage: mechanisms of cell death and potential molecular targets for neuroprotection. Antioxid Redox Signal 2011;14(8):1505–17.
20. Kilgannon JH, Jones AE, Shapiro NI, et al. Association between arterial hyperoxia following resuscitation from cardiac arrest and in-hospital mortality. JAMA 2010;303:2165–71.
21. Fukuda S, Warner DS. Cerebral protection. Br J Anaesth 2007;99:10–7.
22. Sundgreen C, Larsen FS, Herzog TM, et al. Autoregulation of cerebral blood flow in patients resuscitated from cardiac arrest. Stroke 2001;32:128–32.
23. Torbey MT, Selim M, Knorr J, et al. Quantitative analysis of the loss of distinction between gray and white matter in comatose patients after cardiac arrest. Stroke 2000;31:2163–7.
24. Fujioka M, Okuchi K, Sakaki T, et al. Specific changes in human brain following reperfusion after cardiac arrest. Stroke 1994;25:2091–5.
25. Morimoto Y, Kemmotsu O, Kitami K, et al. Acute brain swelling after out-of-hospital cardiac arrest: pathogenesis and outcome. Crit Care Med 1993;21:104–10.
26. Laurent I, Monchi M, Chiche JD, et al. Reversible myocardial dysfunction in survivors of out-of-hospital cardiac arrest. J Am Coll Cardiol 2002;40:2110–6.
27. El-Menyar AA. The resuscitation outcome: revisit the story of the stony heart. Chest 2005;128:2835–46.
28. Trzeciak S, Jones AE, Kilgannon JH, et al. Significance of arterial hypotension after resuscitation from cardiac arrest. Crit Care Med 2009;37:2895–904.
29. Kilgannon JH, Roberts BW, Reihl LR, et al. Early arterial hypotension is common in the post-cardiac arrest syndrome and associated with increased in-hospital mortality. Resuscitation 2008;79:410–6.
30. Ruiz-Bailen M, Aguayo de Hoyos E, Ruiz-Navarro S, et al. Reversible myocardial dysfunction after cardiopulmonary resuscitation. Resuscitation 2005;66:175–81.
31. Kern KB. Postresuscitation myocardial dysfunction. Cardiol Clin 2002;20:89–101.
32. Spaulding CM, Joly LM, Rosenberg A, et al. Immediate coronary angiography in survivors of out-of-hospital cardiac arrest. N Engl J Med 1997;336:1629–33.
33. Berg RA, Hemphill R, Abella BS, et al. Part 5: adult basic life support: 2010 American Heart Association Guidelines for Cardiopulmonary Resuscitation and Emergency Cardiovascular Care. Circulation 2010;122:S685–705.
34. Kurkciyan I, Meron G, Sterz F, et al. Pulmonary embolism as a cause of cardiac arrest: presentation and outcome. Arch Intern Med 2000;160:1529–35.
35. Hess EP, Campbell RL, White RD. Epidemiology, trends, and outcome of out-of-hospital cardiac arrest of non-cardiac origin. Resuscitation 2007;72:200–6.

36. Vereczki V, Martin E, Rosenthal RE, et al. Normoxic resuscitation after cardiac arrest protects against hippocampal oxidative stress, metabolic dysfunction, and neuronal death. J Cereb Blood Flow Metab 2006;26:821–35.
37. Balan IS, Fiskum G, Hazelton J, et al. Oximetry-guided reoxygenation improves neurological outcome after experimental cardiac arrest. Stroke 2006;37:3008–13.
38. Kuisma M, Boyd J, Voipio V, et al. Comparison of 30 and the 100% inspired oxygen concentrations during early post-resuscitation period: a randomised controlled pilot study. Resuscitation 2006;69:199–206.
39. Ventilation with lower tidal volumes as compared with traditional tidal volumes for acute lung injury and the acute respiratory distress syndrome. The Acute Respiratory Distress Syndrome Network. N Engl J Med 2000;342:1301–8.
40. Tremblay LN, Slutsky AS. Ventilator-induced lung injury: from the bench to the bedside. Intensive Care Med 2006;32:24–33.
41. Putensen C, Theuerkauf N, Zinserling J, et al. Meta-analysis: ventilation strategies and outcomes of the acute respiratory distress syndrome and acute lung injury. Ann Intern Med 2009;151:566–76.
42. Curley G, Kavanagh BP, Laffey JG. Hypocapnia and the injured brain: more harm than benefit. Crit Care Med 2010;38:1348–59.
43. Carr BG, Matthew Edwards J, Martinez R. Regionalized care for time-critical conditions: lessons learned from existing networks. Acad Emerg Med 2010;17:1354–8.
44. Mullner M, Sterz F, Binder M, et al. Arterial blood pressure after human cardiac arrest and neurological recovery. Stroke 1996;27:59–62.
45. Langhelle A, Tyvold SS, Lexow K, et al. In-hospital factors associated with improved outcome after out-of-hospital cardiac arrest: a comparison between four regions in Norway. Resuscitation 2003;56:247–63.
46. De Backer D, Biston P, Devriendt J, et al. Comparison of dopamine and norepinephrine in the treatment of shock. N Engl J Med 2010;362:779–89.
47. Rivers EP, Rady MY, Martin GB, et al. Venous hyperoxia after cardiac arrest. Characterization of a defect in systemic oxygen utilization. Chest 1992;102:1787–93.
48. Donnino MW, Miller J, Goyal N, et al. Effective lactate clearance is associated with improved outcome in post-cardiac arrest patients. Resuscitation 2007;75:229–34.
49. Kliegel A, Losert H, Sterz F, et al. Serial lactate determinations for prediction of outcome after cardiac arrest. Medicine (Baltimore) 2004;83:274–9.
50. Jones AE, Shapiro NI, Trzeciak S, et al. Lactate clearance vs central venous oxygen saturation as goals of early sepsis therapy: a randomized clinical trial. JAMA 2010;303:739–46.
51. Cokkinos P. Post-resuscitation care: current therapeutic concepts. Acute Card Care 2009;11:131–7.
52. Vasquez A, Kern KB, Hilwig RW, et al. Optimal dosing of dobutamine for treating post-resuscitation left ventricular dysfunction. Resuscitation 2004;61:199–207.
53. Tennyson H, Kern KB, Hilwig RW, et al. Treatment of post resuscitation myocardial dysfunction: aortic counterpulsation versus dobutamine. Resuscitation 2002;54:69–75.
54. Prondzinsky R, Lemm H, Swyter M, et al. Intra-aortic balloon counterpulsation in patients with acute myocardial infarction complicated by cardiogenic shock: the prospective, randomized IABP SHOCK trial for attenuation of multiorgan dysfunction syndrome. Crit Care Med 2010;38:152–60.
55. Barron HV, Every NR, Parsons LS, et al. The use of intra-aortic balloon counterpulsation in patients with cardiogenic shock complicating acute myocardial

infarction: data from the National Registry of Myocardial Infarction 2. Am Heart J 2001;141:933–9.

56. Hypothermia after Cardiac Arrest Study Group. Mild therapeutic hypothermia to improve the neurologic outcome after cardiac arrest. N Engl J Med 2002;346: 549–56.

57. Bernard SA, Gray TW, Buist MD, et al. Treatment of comatose survivors of out-of-hospital cardiac arrest with induced hypothermia. N Engl J Med 2002;346: 557–63.

58. Benson DW, Williams GR Jr, Spencer FC, et al. The use of hypothermia after cardiac arrest. Anesth Analg 1959;38:423–8.

59. Bernard S. Hypothermia after cardiac arrest: expanding the therapeutic scope. Crit Care Med 2009;37:S227–33.

60. Rittenberger JC, Guyette FX, Tisherman SA, et al. Outcomes of a hospital-wide plan to improve care of comatose survivors of cardiac arrest. Resuscitation 2008;79:198–204.

61. Bernard SA, Jones BM, Horne MK. Clinical trial of induced hypothermia in comatose survivors of out-of-hospital cardiac arrest. Ann Emerg Med 1997;30: 146–53.

62. Hachimi-Idrissi S, Corne L, Ebinger G, et al. Mild hypothermia induced by a helmet device: a clinical feasibility study. Resuscitation 2001;51:275–81.

63. Arrich J. Clinical application of mild therapeutic hypothermia after cardiac arrest. Crit Care Med 2007;35:1041–7.

64. Jacobshagen C, Pax A, Unsold BW, et al. Effects of large volume, ice-cold intravenous fluid infusion on respiratory function in cardiac arrest survivors. Resuscitation 2009;80:1223–8.

65. Don CW, Longstreth WT Jr, Maynard C, et al. Active surface cooling protocol to induce mild therapeutic hypothermia after out-of-hospital cardiac arrest: a retrospective before-and-after comparison in a single hospital. Crit Care Med 2009; 37:3062–9.

66. Larsson IM, Wallin E, Rubertsson S. Cold saline infusion and ice packs alone are effective in inducing and maintaining therapeutic hypothermia after cardiac arrest. Resuscitation 2010;81:15–9.

67. Kilgannon JH, Roberts BW, Stauss M, et al. Use of a standardized order set for achieving target temperature in the implementation of therapeutic hypothermia after cardiac arrest: a feasibility study. Acad Emerg Med 2008;15:499–505.

68. Akata T, Setoguchi H, Shirozu K, et al. Reliability of temperatures measured at standard monitoring sites as an index of brain temperature during deep hypothermic cardiopulmonary bypass conducted for thoracic aortic reconstruction. J Thorac Cardiovasc Surg 2007;133:1559–65.

69. Polderman KH. Mechanisms of action, physiological effects, and complications of hypothermia. Crit Care Med 2009;37:S186–202.

70. Polderman KH. Application of therapeutic hypothermia in the intensive care unit. Opportunities and pitfalls of a promising treatment modality–Part 2: Practical aspects and side effects. Intensive Care Med 2004;30:757–69.

71. Reynolds JC, Callaway CW, El Khoudary SR, et al. Coronary angiography predicts improved outcome following cardiac arrest: propensity-adjusted analysis. J Intensive Care Med 2009;24:179–86.

72. Wolfrum S, Pierau C, Radke PW, et al. Mild therapeutic hypothermia in patients after out-of-hospital cardiac arrest due to acute ST-segment elevation myocardial infarction undergoing immediate percutaneous coronary intervention. Crit Care Med 2008;36:1780–6.

73. Batista LM, Lima FO, Januzzi JL Jr, et al. Feasibility and safety of combined percutaneous coronary intervention and therapeutic hypothermia following cardiac arrest. Resuscitation 2010;81:398–403.
74. Morrison LJ, Deakin CD, Morley PT, et al. Part 8: advanced life support: 2010 international consensus on cardiopulmonary resuscitation and emergency cardiovascular care science with treatment recommendations. Circulation 2010; 122:S345–421.
75. Kudenchuk PJ, Cobb LA, Copass MK, et al. Amiodarone for resuscitation after out-of-hospital cardiac arrest due to ventricular fibrillation. N Engl J Med 1999; 341:871–8.
76. Hebert PC, Wells G, Blajchman MA, et al. A multicenter, randomized, controlled clinical trial of transfusion requirements in critical care. Transfusion requirements in critical care investigators, Canadian Critical Care Trials Group. N Engl J Med 1999;340:409–17.
77. Netzer G, Liu X, Harris AD, et al. Transfusion practice in the intensive care unit: a 10-year analysis. Transfusion 2010;50:2125–34.
78. Nielsen N, Sunde K, Hovdenes J, et al. Adverse events and their relation to mortality in out-of-hospital cardiac arrest patients treated with therapeutic hypothermia. Crit Care Med 2011;39:57–64.
79. Hui AC, Cheng C, Lam A, et al. Prognosis following postanoxic myoclonus status epilepticus. Eur Neurol 2005;54:10–3.
80. Caviness JN, Brown P. Myoclonus: current concepts and recent advances. Lancet Neurol 2004;3:598–607.
81. Randomized clinical study of thiopental loading in comatose survivors of cardiac arrest. Brain Resuscitation Clinical Trial I Study Group. N Engl J Med 1986;314: 397–403.
82. Longstreth WT Jr, Fahrenbruch CE, Olsufka M, et al. Randomized clinical trial of magnesium, diazepam, or both after out-of-hospital cardiac arrest. Neurology 2002;59:506–14.
83. Finfer S, Chittock DR, Su SY, et al. Intensive versus conventional glucose control in critically ill patients. N Engl J Med 2009;360:1283–97.
84. Losert H, Sterz F, Roine RO, et al. Strict normoglycaemic blood glucose levels in the therapeutic management of patients within 12h after cardiac arrest might not be necessary. Resuscitation 2008;76:214–20.
85. Oksanen T, Skrifvars MB, Varpula T, et al. Strict versus moderate glucose control after resuscitation from ventricular fibrillation. Intensive Care Med 2007;33:2093–100.
86. Zeiner A, Holzer M, Sterz F, et al. Hyperthermia after cardiac arrest is associated with an unfavorable neurologic outcome. Arch Intern Med 2001;161:2007–12.
87. Iwami T, Kawamura T, Hiraide A, et al. Effectiveness of bystander-initiated cardiac-only resuscitation for patients with out-of-hospital cardiac arrest. Circulation 2007;116:2900–7.
88. Nichol G, Soar J. Regional cardiac resuscitation systems of care. Curr Opin Crit Care 2010;16:223–30.
89. Callaway CW, Schmicker R, Kampmeyer M, et al. Receiving hospital characteristics associated with survival after out-of-hospital cardiac arrest. Resuscitation 2010;81:524–9.
90. Hartke A, Mumma BE, Rittenberger JC, et al. Incidence of re-arrest and critical events during prolonged transport of post-cardiac arrest patients. Resuscitation 2010;81:938–42.

Rapid Response Systems: Identification and Management of the "Prearrest State"

Michael T. McCurdy, MD[a,b,*], Samantha L. Wood, MD[c]

KEYWORDS

- Rapid response • Medical emergency team
- Patient monitoring • Cardiac arrest

Cardiac arrest occurs in up to 5 out of every 1000 adult hospital admissions.[1] Despite aggressive postresuscitation management, in-hospital cardiac arrest (IHCA) is associated with poor outcomes. In a review of 49,130 patients with IHCA, 84% died before hospital discharge or suffered severe neurologic disability, with 55.2% dying during the acute event.[2] Disappointingly, rates of survival to hospital discharge for IHCA patients have not changed over the last several decades.[1,3,4] Although IHCA is more common in children, they fare slightly better; cardiac arrest occurs in 7 to 30 out of every 1000 pediatric admissions,[5–7] and survival to hospital discharge is 25% to 50%.[8]

Signs of deterioration usually precede IHCA,[9–14] and over half of cases are preventable.[15,16] Care for deteriorating ward patients awaiting intensive care unit (ICU) transfer is frequently inadequate.[17] The improvements in morbidity and mortality attributed to early, aggressive intervention in sepsis,[18] trauma,[19] stroke,[20] and ST-elevation myocardial infarction[21] have led to a paradigm shift in how to best care for other critically ill patients as well. Rapid response systems (RRS) represent one way to intervene early on deteriorating patients in an attempt to prevent cardiac arrest and its dismal outcome.

The authors have nothing to disclose.

[a] Division of Pulmonary & Critical Care Medicine, Department of Medicine, University of Maryland School of Medicine, 110 South Paca Street, 2nd Floor, Baltimore, MD 21201, USA
[b] Department of Emergency Medicine, University of Maryland School of Medicine, Baltimore, MD, USA
[c] Combined Emergency Medicine/Internal Medicine/Critical Care Program, University of Maryland Medical Center, 110 South Paca Street, Suite 200, Baltimore, MD 21201, USA
* Corresponding author. Division of Pulmonary & Critical Care Medicine, Department of Medicine, University of Maryland School of Medicine, 110 South Paca Street, 2nd Floor, Baltimore, MD 21201.
E-mail address: DrMcCurdy@gmail.com

Emerg Med Clin N Am 30 (2012) 141–152
doi:10.1016/j.emc.2011.09.012
0733-8627/12/$ – see front matter © 2012 Elsevier Inc. All rights reserved.

THE RAPID RESPONSE SYSTEM

An RRS should provide emergent assessment and care for sick patients who require a higher level of care. The system can be divided into "afferent" and "efferent" limbs. The afferent limb refers to monitoring the patient, detecting crisis, and activating the team. The RRS generally includes a protocol for monitoring patients and a list of "calling criteria." Calling criteria vary among institutions and may include vital-sign abnormalities, changes in mental status, threatened airway, or other signs of deterioration. When a patient meets calling criteria, system activation is optional or mandatory. Most systems encourage nurses to activate the system when concerned about potential patient deterioration regardless of whether calling criteria are met.

Once activated, a team of health care providers presents immediately to the patient's bedside to address the crisis; this team represents the efferent limb of the RRS. There are several types of responding teams, including medical emergency teams (METs), rapid response teams (RRTs), and critical care outreach (CCO) teams. A 2006 consensus conference suggested using the term "medical emergency team" for teams that are generally led by physicians and have the ability to: (1) prescribe therapy; (2) place central vascular lines; (3) initiate ICU-level care at the bedside; and (4) perform advanced airway management. The conference suggested the use of the term 'rapid response team' to describe a team without all 4 of those abilities that performs a preliminary evaluation of a patient and summons additional help or facilitates transfer to a higher level of care if warranted. "Critical care outreach team" implies an outreach component such as proactively visiting hospital wards to identify patients at risk for decompensation.[22]

Research on RRSs has focused primarily on the afferent limb, whereas studies assessing the efficacy of the efferent limb are sparse. This difference can be attributed to the ease of analyzing the afferent limb as compared with the complexity of studying the efferent limb. For example, tracking RRS activation is fairly straightforward: teams are either activated or not. On the other hand, the efferent limb is exceedingly difficult to study because of the numerous variables involving different types of RRSs (eg, MET, RRT, CCO), patient populations (eg, inner city, rural), disease processes (eg, IHCA, hypotension, respiratory distress), care delivered (eg, antibiotics, fluids, vasopressors, intubation), and hospital resources (eg, nursing-to-patient ratios, ICU bed availability, access to ancillary services). Because of the paucity of data on the efferent limb, this review focuses exclusively on the afferent limb of the RRS.

THE AFFERENT LIMB

The afferent limb of the typical RRS comprises several steps. First, a patient clinically deteriorates. Second, nursing staff detects the deterioration following patient assessment or monitoring. Third, nursing staff makes a decision to activate the team. Fourth, the team is activated. Each of these seemingly simple steps presents challenges to the effective and efficient functioning of the RRS.

Antecedents to IHCA

Warning signs precede 60% to 84% of IHCAs[9–14] and are predictive of in-hospital, 30-day, and 1-year mortality.[12,23–25] Most studies refer to these detectable signs of patient deterioration as "antecedents" or "abnormal indices," and include vital sign abnormalities, changes in Glasgow Coma Scale (GCS) score, or other changes in patient condition.

The majority of hospitalized patients remain stable throughout their stay,[23,26] and most of those who develop an abnormal vital sign or other concerning clinical derangement will not experience cardiac arrest or death. In one prospective study of ward patients, 66.7% of observed vital-sign abnormalities spontaneously resolved and an additional 21.6% resolved with treatment. However, presence of a single abnormality was associated with a significant increase in mortality, and mortality risk further increased with every additional abnormality.[23] Another study prospectively evaluated "abnormal indices" in medical and surgical patients at a Veterans Affairs Hospital. Thirty-five percent of those with at least one abnormality, compared with 2.5% of patients without any, later experienced cardiac arrest, death, or unexpected ICU transfer.[12] Use of an "abnormal index" oversimplifies a patient's true risk for cardiac arrest. However, vital signs and other basic findings, such as GCS score, help to grossly estimate a patient's risk of IHCA, death, or ICU transfer.

Antecedents to IHCA provide an opportunity for intervention, but they must be identified early enough to correct the underlying problem. Fortunately, adequate time usually exists to intervene before patient deterioration.[11,23] In one study, 48% of non-"Do Not Resuscitate" (DNR) ward patients exhibited abnormal vital signs in the 8 to 48 hours prior to death.[27] Patients with abnormal indices 8 hours preceding arrest have higher in-hospital mortality (92% vs 81%), notwithstanding the higher likelihood that patients with early abnormal vital signs are on monitored units and receive earlier defibrillation.[28,29] Physicians frequently document concern for patient deterioration hours to days before requiring an unexpected ICU transfer.[30] This alarming finding may result from: (1) physician failure to recognize the prognostic significance of concerning data; (2) institution of inadequate interventions; or (3) failure to either get help or successfully transfer the patient to a higher level of care. Regardless of the reason, physician suspicion of patient deterioration is a harbinger of the eventual need for ICU transfer, and sufficient time often exists for a meaningful preventive intervention if the physician acts on such clinical suspicion.

Monitoring

Identification of appropriate RRS monitoring parameters is the subject of substantial debate. Although the policies of most hospitals include monitoring of vital signs and mental status, the specific parameters used to activate the RRS vary widely. In accordance with standards established at a recent RRS consensus conference, the afferent limb should, at a minimum, monitor heart rate, blood pressure, respiratory rate, temperature, and pulse oximetry. Airway patency, behavior change, capillary refill, urine output, basic chemistry and hematology results, and clinical observations are listed as additional possible monitoring parameters.[9] In these studies, it is noteworthy that telemetry analysis is not included as a routine monitoring parameter in patients without dysrhythmias or suspected acute coronary syndrome.[31]

Determining the proper frequency of monitoring is also a significant challenge. Continuous monitoring is associated with improved outcome in patients with IHCA,[32] whereas less frequent monitoring may delay the detection of impending instability. RRSs receive significantly more calls during the day and from monitored units, reinforcing the concept that more intensive patient monitoring may increase the detection of critical events.[33] Because good outcomes in critically ill patients depend on how rapidly proper treatment is initiated, it logically follows that delay of RRS activation is associated with increased mortality.[34]

Although common sense and some studies suggest that more monitoring improves patient outcomes, data do not consistently support this assertion.[35–37] Patient monitoring is also limited by practical concerns. Nursing resources, bed availability, and cost may prohibit increased monitoring. Technological limitations also present challenges; one study showed that 40.6% of vital-sign abnormalities detected with continuous monitoring in a step-down unit were artifacts.[26] Accurate vital signs are sometimes challenging to obtain (eg, using a too-small blood pressure cuff in an obese patient will result in an inaccurate blood pressure measurement), and an inappropriate emphasis on absolute values rather than relative changes may limit monitoring utility.[38,39] The RRS consensus conference acknowledges that the ideal monitoring frequency is still a matter of debate. The current recommendation is for individualized monitoring plans for all patients, as long as indices are checked at least every 6 to 12 hours.[9]

RRS Activation

Since no standardized early warning score exists, different institutions employ various scoring systems to activate the RRS. Regardless of the type of scoring system utilized, the decision to active the RRS based on a score is ultimately the responsibility of the bedside clinician. For example, a clinician may determine that despite the presence of an abnormal vital sign, the patient does not warrant further evaluation. Whereas other activation criteria can be quite subjective (eg, patient does not "look good"). Although many "track and trigger" systems have been developed to guide this decision making process[40] none is sufficiently reliable to be adopted as the standard means of assessing the likelihood of clinical deterioration in either adults or children.[41–43]

The simplest type of track and trigger system is the single-parameter track and trigger system (SPTTS). In this system, a single vital sign or clinical abnormality outside a specified range prompts RRS activation. A 2008 review examined 30 different SPTTSs by retrospectively applying their criteria to a large database of patients' admission vital signs to evaluate their effectiveness in predicting in-hospital mortality.[44] Specificity ranged from 68.1% to 98.1%, but sensitivity was only 7.1% to 52.8%.

Multiple-parameter track and trigger systems require more than one abnormality for team activation. For example, the Patient-at-Risk score requires either 3 abnormal indices or decreased mental status plus tachycardia or tachypnea for system activation.[45] Sensitivity and specificity for ICU admission were poor (27% and 57%, respectively).[40]

Aggregate-weighted track and trigger systems (AWTTSs) calculate a score based on the degree to which a patient's vital signs are abnormal. One frequently cited AWTTS is the Modified Early Warning Score (MEWS). The MEWS assigns points based on the degree of derangement of systolic blood pressure, heart rate, respiratory rate, temperature, and mental status, with an elevated score correlating with increased risk of death and ICU admission.[46] The MEWS accurately identifies patients at risk for deterioration when a score for age is included; unfortunately, its application to acute medical admissions has not been shown to change outcomes.[47] Dozens of other AWTTs exist, but a recent review concluded that most did not perform well.[48] Hospitals continue to use a variety of scoring systems, but clearly more research is needed to identify the best-performing scoring system.

Several barriers to nursing activation of the RRS exist. Nurses may be reluctant to call because they frequently witness patients who briefly exhibit abnormal signs that spontaneously normalize.[49] In addition, nurses may not know whom to contact (eg, RRS vs primary team) in the event of patient decompensation or fear being reprimanded if a call is later deemed unnecessary.[50] RRS activation rates improve with supportive response by the RRS team and with increased nursing education,[51,52] expertise, and patient familiarity. Mandatory RRS activation for all patients meeting criteria also facilitates improved nursing activation.[53] The relationship between nurse workload and RRS activation is unclear, as studies have shown both increased and decreased activation during busy shifts.[54]

As an alternative to nurse-triggered RRS activation, one study confirmed the feasibility of vital-sign data entry into a Personal Digital Assistant (PDA) that calculates an early-warning score. This score is then transmitted to physicians who can access the information online from anywhere in the hospital.[55] Another study assessed the utility of continuously calculating an "instability index value"; when this value exceeded a certain cutoff, an alarm alerted nursing staff to determine the need for RRS activation.[56] Although this system was associated with a decrease in episodes of patient instability, its ability to alter outcomes and cost compared with simply increasing nursing staffing level is unknown.[57]

Although "family concern" is frequently included in protocols as a trigger for nursing activation of the RRS and often portends a decline in clinical status, experience with direct activation of the RRS by a patient's family is limited. Educational programs have attempted to encourage family members to directly activate the RRS by calling a phone number if they have any concern about the patient's status. However, direct activation remains rare and is frequently prompted by pain control or communication issues rather than a patient's clinical condition.[55,58–60]

Criteria for RRS activation need to be more clearly defined to support decision making. The heterogeneity of early-warning scores limits widespread implementation, and difficulty exists in effectively identifying the most accurate one. As of yet, no system has proved its ability to adequately substitute for the bedside clinician's vigilance in preventing a patient's clinical deterioration.

RRS Efficacy

Outcome data for RRSs vary widely. In adults, some studies demonstrate reductions in both IHCA and mortality,[61,62] others demonstrate reductions in IHCA without a significant change in mortality,[63–66] and still others show no significant differences in either IHCA or mortality.[59,67,68] One study showed decreased mortality in surgical patients but increased mortality in medical patients after RRS implementation.[69] Pediatric studies show decreases in IHCA only,[5] decreases in IHCA and mortality,[70,71] reductions in pulmonary arrest requiring intubation but no changes in IHCA or mortality,[72] and no significant decreases in IHCA or mortality.[73]

The inconsistent conclusions of these studies likely result from methodological design flaws. Most are limited by historical controls, lack of randomization, inclusion of DNR patients, and lack of standardized calling criteria and interventions. The International Liaison Committee on Resuscitation (ILCOR) has since called for consistency and comparability of relevant collected and reported data regarding RRSs.[74]

Two randomized trials assessing the effect of RRSs yielded conflicting results. One assessed the efficacy of a phased introduction of a nurse-led CCO service that provided education on caring for critically ill patients and responded to emergent calls prompted by a Patient-at-Risk score. Hospital wards randomized to CCO implementation reduced mortality compared with controls.[75] The MERIT study, which randomized 23 Australian hospitals to either MET implementation or control, demonstrated significant improvements in both the intervention and control arms, thus yielding no differences in mortality, IHCA, or unplanned ICU admission at 6 months between the arms.[76] The findings of the MERIT study were affected by contamination between the groups: RRSs in the intervention hospitals were often not activated, and preexisting cardiac arrest teams in control hospitals were frequently activated before actual arrest. In addition, because the primary outcome was much lower than expected, the study was underpowered to detect statistical significance. Therefore, a post hoc analysis of the MERIT database attempted to distinguish why before-and-after trials show improved outcomes in hospitals implementing RRSs whereas the randomized MERIT study showed no significant difference between treatment arms. Although fraught with the typical limitations of a post hoc review of data from both intervention and control hospitals, the reanalysis of the MERIT trial identified early RRS activation (ie, calling for help before cardiac arrest) as the primary determinant of lower rates of cardiac arrest and unexpected death.[77]

Follow-up studies involving MERIT hospitals offer possible explanations for the initial negative results. For example, one participating hospital continued to follow these outcomes beyond the 6-month study period and found significantly decreased 2- and 4-year IHCA and mortality with increased MET activation.[78] The investigators argued that hospital culture and "institutional inertia" impede rapid policy changes and that MET efficacy may only be evident once hospital culture has time to adapt. However, one study of a "mature" MET system demonstrated the persistence of preventable cardiac arrests even after 16 years from its implementation.[79] Experience dictates that successful MET systems may not feasibly achieve a "zero rate" of preventable IHCA.

A 2010 meta-analysis of 18 studies including over 1.2 million hospital admissions assessed the effects of RRS implementation.[80] Overall, RRSs were associated with a 33.8% reduction in non-ICU adult IHCA. Mortality data varied widely among studies, but no overall effect was demonstrated in adults, prompting concern that RRS implementation simply shifts patients who will likely die during their hospitalizations from the ward to the ICU. Pediatric mortality from IHCA, however, was reduced by 37.7%. The lower mortality rate was disproportionately large relative to the lower cardiac arrest rate, raising doubt that decreased deaths were due to RRS interventions. This study concluded that there was not robust evidence to support the ability of RRSs to reduce in-hospital mortality. It also noted that study results over time trended toward the null hypothesis, raising questions about initial publication bias.

One inconsistency common to several studies is that mortality rates decline out of proportion to decreases in cardiac arrests.[62,70,71] For example, 6-month periods before and after implementation of an RRT in a Colorado hospital showed a decrease in "code blue" calls from 70 to 55, indicating 15 fewer cardiac arrests; however, this study also reported a significant decrease in mortality rate "equivalent to 75 lives saved."[81]

In summary, the data on RRS efficacy vary. Although some large studies fail to show convincing results, others support RRS implementation when the system promotes earlier calls. Further quality studies undoubtedly are needed to clarify what specific aspects of the RRS are linked to improvement in meaningful outcomes.

CONTROVERSY

RRSs represent a highly controversial issue, and opinion pieces abound in the medical literature. RRS supporters urge aggressive monitoring and evaluation.[82] Skeptics express concern that the rapid institution of RRSs may inhibit study and implementation of alternative and potentially superior ways to improve patient safety such as educational initiatives, increased nursing staff, automated monitoring systems, or hospitalist presence on the floor.[83] Concern also exists that the RRS may temporarily mask underlying deficiencies in medical care for hospitalized patients, such as insufficient physician presence, patient admission to an inappropriate level of care, and inefficient transfer of patients to a higher level of care.[84,85] Others argue for a moderate approach, acknowledging that RRSs are not supported by conclusive data, but asserting that they are currently the best method to manage deteriorating patients.[86] By taking an individualized approach to each patient, RRSs may optimize the use of hospital resources by considering the appropriateness of invasive interventions in individuals unlikely to benefit from such care and by pursuing aggressive measures in those who will.[77]

The major conflict surrounding RRSs reflects a problem commonly encountered in medicine: how to reconcile the intuitive, logical appeal of an intervention with inconsistent and inconclusive evidence. This problem is perhaps most apparent in the Institute for Healthcare Improvement's (IHI) 100,000 Lives Campaign, which challenged hospitals to prevent accidental deaths by pursuing 6 initiatives for patient safety. Although the campaign's success was questioned,[87,88] the IHI supported its RRS advocacy by highlighting the shortcomings of the MERIT study and argued against "enforcing standards of evidence that in this case ignore accumulated reports, time-series data, common sense, and sound logic."[89] Explicitly or implicitly, policy continues to support RRSs, as evidenced by the Joint Commission's recent patient safety goals. These goals include a recommendation that hospitals "select a suitable method that enables health care staff members to directly request additional assistance from a specially trained individual(s) when the patient's condition appears to be worsening."[90]

SUMMARY

Bridging the divide between evidence-based and commonsense medical decision making is challenging, especially when randomized, controlled study of the intervention is difficult and blinding is impossible. The benefit of RRSs is that intuitive and supportive data exist, but the institution of an RRS is not a panacea for IHCA or unexpected deaths. RRS implementation should be one component of an effort to improve patient safety that includes adequate nursing education and staffing, availability and involvement of a patient's primary caregivers, and hospital provision of sufficient resources and efficiency. This coordinated approach facilitates appropriate admission triage decisions and effective monitoring of stable patients, as well as rapid evaluation, treatment, and transfer when necessary.

REFERENCES

1. Sandroni C, Nolan J, Cavallaro F, et al. In-hospital cardiac arrest: incidence, prognosis and possible measures to improve survival. Intensive Care Med 2007;33(2): 237–45.
2. Larkin GL, Copes WS, Nathanson BH, et al. Pre-resuscitation factors associated with mortality in 49,130 cases of in-hospital cardiac arrest: a report from the National Registry for Cardiopulmonary Resuscitation. Resuscitation 2010;81(3): 302–11.
3. Ebell MH, Becker LA, Barry HC, et al. Survival after in-hospital cardiopulmonary resuscitation. A meta-analysis. J Gen Intern Med 1998;13(12):805–16.
4. Ehlenbach WJ, Barnato AE, Curtis JR, et al. Epidemiologic study of in-hospital cardiopulmonary resuscitation in the elderly. N Engl J Med 2009; 361(1):22–31.
5. Brilli RJ, Gibson R, Luria JW, et al. Implementation of a medical emergency team in a large pediatric teaching hospital prevents respiratory and cardiopulmonary arrests outside the intensive care unit. Pediatr Crit Care Med 2007;8(3):236–46 [quiz: 247].

6. Reis AG, Nadkarni V, Perondi MB, et al. A prospective investigation into the epidemiology of in-hospital pediatric cardiopulmonary resuscitation using the international Utstein reporting style. Pediatrics 2002;109(2):200–9.

7. Suominen P, Olkkola KT, Voipio V, et al. Utstein style reporting of in-hospital paediatric cardiopulmonary resuscitation. Resuscitation 2000;45(1):17–25.

8. Topjian A, Berg RA, Nadkarni VM. Pediatric cardiopulmonary arrest and resuscitation. In: Vincent JL, editor. 2008 Yearbook of intensive care and emergency medicine. Berlin, Heidelberg, New York: Springer-Verlag; 2008.

9. DeVita MA, Smith GB, Adam SK, et al. "Identifying the hospitalised patient in crisis"—a consensus conference on the afferent limb of rapid response systems. Resuscitation 2010;81(4):375–82.

10. Franklin C, Mathew J. Developing strategies to prevent in-hospital cardiac arrest: analyzing responses of physicians and nurses in the hours before the event. Crit Care Med 1994;22(2):244–7.

11. Kause JS, Smith G, Prytherch D, et al. A comparison of antecedents to cardiac arrests, deaths, and emergency intensive care admissions in Australia and New Zealand, and the United Kingdom– the ACADEMIA study. Resuscitation 2004;62:275–82.

12. Lighthall GK, Markar S, Hsiung R. Abnormal vital signs are associated with an increased risk for critical events in US veteran inpatients. Resuscitation 2009; 80(11):1264–9.

13. Schein RM, Hazday N, Pena M, et al. Clinical antecedents to in-hospital cardiopulmonary arrest. Chest 1990;98(6):1388–92.

14. Smith AF, Wood J. Can some in-hospital cardio-respiratory arrests be prevented? A prospective survey. Resuscitation 1998;37:133–7.

15. Hodgetts TJ, Kenward G, Vlackonikolis I, et al. Incidence, location and reasons for avoidable in-hospital cardiac arrest in a district general hospital. Resuscitation 2002;54(2):115–23.

16. McGloin H, Adam SK, Singer M. Unexpected deaths and referrals to intensive care of patients on general wards. Are some cases potentially avoidable? J R Coll Physicians Lond 1999;33(3):255–9.

17. McQuillan P, Pilkington S, Allan A, et al. Confidential inquiry into quality of care before admission to intensive care. BMJ 1998;316(7148):1853–8.

18. Rivers E, Nguyen B, Havstad S, et al. Early goal-directed therapy in the treatment of severe sepsis and septic shock. N Engl J Med 2001;345(19): 1368–77.

19. Santy P, Moulinier M, Marquis D. Shock traumatique dans les blessures de guerre, analysis d'observations. Bull Med Soc Chir 1918;44:205 [in French].

20. Tissue plasminogen activator for acute ischemic stroke. The National Institute of neurological disorders and stroke rt-PA Stroke Study Group. N Engl J Med 1995; 333(24):1581–7.

21. Boersma E, Maas AC, Deckers JW, et al. Early thrombolytic treatment in acute myocardial infarction: reappraisal of the golden hour. Lancet 1996;348(9030): 771–5.

22. Devita MA, Bellomo R, Hillman K, et al. Findings of the first consensus conference on medical emergency teams. Crit Care Med 2006;34(9):2463–78.

23. Buist M, Bernard S, Nguyen TV, et al. Association between clinically abnormal observations and subsequent in-hospital mortality: a prospective study. Resuscitation 2004;62(2):137–41.

24. Goldhill DR, McNarry AF. Physiological abnormalities in early warning scores are related to mortality in adult inpatients. Br J Anaesth 2004;92(6):882–4.

25. Goldhill DR, White SA, Sumner A. Physiological values and procedures in the 24 h before ICU admission from the ward. Anaesthesia 1999;54(6):529–34.
26. Hravnak M, Edwards L, Clontz A, et al. Defining the incidence of cardiorespiratory instability in patients in step-down units using an electronic integrated monitoring system. Arch Intern Med 2008;168(12):1300–8.
27. Hillman KM, Bristow PJ, Chey T, et al. Antecedents to hospital deaths. Intern Med J 2001;31(6):343–8.
28. Matot I, Shleifer A, Hersch M, et al. In-hospital cardiac arrest: is outcome related to the time of arrest? Resuscitation 2006;71(1):56–64.
29. Skrifvars MB, Nurmi J, Ikola K, et al. Reduced survival following resuscitation in patients with documented clinically abnormal observations prior to in-hospital cardiac arrest. Resuscitation 2006;70(2):215–22.
30. Hillman KM, Bristow PJ, Chey T, et al. Duration of life-threatening antecedents prior to intensive care admission. Intensive Care Med 2002;28(11):1629–34.
31. Dhillon SK, Rachko M, Hanon S, et al. Telemetry monitoring guidelines for efficient and safe delivery of cardiac rhythm monitoring to noncritical hospital inpatients. Crit Pathw Cardiol 2009;8(3):125–6.
32. Herlitz J, Bang A, Aune S, et al. Characteristics and outcome among patients suffering in-hospital cardiac arrest in monitored and non-monitored areas. Resuscitation 2001;48(2):125–35.
33. Galhotra S, DeVita MA, Simmons RL, et al. Impact of patient monitoring on the diurnal pattern of medical emergency team activation. Crit Care Med 2006; 34(6):1700–6.
34. Downey AW, Quach JL, Haase M, et al. Characteristics and outcomes of patients receiving a medical emergency team review for acute change in conscious state or arrhythmias. Crit Care Med 2008;36(2):477–81.
35. Moller JT, Johannessen NW, Espersen K, et al. Randomized evaluation of pulse oximetry in 20,802 patients: II. Perioperative events and postoperative complications. Anesthesiology 1993;78(3):445–53.
36. Taenzer AH, Pyke JB, McGrath SP, et al. Impact of pulse oximetry surveillance on rescue events and intensive care unit transfers: a before-and-after concurrence study. Anesthesiology 2010;112(2):282–7.
37. Watkinson PJ, Barber VS, Price JD, et al. A randomised controlled trial of the effect of continuous electronic physiological monitoring on the adverse event rate in high risk medical and surgical patients. Anaesthesia 2006;61(11):1031–9.
38. Edelson DP. A weak link in the rapid response system. Arch Intern Med 2010; 170(1):12–3.
39. Winters ME, McCurdy MT, Zilberstein J. Monitoring the critically ill emergency department patient. Emerg Med Clin North Am 2008;26(3):741–57, ix.
40. Jansen JO, Cuthbertson BH. Detecting critical illness outside the ICU: the role of track and trigger systems. Curr Opin Crit Care 2010;16(3):184–90.
41. Subbe CP. Better ViEWS ahead? It is high time to improve patient safety by standardizing Early Warning Scores. Resuscitation 2010;81(8):923–4.
42. Chapman SM, Grocott MP, Franck LS. Systematic review of paediatric alert criteria for identifying hospitalised children at risk of critical deterioration. Intensive Care Med 2010;36(4):600–11.
43. Gao H, McDonnell A, Harrison DA, et al. Systematic review and evaluation of physiological track and trigger warning systems for identifying at-risk patients on the ward. Intensive Care Med 2007;33(4):667–79.
44. Smith GB, Prytherch DR, Schmidt PE, et al. A review, and performance evaluation, of single-parameter "track and trigger" systems. Resuscitation 2008;79(1):11–21.

45. Goldhill DR, Worthington L, Mulcahy A, et al. The patient-at-risk team: identifying and managing seriously ill ward patients. Anaesthesia 1999;54(9):853–60.
46. Subbe CP, Slater A, Menon D, et al. Validation of physiological scoring systems in the accident and emergency department. Emerg Med J 2006;23(11):841–5.
47. Subbe CP, Davies RG, Williams E, et al. Effect of introducing the Modified Early Warning score on clinical outcomes, cardio-pulmonary arrests and intensive care utilisation in acute medical admissions. Anaesthesia 2003;58(8):797–802.
48. Smith GB, Prytherch DR, Schmidt PE, et al. Review and performance evaluation of aggregate weighted 'track and trigger' systems. Resuscitation 2008;77(2):170–9.
49. Buist MD, Shearer W. Rapid response systems: a mandatory system of care or an optional extra for bedside clinical staff. Jt Comm J Qual Patient Saf 2010;36(6): 263–5, 241.
50. Shapiro SE, Donaldson NE, Scott MB. Rapid response teams seen through the eyes of the nurse. Am J Nurs 2010;110(6):28–34 [quiz: 35–6].
51. Maupin JM, Roth DJ, Krapes JM. Use of the modified early warning score decreases code blue events. Jt Comm J Qual Patient Saf 2009;35(12):598–603.
52. Mitchell IA, McKay H, Van Leuvan C, et al. A prospective controlled trial of the effect of a multi-faceted intervention on early recognition and intervention in deteriorating hospital patients. Resuscitation 2010;81(6):658–66.
53. Jones CM, Bleyer AJ, Petree B. Evolution of a rapid response system from voluntary to mandatory activation. Jt Comm J Qual Patient Saf 2010;36(6):266–70, 241.
54. Jones L, King L, Wilson C. A literature review: factors that impact on nurses' effective use of the Medical Emergency Team (MET). J Clin Nurs 2009;18(24): 3379–90.
55. Smith GB, Prytherch DR, Schmidt P, et al. Hospital-wide physiological surveillance—a new approach to the early identification and management of the sick patient. Resuscitation 2006;71(1):19–28.
56. Hravnak M, DeVita M, Clontz A, et al. Cardiorespiratory instability before and after implementing an integrated monitoring system. Crit Care Med 2011;39(1):65–72.
57. Arroliga A, Sanchez J, Sikka P. Monitoring the ill: is this another measurement or will it change outcomes? Crit Care Med 2011;39(1):202–3.
58. Bogert S, Ferrell C, Rutledge DN. Experience with family activation of rapid response teams. Medsurg Nurs 2010;19(4):215–22 [quiz: 223].
59. Bristow PJ, Hillman KM, Chey T, et al. Rates of in-hospital arrests, deaths and intensive care admissions: the effect of a medical emergency team. Med J Aust 2000;173(5):236–40.
60. Ray EM, Smith R, Massie S, et al. Family alert: implementing direct family activation of a pediatric rapid response team. Jt Comm J Qual Patient Saf 2009;35(11): 575–80.
61. Bellomo R, Goldsmith D, Uchino S, et al. A prospective before-and-after trial of a medical emergency team. Med J Aust 2003;179(6):283–7.
62. Buist MD, Moore GE, Bernard SA, et al. Effects of a medical emergency team on reduction of incidence of and mortality from unexpected cardiac arrests in hospital: preliminary study. BMJ 2002;324(7334):387–90.
63. Baxter AD, Cardinal P, Hooper J, et al. Medical emergency teams at The Ottawa Hospital: the first two years. Can J Anaesth 2008;55(4):223–31.
64. Dacey MJ, Mirza ER, Wilcox V, et al. The effect of a rapid response team on major clinical outcome measures in a community hospital. Crit Care Med 2007;35(9): 2076–82.
65. DeVita M. Use of medical emergency team responses to reduce cardiopulmonary arrests. Qual Saf Health Care 2004;13:251–4.

66. Jones D, Bellomo R, Bates S, et al. Long term effect of a medical emergency team on cardiac arrests in a teaching hospital. Crit Care 2005;9(6):R808–15.
67. Chan PS, Khalid A, Longmore LS, et al. Hospital-wide code rates and mortality before and after implementation of a rapid response team. JAMA 2008; 300(21):2506–13.
68. Kenward G, Castle N, Hodgetts T, et al. Evaluation of a medical emergency team one year after implementation. Resuscitation 2004;61(3):257–63.
69. Jones D, Opdam H, Egi M, et al. Long-term effect of a medical emergency team on mortality in a teaching hospital. Resuscitation 2007;74(2):235–41.
70. Sharek PJ, Parast LM, Leong K, et al. Effect of a rapid response team on hospital-wide mortality and code rates outside the ICU in a Children's Hospital. JAMA 2007;298(19):2267–74.
71. Tibballs J, Kinney S. Reduction of hospital mortality and of preventable cardiac arrest and death on introduction of a pediatric medical emergency team. Pediatr Crit Care Med 2009;10(3):306–12.
72. Hunt EA, Zimmer KP, Rinke ML, et al. Transition from a traditional code team to a medical emergency team and categorization of cardiopulmonary arrests in a children's center. Arch Pediatr Adolesc Med 2008;162(2):117–22.
73. Zenker P, Schlesinger A, Hauck M, et al. Implementation and impact of a rapid response team in a children's hospital. Jt Comm J Qual Patient Saf 2007;33(7):418–25.
74. Peberdy MA, Cretikos M, Abella BS, et al. Recommended guidelines for monitoring, reporting, and conducting research on medical emergency team, outreach, and rapid response systems: an Utstein-style scientific statement: a scientific statement from the International Liaison Committee on Resuscitation (American Heart Association, Australian Resuscitation Council, European Resuscitation Council, Heart and Stroke Foundation of Canada, InterAmerican Heart Foundation, Resuscitation Council of Southern Africa, and the New Zealand Resuscitation Council); the American Heart Association Emergency Cardiovascular Care Committee; the Council on Cardiopulmonary, Perioperative, and Critical Care; and the Interdisciplinary Working Group on Quality of Care and Outcomes Research. Circulation 2007;116(21):2481–500.
75. Priestley G, Watson W, Rashidian A, et al. Introducing Critical Care Outreach: a ward-randomised trial of phased introduction in a general hospital. Intensive Care Med 2004;30(7):1398–404.
76. Hillman K, Chen J, Cretikos M, et al. Introduction of the medical emergency team (MET) system: a cluster-randomised controlled trial. Lancet 2005;365(9477): 2091–7.
77. Chen J, Bellomo R, Flabouris A, et al. The relationship between early emergency team calls and serious adverse events. Crit Care Med 2009;37(1):148–53.
78. Santamaria J, Tobin A, Holmes J. Changing cardiac arrest and hospital mortality rates through a medical emergency team takes time and constant review. Crit Care Med 2010;38(2):445–50.
79. Galhotra S, DeVita MA, Simmons RL, et al. Mature rapid response system and potentially avoidable cardiopulmonary arrests in hospital. Qual Saf Health Care 2007;16(4):260–5.
80. Chan PS, Jain R, Nallmothu BK, et al. Rapid response teams: a systematic review and meta-analysis. Arch Intern Med 2010;170(1):18–26.
81. Braaten J, Levin S, O'Rourke PT, et al. Saving lives at Centura. A Colorado System has developed a rapid-response team for critically ill patients. Health Prog 2006;87(6):64–7.
82. Berwick DM. The science of improvement. JAMA 2008;299(10):1182–4.

83. Winters BD, Pham J, Pronovost PJ. Rapid response teams—walk, don't run. JAMA 2006;296(13):1645–7.
84. Litvak E, Pronovost PJ. Rethinking rapid response teams. JAMA 2010;304(12): 1375–6.
85. Pickoff RM. Are rapid response teams simply a bandage on a bigger problem? Physician Exec 2006;32(3):36–8.
86. DiGiovine B. Rapid response teams: let us pick up the pace. Crit Care Med 2010; 38(2):700–1.
87. Ross TK. A second look at 100 000 Lives Campaign. Qual Manag Health Care 2009;18(2):120–5.
88. Wachter RM, Pronovost PJ. The 100,000 Lives Campaign: a scientific and policy review. Jt Comm J Qual Patient Saf 2006;32(11):621–7.
89. Berwick DM, Hackbarth AD, McCannon CJ. IHI replies to "The 100,000 Lives Campaign: a scientific and policy review". Jt Comm J Qual Patient Saf 2006; 32(11):628–30 [discussion: 631–3].
90. Approved: 2010 National Patient Safety Goals. Some changes effective immediately. Jt Comm Perspect 2009;29(10):1, 20–31.

Pediatric Resuscitation and Cardiac Arrest

William A. Woods, MD

KEYWORDS

- Pediatrics • Cardiopulmonary resuscitation • Emergencies
- Critical care • Cardiac arrest

Cardiac arrest (CA) in children is, fortunately, a relatively infrequent event. Because adults are just "big children," many of the principles discussed in this article also apply to adults. Whereas the majority of articles in this issue focus on care specific to adults, this article highlights the issues specific to the critical care and resuscitation of children. The article reviews the causes and conditions associated with pediatric CA and pediatric care in the prearrest phase, and updates and reviews pediatric resuscitation for CA, including the 2010 updates by the American Heart Association (AHA). Where controversy exists, alternative recommendations by the International Liaison Committee on Resuscitation (ILCOR) and the European Resuscitation Committee (ERC) are discussed. Finally, topics that may be of special interest are presented. A recurring theme throughout this article is that, though infrequent, presentations and complications during pediatric CA are predictable, and expected challenges can be minimized through effective planning and education prior to patient presentation.

EPIDEMIOLOGY OF PEDIATRIC CARDIAC ARREST

Pediatric CA victims constitute a minor patient population in the emergency department (ED). Unfortunately, this can lead to unfamiliarity of staff with proper procedures for pediatric CA. The review by Babl and colleagues[1] describes the prehospital experience in Boston for 1 year; there were a total of 130,000 emergency medical services (EMS) dispatches with 59,000 patient transports. Pediatric transports totaled only 5280 (8.9%) for the year with 13 children requiring cardiopulmonary resuscitation and 15 requiring intubation. In-hospital arrests are also relatively infrequent. The PECARN study by Moler and colleagues[2,3] included 353 in-hospital and 138 out-of-hospital pediatric arrests from 15 hospitals over an 18-month period. On average, the rate of pediatric CA was 15 in-hospital and 6 out-of-hospital arrests per hospital per year. The most common presenting rhythm for in-hospital arrest was bradycardia

Funding: None.
The authors have nothing to disclose.
Department of Emergency Medicine, University of Virginia, PO Box 800699, Charlottesville, VA 22908-0699, USA
E-mail address: waw9h@virginia.edu

Emerg Med Clin N Am 30 (2012) 153–168
doi:10.1016/j.emc.2011.09.013
0733-8627/12/$ – see front matter © 2012 Elsevier Inc. All rights reserved.

emed.theclinics.com

while asystole was most common during out-of-hospital arrests. Ventricular fibrillation or tachycardia (VF/VT) was the presenting electrical rhythm in only 10% of in-hospital arrests. Only 19% developed VF/VT sometime during the arrest phase.

A review of the epidemiology of pediatric CA can serve as a framework for planning and preparation for pediatric CA victims. In the 1990s Schindler and colleagues[4] and Sirbaugh and colleagues[5] found the most common cause of pediatric CA to be sudden infant death syndrome (SIDS). These classic studies were done in the mid to late 1990s before the successful "Back to Sleep" campaign.[6] Subsequently, the number of deaths due to SIDS has decreased dramatically, with more recent work by Moler and colleagues[2] showing a drop in the percentage of arrests caused by SIDS. The most common reasons EMS crews will arrive to find a child in cardiopulmonary arrest are trauma, drowning, sepsis, respiratory arrest, and cardiac abnormalities.[4,5]

Even after initiation of the "Back to Sleep" education program, pediatric out-of-hospital CA remained much more common in younger children. Nearly one-third of the children in Moler's out-of-hospital arrest series were younger than 1 year with a survival rate of 30%. Another third of victims were age 1 to 8 years, and survival was 50% in this population. Survival in the third of victims aged 8 through 18 was 36%.[2]

Analysis of pediatric CA in the ED pediatric patient population is typically included in studies evaluating all in-hospital pediatric arrests. While inpatient pediatric CA has some of the same causes as out-of-hospital arrest, it is more commonly a result of respiratory failure/asphyxia. Children suffering an in-hospital CA are more likely to have an underlying medical condition (88% for in-hospital vs 49% for out-of-hospital) and to be younger.[2,3] The average ages are 0.9 and 2.9 years old for in-hospital CA and out-of-hospital, respectively. The most common chronic medical conditions are prenatal conditions, congenital heart disease, and lung or airway disease.

In summary, pediatric CA is an infrequent event that occurs most commonly in children younger than 1 year. Outcomes are best in the 1- to 8-year-old population. Unlike CA in adults, causes are frequently attributable to respiratory failure or trauma; VF/VT occurs infrequently either as an initial rhythm or during resuscitation efforts. Thus, though used infrequently, those that care for children with CA must have a broad skill set because children with CA should not be expected to respond as readily to only closed-chest compressions and early defibrillation, as may occur in adults.

PREVENTION OF CARDIAC ARREST (PREARREST)

In a comparison between in-hospital CA and out-of-hospital CA it was noted that of 37 pediatric CA due to trauma, 22 occurred in-hospital.[3] In addition, 112 of the 149 pediatric CA due to respiratory failure were in-hospital.[3] As these results demonstrate, children may continue to deteriorate after presentation to medical care. The landmark study by Gausche and colleagues[7] did not demonstrate a survival benefit with paramedic intubation in comparison with bag-valve-mask ventilation in 830 children requiring advanced life support. The text also presents a description of the subgroups and although the results did not achieve statistical significance, it is difficult not to wonder whether expert clinical judgment can improve the survival of many children requiring advanced life support. Acknowledging that children may continue to deteriorate after reaching ED care, what interventions may decrease the risk of subsequent CA?

As a first step, emergency physicians should be familiar with emergency interventions that may be required for the children suffering CA who have an underlying medical condition. Though often daunting to the emergency physician, the easiest preexisting condition to review is inborn errors of metabolism. The emergency treatment of the metabolic disarray resulting from essentially all inborn errors of metabolism requires maintaining serum glucose levels and intravascular volume status while temporarily suspending oral food intake by the child.[8] The most notable exception to this rule is congenital adrenal insufficiency, which may present with hyperkalemia and may require stress-dose corticosteroids.

Children with congenital heart disease may require emergency care for several reasons. First, the child with an undiagnosed ductal-dependent lesion may present early in the newborn period with central or peripheral cyanosis as the ductus arteriosis closes. Treatment involves the early initiation of a prostaglandin infusion to reopen the ductus arteriosis and intensive care admission for definitive therapy. Complications of prostaglandin infusion include apnea, hyperthermia, and irritability. Prophylactic intubation may be considered, especially in consultation with the receiving intensivist. The decision may depend on duration of transport, if necessary, and skill of transport personnel.

Second, children who have undergone surgical repair of congenital heart disease have an increased risk of sudden death from dysrhythmias. This risk is more common in those with more complex primary lesions, and may not occur in those with atrial septal and some ventricular septal defect repairs.[9] In addition, there are no clear data to define how long this risk persists. Thus, it is advisable to consider cardiology consultation in those children with surgically corrected congenital heart disease who present with significant chest pain or palpitations. All of these children with evidence of dysrhythmia on their ED electrocardiogram require cardiology consultation.

Third, children with partially corrected congenital heart disease may present with an alteration in their shunt fraction, or a change in the percentage of their cardiac output directed toward the pulmonary artery. These children may have an increase in their pulmonary blood flow, such as if volume overloaded from decreased compliance or malabsorption of their home diuretic. Such children may have too little pulmonary blood flow if their Blalock-Taussig shunt clots during mild dehydration or if the cardiac output drops because of chronic hypoxia in the child with partial correction. Children with a decrease in room air oxygen saturations may benefit from intravenous fluids if they have a decrease in pulmonary blood flow, or may benefit from diuresis and positive-pressure ventilation if they have an increased pulmonary blood flow. Obtaining a chest radiograph and comparing with an old radiograph will help the emergency physician decide if the child has a decrease or increase in his or her pulmonary blood flow (decreased pulmonary vascularity or increased pulmonary vascularity, respectively, compared with baseline). Children who become more hypoxic with agitation in the ED may benefit from a small dose of intranasal fentanyl prior to intravenous cannulation to prevent cardiovascular deterioration during attempts at peripheral vascular access.

Finally, children who have undergone cardiac transplantation may present to the ED with episodes of acute rejection.[10] Unfortunately, the symptoms of acute rejection are vague, and diagnostic studies do not have high enough positive and negative predictive value to allow the emergency physician to exclude the diagnosis of acute rejection. Thus, it is reasonable to consult a child's cardiologist, especially if the child's symptoms are nonspecific (especially nausea), if he or she has an increase in liver function studies or shows signs of dehydration.

Children with severe acute exacerbations of bronchospasm require aggressive therapy. Early administration of corticosteroids is recommended.[11,12] While frequent β-agonist dosing has been the mainstay of therapy, the optimal bronchodilator regimen continues to be controversial. It is unclear whether continuous albuterol therapy is more effective than sequential bolus dosing. Ipratropium is a potent bronchodilator alone, and its use can decrease the admission rate among children with acute bronchospasm.[13-15] Rodrigo and Rodrigo[16] reviewed the data on multiple dosing of ipratropium. This review argues that multiple doses of ipratropium in the ED can decrease the admission rate for those with severe asthma exacerbations, with a number needed to treat of 5 to 11.

Treatment options for the child with bronchiolitis are limited. The key to early care of these children is good supportive care: frequent effective nasal suction, supplemental oxygen as needed, and repositioning for optimal air exchange. It is always tempting to try a diagnostic and therapeutic trial of albuterol in children with bronchiolitis, as viral respiratory infections are the most common trigger for acute bronchospasm in children. Bronchodilator therapy should not be continued without objective findings of clinical improvement. The role in the ED of therapies such as nebulized hypertonic saline and high-flow humidified intranasal cannula is evolving.[17,18]

Sepsis protocols are proving to be beneficial in improving outcomes in adults with sepsis syndromes. There is no reason to think that the outcome of children with sepsis cannot be improved by aggressive, systematic care with attention to clinical details. Clinically identifying sepsis in young children and determining resuscitation end points may be challenging, as children in "warm shock" may have bounding peripheral pulses and an adequate blood pressure. Serial, careful clinical examinations are vital. Physicians should pay attention to relative changes in vital signs, mental status, relative change in pulse character and perfusion, as well as respiratory rate and effort. The clinician should suspect that tachypnea is a compensatory effort due to metabolic acidosis. Early dosing with antipyretics is indicated to attempt to separate examination findings resulting from fever from those due to sepsis. Aggressive fluid resuscitation is indicated for septic shock. Young children may require up to 80 to 100 mL/kg of isotonic solution during their initial resuscitation phase.

Fortunately, care of the newborn infant is typically not complicated. Keys to successful transition to extrauterine life are: adequately stimulate and dry; adequately position for easy respiration; and ensure an adequately warm environment. The AHA recommends not separating the newborn from the mother if a term gestation is crying and/or breathing and has good muscle tone.[19] Airway suctioning need only be performed for excessive secretions. If performed, care must be taken to detect any episode of bradycardia that may result from stimulation of the posterior nasopharynx. The pulse at the base of the umbilical stump is the most reliable location to palpate a pulse in a newborn.

Guidelines for newborn resuscitation have changed over recent years to deemphasize the use of oxygen in the resuscitation of a newborn.[19] Most newborns, even those requiring some bag-valve mask ventilation, can be effectively treated with room air. In fact, room air or blended oxygen is recommended for normal newborn resuscitation in the AHA 2010 Guidelines.[19] If supplemental oxygen is supplied, the concentration should be aggressively weaned as soon as is practical. It is reasonable to consider withholding resuscitation efforts if a newborn is so premature that the eyelids are still fused; otherwise the emergency physician should consider the child of viable age and attempt resuscitation. It is appropriate to stop resuscitation efforts if there is no detectable heart rate after 10 minutes of resuscitation efforts.[19] However, this decision should also consider the presumed etiology of the arrest of the newborn.

CARE OF THE CHILD IN CARDIAC ARREST

In 2010, the ILCOR, AHA, and ERC provided updates to the 2005 recommendations.[20-22] **Box 1** summarizes the new changes in the 2010 AHA recommendations.[19,20] Optimal care of the child in CA demands a prepared system and skilled

---

Box 1
Changes to the 2010 AHA Guidelines for resuscitation and emergency care of children

Resuscitation techniques:

  Retraining is emphasized to ensure familiarity with equipment

  Cricoid pressure is deemphasized as a method to prevent aspiration during intubation attempts

  Minimizing rescuer fatigue is emphasized to maintain the quality of chest compressions

  Chest compressions without ventilation is encouraged in cases of nonasphyxial arrest during bystander rescue (more common in adults)

Medications:

  Medication dosing is controversial: use of lean body weight versus actual body weight is unknown

  The dose of intratracheal administration of medications should, in general be 2 to 3 times the intravenous dose

  The dose of intratracheal administration of epinephrine is suggested to be 10 times the intravenous dose.

  The dose of intratracheal administration of atropine is increased to 0.04–0.06 mg/kg

  The routine use of sodium bicarbonate is discouraged during resuscitation

  The routine use of calcium is discouraged during resuscitation

  The role of vasopressin is not clear, but there is more support for its use during refractory CA

  Lidocaine use is no longer specifically recommended for the treatment of VF/VT

Protocols:

  With refractory bradycardia, epinephrine and isoproterenol infusions are no longer advocated

  Adenosine may have a role in the treatment of wide complex tachycardia

  Postresuscitation hyperoxemia should be avoided

  There is no longer a lower age limit to the use of automated external defibrillators

Special resuscitation situations:

  The AHA gives treatment and protocol suggestions for children with:

    Septic shock

    Single-ventricle anatomy

    Pulmonary hypertension

---

providers who are familiar with guidelines and equipment. An optimally prepared system should have appropriate equipment, and organizational and consultation patterns in place before the arrival of the critically ill child. To aid preparation the American Academy of Pediatrics (AAP), the American College of Emergency Physicians (ACEP), and the Emergency Nurses Association produced a joint policy statement that can be used as a starting reference to ensure an optimally prepared system for those who provide emergency care for children.[23]

The 2010 recommendations from AHA and ILCOR recognize the importance of rapid intervention and aggressive implementation of resuscitation protocols.[20,21,24] Medical emergency teams or rapid response teams are gaining favor for inpatient units because use of these teams brings aggressive skilled resources to the bedside.[25] Literature continues to support the conventional teaching that rapidly and effectively declaring an emergency is often the biggest barrier to effective resuscitation.[26]

EQUIPMENT

The aforementioned collaborative policy statement defines the equipment needed to obtain vascular access in children of all sizes.[23] Vascular access is essential for optimal pediatric resuscitation. Peripheral venous access is relatively easy to obtain and has the advantage of low-resistance catheters that allow rapid infusion of isotonic solution or blood products. The easiest veins to cannulate include the antecubital fossa, the dorsum of the hand, and the scalp (using a rubber band tourniquet with a tab of tape to ease removal).

Central venous access is typically more difficult to obtain in the young child. Preambulatory children may have relatively smaller femoral veins, as the metabolic requirement of the lower extremities is lower than a walking age child. When performing a blind attempt at femoral venous access in adults, classic teaching says that the femoral vein is one-third of the distance from the symphysis pubis toward the anterior superior iliac spine. In young children the femoral vein may be closer to halfway between the symphysis pubis and anterior superior iliac spine. ED ultrasound assists emergency physicians in central venous cannulation of adults and should be helpful in infants and children, although data are not yet convincing.[27] Once obtained, central venous catheters can be used for higher-dose infusions of vasoactive agents.

Intraosseous (IO) catheters are relatively simple to place, have landmarks unaltered by volume status, and can be used to administer all drugs commonly used during a resuscitation. The relatively new intraosseous catheter drills are much more elegant and problem free than previous manual IO catheters. IO catheters can be used for volume resuscitation, vasoactive infusions, and most laboratory studies. When training practitioners to use IO needles it is imperative to emphasize that fluid may not infuse easily. In fact, a syringe on a 3-way stopcock to provide a bolus of fluid is frequently required. **Box 2** lists the most commonly used sites for IO catheter placement. Educators must also train providers on acceptable methods to secure the catheter, to prevent dislodging the catheter during resuscitation efforts.

Airway equipment should include masks, airway adjuncts, and intubation equipment appropriate for all sizes of children. Providers differ on the choice of

---

Box 2
Sites and contraindications of IO catheter placement

Site of placement

    Proximal medial tibia

    Distal medial tibia

    Distal medial femur

    Anterolateral proximal humerus

Contraindication to placement

    Fracture of the same bone

    Previous intraosseous needle placement attempt in the same bone

    Cellulitis overlying placement site

    Osteogenesis imperfecta

laryngoscope blades (curved, straight, and so forth) when intubating children. Many experts will use a straight blade when intubating young children because of the anterior larynx and floppy epiglottis. As devices such as video-assisted intubating laryngoscopes are becoming more widely available, further research will be needed to determine the optimal equipment for securing the pediatric airway in the critically unstable child. The 2010 AHA Pediatric Advance Life Support Guidelines do not comment on laryngoscope choices. Providers should use the laryngoscope they are most comfortable with during pediatric intubations, as first-pass success rates are lower in ED intubations of young children than in adults.[28]

Whereas traditionally uncuffed endotracheal tubes (ETTs) were considered to be preferable in younger children, cuffed and uncuffed ETTs are both acceptable according to the 2010 recommendations.[20–22] A cuffed ETT may be more desirable in cases where a child has high airway resistance or poor lung compliance. Cuffed ETTs have the advantage of smaller air leak in comparison with uncuffed tubes. However, cuffed ETTs are also sized one-half size smaller internal diameter than their uncuffed counterparts. Thus, suction catheters may be more difficult to use in smaller-cuffed tube sizes. If placing cuffed tubes, physicians and respiratory therapy must be properly oriented to accurate cuff inflation pressure, as overfilling the cuff may cause airway injury. It would not be unreasonable to consider cuffed tubes for children older than 1 year, while considering uncuffed tubes for younger children if suctioning will be important. When intubating a child a good rule of thumb is the depth of intubation should be 3 times the tube diameter when measured at the lips. Endotracheal tube placement must be confirmed with exhaled carbon dioxide detection. Acceptable methods include capnography or colorimetry, with continuous capnography being preferable, if available, as it can guide effective chest compressions and signal tube dislodgment. Providers should be oriented to the equipment and understand the scenarios whereby false-positive and false-negative results may occur.

Equipment storage and organization may be unique to many different EDs. However, all providers (physicians and nurses) should be knowledgable of the local organizational system used. A reliable resupply system ensures that proper functioning equipment is fully stocked and not beyond expiration dates, as this equipment will be used relatively infrequently. Staff should have in-house call schedules and referral destinations organized. Transportation teams should be properly educated as to the pediatric critical care that may be required during anticipated transports. Policies and equipment should be in place to estimate a child's weight and to ensure accurate equipment and medication dosing based on that child's size. Reference material should include suggested sizes of ETTs, thoracostomy tubes, and laryngeal mask airways, as well as expected drug doses and rates of infusions. Radiology resources specific to pediatric care should be organized and defined.

It is essential to ensure accurate medication dosing and the ability to deliver appropriate medication doses and infusion rates. Controversy exists over whether to use actual weight or ideal body weight in obese children. In fact, recent recommendations vary between publications on this topic. The AHA recommends basing medication doses on ideal body weight estimates in obese children to prevent drug toxicity.[20] The ILCOR recommends using length-based estimates in trying to approximate lean body mass.[21] Regardless of the method embraced, medication dosing should not exceed adult dosages.

To aid in maintaining dosing accuracy, the author's institution uses a written resource manual to enhance communication between physicians and nurses. Each page of the manual is dedicated to a particular weight, providing the weight-based dose of a medication and the volume to be administered for each drug, and concentration currently available in the ED medication dispensing formulary (eg, midazolam comes in different concentrations in this hospital). If infusions are to be mixed in a central pharmacy, communication and preparation is required to ensure that any vasoactive infusions will be prepared and transported in time to meet clinical requirements. It is important to plan in advance which vasoactive infusions will require a continuous infusion pump versus which can be delivered via intermittent bolus pumps. In the author's institution's ED, all vasoactive infusions are delivered via syringe pump if the child weighs 10 kg or less.

Professional education appears to improve performance during resuscitation.[29–32] There are many sources of professional education: self-directed education, skills practice, high-fidelity simulation, lower-fidelity simulation, Pediatric Advanced Life Support (PALS) courses, and so forth. There is a growing body of literature to suggest that many of these choices can increase care providers' confidence in their ability to perform a skill.[30] There is also a growing body of literature to suggest that many of these choices can increase a provider's recall of information and performance on subsequent tasks using that information.[30] Providers should take an honest, periodic assessment of their skills and recent clinical experiences to determine the appropriate education necessary. An area of research interest is starting to document that outcomes are improved if providers are more experienced.[32] ED leadership should ensure that educational opportunities exist for those that will care for children. Education should also reinforce the clinical examination necessary to identify an impending deterioration, including detection of the typical signs of compensated and decompensated shock.

THE AMERICAN HEART ASSOCIATION GUIDELINES 2010
Chest Compressions and Defibrillation

The 2010 AHA Guidelines on basic life support for adults stress the importance of rapid onset of chest compressions while deemphasizing the benefit of mouth-to-mouth rescue breathing.[33] As many pediatric CA are not a result of a dysrhythmia but rather a respiratory arrest, the AHA recommends chest compressions with ventilations in infants and children.[20] Keys to pediatric chest compressions are to "push fast" (100 compressions per minute) and "push deep" (at least one-third the depth of the chest). For the health care provider the AHA recommends a ratio of compressions to ventilations for lone rescuers of 30:2 and for 2 rescuers of 15:2. Ventilations should be delivered in such a fashion as to minimize any interruption in chest compressions. Rescuers should focus on minimizing common errors: allow the chest to completely recoil between compressions, minimize interruptions of compressions, avoid excessive ventilation, avoid rescuer fatigue, and ensure proper hand placement. The two-thumb encircling hands method is preferred for infants when there are two rescuers present.[20]

Defibrillation for ventricular fibrillation should be done using infant paddles for children less than 10 kg (approximately 1 year).[20,22] If greater than 10 kg the adult size paddles should be used. Biphasic shocks may be preferred, as they are less harmful than monophasic shocks and appear to be at least as equally effective. The initial defibrillation dose for VF is 2 to 4 J/kg. The AHA recommends increasing the second dose to 4 J/kg and considering increasing to a maximum of 10 J/kg or adult maximum dosing.[20] The International Consensus report recommends initial dosing of 2 to 4 J/kg and does not discourage the use of higher doses.[21] The European Resuscitation Council recommends all doses of 4 J/kg.[22] Further research clearly is needed in this area. Cardioversion should be performed with initial doses of 0.5 to 1 J/kg. If unsuccessful, the dose may be increased to 2 J/kg. When considering the use of an automated external defibrillator (AED), standard settings can be used for children older than 8 years. An AED with a dose attenuator is preferred for those aged 1 to 8 years. Manual defibrillation is preferred for patients younger than 1 year. An AED without a dose attenuator can be used for all ages if no other options are available; however, EDs designed to care for children should have manual defibrillators capable of dose adjustment.[34]

Airway Intervention

Effective bag-mask ventilation is a complicated skill. Rescuers should be skilled in airway-positioning maneuvers (jaw lift) and should deliver enough gas (oxygen or room air) volume to just make the chest rise.[20] Excessive ventilation can result in increased intrathoracic pressure with decreased venous return, air trapping with barotrauma, and increased risk of aspiration and regurgitation. Ventilation of the child in CA should be performed with 100% oxygen. After return of spontaneous respiration, the inspired concentration of oxygen should be weaned to achieve saturations of at least 94%.[20,22]

If further airway intervention is required, endotracheal intubation should be performed. A laryngeal mask airway is an option if prolonged bag-mask ventilation and intubation are not possible. Endotracheal tube size may be better estimated by child length than by child weight in obese children; otherwise age-based formulas, weight-based tables, and comparison of external tube diameter with that of the patient's fifth finger are all appropriate initial references.[20] A cuffed ETT should be one-half size smaller than an appropriate uncuffed ETT. Rapid sequence intubation may be performed to eliminate the risk of gastric inflation with bag-mask ventilation. The use of cricoid pressure is not universally supported, and is deemphasized in the 2010 recommendations.[20–22] These recommendations state that cricoid pressure should be performed only if it does not interfere with ventilation or prolong intubation. If gastric inflation occurs, decompression with a nasogastric or orogastric tube may improve oxygenation and ventilation. Venting a gastrostomy tube, if present, can effectively decompress the stomach.

Medication dosing and choice are controversial when intubating a child in or near CA. Based on AHA PALS, medication dosing should be based on actual body weight rather than lean body weight, if using medications to rapidly sedate and provide neuromuscular blockade to ease intubation.[20] Etomidate provides rapid intubating conditions while maintaining hemodynamic status (ie, cardiac and cerebral perfusion pressures).[35–37] A single dose of etomidate has been noted to decrease adrenal function when used in septic adults, and the International Consensus discourages the routine use of etomidate for septic children.[21] Ketamine also provides rapid, predictable sedation while maintaining mean arterial pressure.[37] Traditionally ketamine has been thought to increase intracranial pressure. However, further study is certainly indicated to determine under which physiologic conditions ketamine may cause an increase in intracranial pressure, as some recent data suggest that no significant elevation occurs.[38–40] Succinylcholine has the advantage of rapid neuromuscular blockade of brief duration. As succinylcholine is a depolarizing neuromuscular blocker, clinically significant hyperkalemia may result in children with undiagnosed muscular dystrophy. Thus, rocuronium may also be considered because it is the nondepolarizing neuromuscular blocker with the most rapid onset and briefest duration of action.

Choosing to intubate a child requires a plan to react to expected complications. Complications can include failure to achieve intubation, desaturation, hypotension, bradycardia, vomiting, and laryngospasm.[28,41–43] In anticipation of possible failure to achieve intubation, physicians should always have alternative airway maneuvers and equipment in mind and immediately available. This aspect is particularly important when intubating younger children, as the intubation success rate is lower for young children than teenagers.[28] Hypotension with subsequent CA may occur during intubation.[44] Conventional wisdom states that the use of induction agents can result in hypotension. Various mechanisms have been postulated but remain unproved. Good clinical practice dictates special attention to the child with distributive shock, severe hypovolemic shock, or significant acidosis. If time permits, aggressive volume expansion prior to intubation should be administered, and adrenergic medications should be immediately available prior to intubation.

Once the child is intubated, the emergency physician should carefully consider initial ventilator settings and ventilation strategy. Hyperventilation should be avoided during CA. During the immediate postintubation period, the physician should hand-ventilate the child or work very closely with respiratory therapy to determine the most appropriate ventilator settings for the child who is not yet in CA. While hyperoxemia and hyperventilation are to be avoided, there are clinical scenarios that may require specialized ventilation strategies. Children who are intubated and have a concomitant severe metabolic acidosis will require a very rapid ventilatory rate (ie, at least the preintubation respiratory rate) to provide the necessary compensatory respiratory alkalosis. Sudden, fatal CA may occur with an insufficient minute volume, due to rapid changes in acidemia. Children with bronchospasm or bronchiolitis may require very prolonged exhalation times or slow inhalation periods to allow adequate gas exchange without excessive peak inspiratory pressures. Either venous or arterial blood gases are adequate for assessing the response to the ventilation strategy. **Box 3** describes the mnemonic DOPE for possible causes of a sudden deterioration in an intubated patient's condition.

Fluids and Medications Used in Resuscitation

Early aggressive fluid resuscitation in children may be required in the child with normal blood pressure. As children often maintain systolic blood pressure despite significant volume depletion, the most useful clinical features for detecting dehydration in a young child are absence of tears, dry mucous membranes, prolonged capillary refill, and abnormal general appearance.[45] Isotonic solution, such as normal saline or lactated Ringer solution, can be safely administered in sequential doses of 20 mL/kg. A review of children presenting to the ED in shock noted that children with septic shock received a mean dose of 58 mL/kg of crystalloid while in the ED.[46] Although most children are not overly sensitive to excessive volume resuscitation, common volume-sensitive conditions are children with diabetic ketoacidosis (potential risk of cerebral edema), children with sickle cell disease and suspected acute chest syndrome, and children with partially surgically corrected congenital heart disease with an excess of pulmonary blood flow. When treating children with these acute conditions it is

---

Box 3
DOPE pneumonic for those intubated patients who deteriorate

D Displacement of the tube

O Obstruction of the tube

P Pneumothorax

E Equipment failure

imperative to provide only the resuscitation fluid required to reestablish perfusion while not administering an excessive dose that may increase the risk of complication.

Epinephrine is the most frequent medication administered during resuscitation efforts after CA.[2,3] The α-adrenergic activity of epinephrine increases aortic diastolic and coronary perfusion, due to vasoconstriction. Epinephrine may be administered intravenously, intraosseously, intramuscularly, subcutaneously, or intratracheally. Current recommendations for all intravenous doses during resuscitation are 0.01 mg/kg with a maximum dose of 1 mg.[20] The optimal intratracheal dose is unknown, although the AHA recommend administration of 10 times the intravenous dose if epinephrine is given intratrachially.[20] Sodium bicarbonate and other alkaline solutions may inactivate catecholamines if administered simultaneously. Historically, high-dose epinephrine (10 times typical dose) was considered in cases of refractory CA; however, high-dose epinephrine has fallen out of favor. Epinephrine is recommended for the treatment of pediatric CA (with or without electrical activity), pediatric brady-cardia with a palpable pulse, and anaphylaxis.[12,20] Smaller intravenous doses (5%–10% of intravenous dosing) may be initially administered intravenously to patients with anaphylaxis.[12] Rapid intravenous bolus doses of epinephrine should be avoided in the conscious patient.

Atropine has traditionally been the second most common medication administered during resuscitation efforts after pediatric CA.[2,3] Atropine sulfate accelerates the atrial pacemaker and increases the speed of atrioventricular conduction. Atropine is recom-mended for use in the child with bradycardia with a pulse and with poor perfusion. However, atropine is no longer in the algorithm of pediatric CA, even in the presence of pulseless electrical activity.[20] The minimum dose of atropine is 0.1 mg because smaller doses may cause a paradoxic bradycardia. Dosing of intratracheal atropine is somewhat controversial. The AHA recommends 0.04 to 0.06 mg/kg whereas the European Resuscitation Council recommends 0.03 mg/kg.[20,21]

Sodium bicarbonate is often administered in cases of pediatric CA.[2,3] Current AHA recommendations warn that excessive sodium bicarbonate may impair tissue oxygen delivery and decrease the ventricular fibrillation threshold. It also may induce electro-lyte abnormalities such as hypernatremia, hyperosmolality, hypocalcemia, and hypo-kalemia. Current recommendations state that routine use of sodium bicarbonate is not recommended in the treatment of CA.[20] Sodium bicarbonate, however, may have a role in the treatment of acute intoxications or hyperkalemia.

Vasopressin is an endogenous peptide initially isolated from the posterior pituitary. The V1 receptor in vascular smooth muscle is of the most interest, as stimulation results in vasoconstriction. Trials of vasopressin for the treatment of CA began after it was noted that survivors of CA had substantially higher serum levels of endogenous vasopressin than nonsurvivors. Hypothetical adverse effects of vasopressin include increased myocardial oxygen demand and dysrhythmias, as well as decreasing splanchnic blood flow.[47] Rarely, hyponatremia may result during infusion therapy, typically when being used for sepsis. Current recommendations state that bolus doses can be administered during refractory CA; however, there is insufficient evidence demonstrating that use of vasopressin results in an increased rate of survival to discharge for children.[20] Vasopressin infusions may have a role in the treatment of septic or hemorrhagic shock, but more data are required to demonstrate a benefit in children.[48,49] Vasopressin boluses can be administered via intravenous, intraoss-eous, or endotracheal routes.

Amiodarone may be considered in the treatment of CA due to pediatric VF or VT. The AHA recommends expert consultation before the administration of amiodarone or pro-cainamide in children with tachycardia without shock, hypotension, and acutely altered mental status.[20] Adenosine can also be considered for use in cases of tachycardia. The AHA notes that adenosine may be useful in cases of wide complex tachycardia as long as the child is without known Wolff-Parkinson-White syndrome, the rhythm is regular, and the QRS is monomorphic.[20] Adenosine can be administered in cases of supraventricular tachycardia (SVT); however, the AHA recommends vagal stimulation or Valsalva maneuvers before pharmacologic therapy in cases of stable SVT.[20]

Infusion protocols for vasoactive agents do not differ significantly from adults. In younger children with decompensated shock, epinephrine or norepinephrine infusions are preferred over dopamine. β-Adrenergic actions predominate with epinephrine infusion rates of less than 0.3 μg/kg/min, whereas α-adrenergic actions causing vasoconstriction occur at doses greater than 0.3 μg/kg/min. Norepinephrine is a potent vasoconstrictor used to treat shock, with low systemic vascular resistance.

SPECIAL SITUATIONS
Family Presence During Resuscitation

Current literature and recommendations note that family presence during resuscitation efforts may aid in the grief process for family members of the child undergoing resuscitation.[20–22] This practice is typically more effective if there is an ED team member who can be assigned to the family to answer questions, attend to needs, and pay attention to nonverbal cues from the family. Ideally the team member assigned will be a skilled clinician who can interpret the context of the resuscitative efforts for the family. Preparing an ED for this practice may require orientation sessions with nonclinicians (chaplains, social workers) who may also be assigned to the family. Further instruction should be directed toward staff to anticipate conflicts or likely clarifications that may arise during resuscitation, and plan how to handle them in front of the family. For instance, nurses should practice vocabulary and phrases that will allow for clarification of drug doses while not being perceived by the family as questioning the competence of the team leaders. Similarly, physicians need to be aware that safe practice includes the verification of medication doses, and they should expect such requests for clarification from nursing and pharmacy. Expecting these requests ensures that physicians are more attentive to unusually worded or repetitive questions from staff during the emotional stress of a pediatric CA.

Procedures on the Newly Dead

Occasionally children arrive at the ED in CA after presenting with a history consistent with a contagious illness. Typically the organism of concern is Neisseria meninigitidis, as close family members may require antibiotic prophylaxis. In this scenario, the child is pronounced dead prior to obtaining blood cultures (and/or cerebrospinal fluid cultures). Although individual states may vary, in the Commonwealth of Virginia the Medical Examiner has charge of a body after an unexplained death.[50] Consent from the Medical Examiner would be required before postmortem blood and/or cerebrospinal fluid for culture is obtained. Failure to obtain consent from the Medical Examiner may be considered unlawful. However, obtaining cultures while in the ED should be considered if a delay might occur when the procedure is deferred to the Medical Examiner. Thus, knowledge of local laws and communication with the Medical Examiner is imperative in this scenario.

Disaster Preparation

Branas and colleagues[51] reviewed all of the multiple casualty incidents (MCIs) occurring within the state of Maryland during a 3-year period. An MCI was defined as at least

10 simultaneous victims. Four of the 10 incidents included at least "several" children. Branas' work suggests that 5 or 6 children would seem to be a reasonable maximum number of critically injured children to expect during a "typical" MCI. The New York City Department of Health provides thorough suggestions for infrastructure to plan for multiple injured children.[52] Special pediatric considerations include care for those children who are separated from caregivers (consent issues, identification, emotional care, and so forth), setting up a pediatric safe area for those who are medically clear, and training and equipment in preparation for multiple injured children. Pediatric specific equipment may include medications, decontamination, and transportation equipment. Though infrequent, resources and challenges that will occur during MCIs are predictable. Anticipated challenges ideally can be minimized through pre-event preparation.

Prevention of Pediatric Cardiac Arrest through Advocacy

Emergency physicians are uniquely positioned to view the tragedy of avoidable illness and injury within our society. Many of the deaths in children fall into predictable patterns. For example, with regard to drowning, young children are more likely to drown in bathtubs or after falling into bodies of water when unwitnessed; adolescents aged 15 to 19 are more likely to drown in a rural environment with friends during warm months.[53] What steps are available to advocate and educate to prevent further injury? Rimsza and colleagues[54] reviewed the deaths of children in Arizona in the later 1990s to identify the proportion of preventable deaths. The investigators, from the Arizona Child Fatality Review Program, determined that 29% of all pediatric deaths were preventable.[54] The review identified unintentional injuries that could have been prevented, typically through patient education about appropriate safety procedures. ED teams are very familiar with important safety information, such as pool safety, bicycle helmets, and pediatric motor vehicle restraint recommendations. Parents of patients presenting to the ED are willing to apply educational information provided during the ED visit.[55] The review by Rimsza and colleagues also determined that 253 of the 2983 deaths due to medical causes could have been prevented.[54] The investigators believed that suboptimally prepared EMS and delays in seeking medical care because of lack of health insurance contributed to these deaths. It appears from all available data that emergency physicians can have an impact on children during daily clinical interactions, within our individual medical system, and through the advocacy of our national organizations.

SUMMARY

The AHA, ILCOR, and ERC have recently published updates on pediatric resuscitation. There have been subtle changes to recommended protocols. The most notable shift in the guidelines has been the increased emphasis on provider training and education, and a heightened attention toward the prearrest period. For the emergency physician, these changes point to opportunities to prepare in advance for the critically ill child in order to aggressively bring maximum resources to the bedside of the ill child. Through comprehensive planning, optimal care can be delivered in the most timely fashion.

REFERENCES

1. Babl FE, Vinci RJ, Bauchner H, et al. Pediatric pre-hospital advanced life support care in an urban setting. Pediatr Emerg Care 2001;17:5–9.
2. Moler FW, Donaldson AE, Meert K, et al. Multicenter cohort study of out-of-hospital pediatric cardiac arrest. Crit Care Med 2011;39:141–9.

3. Moler FW, Meert K, Donaldson AE, et al. In-hospital versus out-of-hospital pediatric cardiac arrest: a multicenter cohort study. Crit Care Med 2009;37:2259–67.

4. Schindler MB, Bohn D, Cox PN, et al. Outcome of out-of-hospital cardiac or respiratory arrest in children. N Engl J Med 1996;335:1473–9.

5. Sirbaugh PE, Pepe PE, Shook JE, et al. A prospective, population-based study of the demographics, epidemiology, management, and outcome of out-of-hospital pediatric cardiopulmonary arrest. Ann Emerg Med 1999;33:174–84.

6. American Academy of Pediatrics AAP task force on infant positioning and SIDS: positioning and SIDS. Pediatrics 1992;89:1120–6.

7. Gausche M, Lewis RJ, Stratton SJ, et al. Effect of out-of-hospital pediatric endotracheal intubation on survival and neurological outcome: a controlled clinical trial. JAMA 2000;283:783–90.

8. Baum VC, O'Flaherty JE. Anesthesia for genetic, metabolic, and dysmorphic syndromes of childhood. Philadelphia: Lippincott Williams & Wilkins; 2007.

9. Silka MJ, Hardy BG, Menashe VD, et al. A population-based prospective evaluation of risk of sudden cardiac death after operation for common congenital heart disease. J Am Coll Cardiol 1998;32:245–51.

10. Woods WA, McCulloch MA. Care of the acutely ill pediatric heart transplant recipient. Pediatr Emerg Care 2007;23:721–4.

11. National Heart Lung and Blood Institute. Expert Panel report 3. Guidelines for the diagnosis and management of asthma. Available at: http://www.nhlbi.nih.gov/guidelines/asthma/asthgdln.htm. Accessed March 10, 2011.

12. Vanden Hoek TL, Morrison LJ, Shuster M, et al. Part 12: cardiac arrest in special situations: 2010 American Heart Association guidelines for cardiopulmonary resuscitation and emergency cardiovascular care. Circulation 2010;122:S829–61.

13. Ward MJ, Fentem PH, Roderick Smith WH, et al. Ipratropium bromide in acute asthma. Br Med J 1981;282:598–600.

14. Zorc JJ, Pusic MV, Ogborn J, et al. Ipratropium bromide added to asthma treatment in the pediatric emergency department. Pediatrics 1999;103:748–52.

15. Qureshi F, Pestian J, David P, et al. Effect of nebulized ipratropium on hospitalization rates of children with asthma. N Engl J Med 1998;339:1030–5.

16. Rodrigo GJ, Rodrigo C. The role of anticholinergics in acute asthma treatment: an evidence-based evaluation. Chest 2002;121:1977–87.

17. Mandelberg A, Tal G, Witzling M, et al. Nebulized 3% saline solution treatment in hospitalized infants with viral bronchiolitis. Chest 2003;123:481–7.

18. McKiernan C, Chua LC, Visintainer PF, et al. High flow nasal cannulae therapy in infants with bronchiolitis. J Pediatr 2010;156:634–8.

19. Kattwinkel J, Perlman JM, Aziz K, et al. Part 15: neonatal resuscitation: 2010 American Heart Association guidelines for cardiopulmonary resuscitation and emergency cardiovascular care. Circulation 2010;122:S909–19.

20. Kleinman ME, Chameides L, Schexnayder SM, et al. Part 14: pediatric advanced life support: 2010 American Heart Association guidelines for cardiopulmonary resuscitation and emergency cardiovascular care. Circulation 2010;122:S876–908.

21. de Caen AR, Kleinman ME, Chameides L, et al. Part 10: paediatric basic and advanced life support: 2010 international consensus on cardiopulmonary resuscitation and emergency cardiovascular care science with treatment recommendations. Resuscitation 2010;81S:e213–59.

22. Biarent D, Bingham R, Eich C, et al. European resuscitation council guidelines for resuscitation 2010: Section 6. Paediatric life support. Resuscitation 2010;81:1364–88.

23. American Academy of Pediatrics Committee on Pediatric Emergency Medicine, American College of Emergency Physicians Pediatric Committee, Emergency Nurses Association Pediatric Committee. Joint policy statement—guidelines for care of children in the emergency department. Pediatrics 2009;124: 1233–43.
24. Bhanji F, Mancini ME, Sinz E, et al. Part 16: Education, implementation, and teams: 2010 American Heart Association guidelines for cardiopulmonary resuscitation and emergency cardiovascular care. Circulation 2010;122:S920–33.
25. Brilli RJ, Gibson R, Luria JW, et al. Implementation of a medical emergency team in a large pediatric teaching hospital prevents respiratory and cardiopulmonary arrests outside the intensive care unit. Pediatr Crit Care Med 2007;8:236–46.
26. Hunt EA, Walker AR, Shaffner DH, et al. Simulation of in-hospital pediatric medical emergencies and cardiopulmonary arrests: highlighting the importance of the first 5 minutes. Pediatrics 2008;121:e34–43.
27. Skippen P, Kissoon N. Ultrasound guidance for central vascular access in the pediatric emergency department. Pediatr Emerg Care 2007;23:203–7.
28. Sagarin MJ, Chiang V, Sakles JC, et al. Rapid sequence intubation for pediatric emergency airway management. Pediatr Emerg Care 2002;18:417–23.
29. Baker TW, King W, Soto W, et al. The efficacy of pediatric advanced life support training in emergency medical service providers. Pediatr Emerg Care 2009;25: 508–12.
30. Donoghue AJ, Durbin DR, Nadel FM, et al. Effect of high-fidelity simulation on pediatric advanced support training in pediatric house staff. Pediatr Emerg Care 2009;25:139–44.
31. Nishisaki A, Keren R, Nadkarni V. Does simulation improve patient safety? self-efficacy, competence, operational performance, and patient safety. Anesthesiol Clin 2007;25:225–36.
32. Wang HE, Balasubramani GK, Cook LJ, et al. Out-of-hospital endotracheal intubation experience and patient outcomes. Ann Emerg Med 2010;55:527–37.
33. Berg MD, Schexnayder SM, Chameides L, et al. Part 13: Pediatric basic life support: 2010 American Heart Association guidelines for cardiopulmonary resuscitation and emergency cardiovascular care. Circulation 2010;122:S862–75.
34. Linkk MS, Atkins DL, Passman RS, et al. Part 6: Electrical therapies: automated external defibrillation, cardioversion, and pacing: 2010 American Heart Association guidelines for cardiopulmonary resuscitation and emergency cardiovascular care. Circulation 2010;122:S706–19.
35. Sokolove PE, Price DD, Okada P. The safety of etomidate for emergency rapid sequence intubation of pediatric patients. Pediatr Emerg Care 2000;16:18–21.
36. Zuckerbraun NS, Pitetti RD, Herr SM, et al. Use of etomidate as an induction agent for rapid sequence intubation in a pediatric emergency department. Acad Emerg Med 2006;13:602–9.
37. Jabre P, Combes X, Lapostolle F, et al. Etomidate versus ketamine for rapid sequence intubation in acutely ill patients: a multicentre randomized controlled trial. Lancet 2009;374:293–300.
38. Himmelseher S, Durieux ME. Revising a dogma: ketamine for patients with neurological injury? Anesth Analg 2005;101:524–34.
39. Bar-Joseph G, Guilburd Y, Tamir A, et al. Effectiveness of ketamine in decreasing intracranial pressure in children with intracranial hypertension. J Neurosurg Pediatr 2009;4:40–6.
40. Yehuda YB, Watemberg N. Ketamine increases opening cerebrospinal pressure in children undergoing lumbar puncture. J Child Neurol 2006;21:441–3.

41. Carroll CL, Spinella PC, Corsi JM, et al. Emergent endotracheal intubations in children: be careful if it's late when you intubate. Pediatr Crit Care Med 2010; 11:343–8.
42. Ehrlich PF, Seidman PS, Atallah O, et al. Endotracheal intubation in rural pediatric trauma patients. J Pediatr Surg 2004;39:1376–80.
43. Nishisaki A, Marwaha N, Kasinathan V, et al. Airway management in pediatric patients at referring hospitals compared to a receiving tertiary pediatric ICU. Resuscitation 2011;82:386–90.
44. Sagarin MJ, Barton ED, Chng YM, et al. Airway management by US and Canadian emergency medicine residents: a multicenter analysis of more than 6,000 endotracheal intubation attempts. Ann Emerg Med 2005;46:328–36.
45. Manthous CA. Avoiding circulatory complications during endotracheal intubation and initiation of positive pressure ventilation. J Emerg Med 2010;38:622–31.
46. Gorelick MH, Shaw KN, Murphy KO. Validity and reliability of clinical signs in the diagnosis of dehydration in children. Pediatrics 1997;99:e6.
47. Fisher JD, Nelson DG, Beyerdorf H, et al. Clinical spectrum of shock in the pediatric emergency department. Pediatr Emerg Care 2010;26:622–5.
48. Holt NF, Haspel KL. Vasopressin: a review of therapeutic applications. J Cardiothorac Vasc Anesth 2010;2:330–47.
49. Choong K, Bohn D, Fraser DD, et al. Vasopressin in pediatric vasodilatory shock: a multicenter randomized controlled trial. Am J Respir Crit Care Med 2009;180: 632–9.
50. Va Code § 32.1-283. Available at: http://leg1.state.va.us/000/cod/32.1-283.HTM. Accessed March 10, 2011.
51. Branas CC, Sing RF, Perron AD. A case series analysis of mass casualty incidents. Prehosp Emerg Care 2000;4:299–304.
52. New York City Department of Health and Mental Hygiene. Pediatric disaster toolkit: hospital guidelines for pediatrics during disasters. 2nd edition. Available at: http://www.nyc.gov/html/doh/html/bhpp/bhpp-focus-ped-toolkit.html. Accessed March 10, 2011.
53. Quan L, Cummings P. Characteristics of drowning by different age groups. Inj Prev 2003;9:163–8.
54. Rimsza ME, Schackner RA, Bowen KA, et al. Can child deaths be prevented? The Arizona child fatality review program experience. Pediatrics 2002;110:e11.
55. Posner JC, Hawkins LA, Garcia-Espana F, et al. A randomized, clinical trial of a home safety intervention based in and emergency department setting. Pediatrics 2004;113:1603–8.

Cardiac Arrest in Special Populations

Jeffrey D. Ferguson, MD, NREMT-P[a,b,*], Jocelyn De Guzman, MD[c,d]

KEYWORDS

- Cardiac arrest • Traumatic injury • Asthma • Pregnancy
- Poisoning • Toxicology • Electrical injury • Submersion injury

The following situations present unique challenges in resuscitation of the patient in cardiac arrest. Specific situations were chosen for inclusion based on their likelihood of presentation to the emergency department. These situations not only require modifications to basic adult resuscitation, they house the potential for severe time and resource use. The decision to apply these modifications to standard care for the cardiac arrest patient may be obvious in some cases or may be applied due to suspicion from the presenting medical history, history of present illness, or physical examination. Some of the therapeutic interventions discussed here are applicable to the patient in a near arrest condition and may be considered to prevent progression to cardiovascular collapse in the gravely ill patient. With rare exception, general care of any cardiac arrest patient should include continuous high-quality chest compressions and appropriate airway and ventilatory management.

TRAUMATIC INJURY

Multiple pathologies can lead to cardiac arrest in the setting of traumatic injury and may occur individually or in combination. Etiologies include: severe head injury, hypoxia (airway obstruction or disruption, pulmonary contusion, hemothorax, or pneumothorax), distributive shock (spinal cord injury), or diminished cardiac output (exsanguination, tension pneumothorax, pericardial tamponade, or myocardial contusion).

In cases of traumatic arrest where a clear etiology is not readily apparent, an Airway-Breathing-Circulation (ABC) approach to heroic interventions may be reasonable.

The authors have nothing to disclose.

[a] Department of Emergency Medicine, Brody School of Medicine, East Carolina University, 3ED-330 PCMH ED Tower, Greenville, NC 27834, USA

[b] EastCare Critical Care Transport, Pitt County Memorial Hospital, Greenville, NC, USA

[c] Department of Emergency Medicine, Brody School of Medicine, East Carolina University, Greenville, NC, USA

[d] Disaster Services, Pitt County Memorial Hospital, Greenville, NC, USA

* Corresponding author. Department of Emergency Medicine, Brody School of Medicine, East Carolina University, 3ED-330 PCMH ED Tower, Greenville, NC 27834.

E-mail address: fergusonjef@ecu.edu

Emerg Med Clin N Am 30 (2012) 169–178

doi:10.1016/j.emc.2011.09.014

0733-8627/12/$ – see front matter © 2012 Elsevier Inc. All rights reserved.

emed.theclinics.com

Unfortunately, the prognosis of out-of-hospital cardiac arrest due to trauma is poor, particularly in the setting of blunt injury. Cervical spinal immobilization should be maintained throughout resuscitation unless there is a clear mechanism of injury that excludes the potential for spinal injury.

The airway should be immediately assessed and stabilized. Conventional direct laryngoscopy and endotracheal intubation remain the standard of care for definitive airway control. Rates for successful endotracheal tube placement may be augmented with cricoid maneuvers such as Sellick; backward, upwards, rightwards pressure (BURP); or 2-handed laryngoscopy or with tube introducers like the gum elastic bougie.[1–4] Video or optical laryngoscopic modalities have shown promise for successful airway management with decreased times for tube placement and minimizing cervical spine manipulation.[1,5–7] Supraglottic blind insertion airway devices (King LT [King Systems, Noblesville, IN, USA] LMA [LMA North America, Inc, San Diego, CA, USA], and others) may also be useful in difficult airway or failed intubation.[8] These devices may also be in place as part of prehospital resuscitation efforts. In these cases, the decision to remove them and attempt endotracheal intubation should be guided by the ability to oxygenate, ventilate, and prevent aspiration. Surgical cricothyrotomy equipment should be readied at the earliest identification of a potentially difficult airway and should proceed if the previously described methods are ineffective at airway control.

Following trauma, ventilation difficulty may be the result of pneumothorax, hemothorax, or gastric distention. For patients in extremis, bilateral needle decompression or tube thoracostomies should be empirically performed. Orogastric tube placement should also be performed if gastric distention is suspected based on physical examination, poor ventilator compliance after pleural decompression, or if a history of prolonged or aggressive bag valve mask use was present before airway control.

External hemorrhage control should be performed to prevent additional volume depletion. This may occur through a combination of clamping visible vessels, tourniquet application to extremities with severe wounds, and pressure application with or without commercially available hemostatic agents. If used, nongranular, low heat-generating hemostatic products are recommended.[9,10] Large-bore peripheral venous access should be obtained with rapid infusion of 2 L of isotonic crystalloid followed by uncross-matched packed red blood cells if available. Peripheral access remains superior for infusion rates required in traumatic arrest; however, intraosseous and central lines should be placed if peripheral access is difficult to obtain. Needle pericardiocentesis may be therapeutic for pericardial tamponade; however, it will likely prove only to be a temporizing measure.

If definitive surgical intervention is readily available, a subset of patients may benefit from resuscitative thoracotomy. A proposed subset includes any witnessed post-traumatic arrest in the emergency department, arrest less than 5 minutes for penetrating cardiac injury, less than 15 minutes for penetrating thoracic injury, or any exsanguinating abdominal vascular injury where secondary signs of life are present (eg, pupillary reflexes, spontaneous movement, organized electrocardiographic (ECG) activity).[11] While these indications have not been universally accepted, subsequent literature affirms high mortality rates in patients who undergo emergency department thoracotomy, particularly for blunt trauma.[12,13] Internal cardiac massage and defibrillation, relief of pericardial tamponade, direct control of cardiac or thoracic hemorrhage, and cross-clamping of the aorta can be performed during the thoracotomy; however, these interventions require a high degree of technical skill, and should only be attempted by experienced providers.

Ventricular fibrillation (VF) and ventricular tachycardia (VT) should be defibrillated immediately upon their recognition. Advanced cardiac life support (ACLS) algorithms for these and other dysrhythmias should be considered, with the likelihood of successful chemical conversion of these being small if their underlying etiology is hypovolemia.

The use of bedside ultrasound may provide rapid diagnosis of many of the conditions discussed previously in the hands of an experienced practitioner. There is, however, no evidence to support delaying the previously described empiric interventions for ultrasonography in the setting of traumatic arrest.

ASTHMA

There were 1.75 million asthma-related emergency department visits and nearly 3500 deaths in 2007.[14] There are 2 general scenarios for which cardiac arrest can occur. The first is a severe exacerbation that progresses rapidly to arrest. The second is when a patient experiencing an exacerbation is already receiving maximal therapy and deteriorates to arrest. This section addresses the first scenario; however, therapies discussed may be applied in either situation if not already in place.

The primary therapies in treating asthma-induced arrest are aimed at overcoming hypoxia and bronchoconstriction. To that end, endotracheal intubation should be rapidly established. The largest possible endotracheal tube should be inserted to limit air flow resistance through the airway adjunct. In most adults, an 8 mm or 9 mm diameter tube can be used. Ventilation techniques should avoid breath stacking or auto-positive end-expiratory pressure (PEEP) situations caused by the prolonged expiratory phase inherent to bronchospastic conditions.[15,16] A proposed ventilatory strategy includes a tidal volume of 6 to 8 mL/kg with a slower ventilatory rate, short inspiratory times (80–100 mL/min), and inspiratory to expiratory times of 1:4 or 1:5.[17]

Nebulized beta-2 agonists can be administered continuously (albuterol 10–15 mg/h or equivalent) or intermittently (2.5–5 mg every 20 minutes) through the endotracheal tube.[18] Nebulized anticholinergic agents (ipatroprium bromide 0.5 mg) may have added benefit with albuterol, but the onset of action is delayed as much as 20 minutes.[18] Corticosteroids should be administered early; however, they have a delayed onset of action (6–12 hours) and will likely only benefit the patient if resuscitation is successful.[17]

While external compression of the thorax during the expiratory phase to maximize exhalation has been proposed, its use remains controversial and is difficult to coordinate during compressions of cardiopulmonary resuscitation (CPR).[19] Needle or tube thoracostomy decompression should be performed if pneumothorax is suspected based on worsening ventilatory compliance or lateralizing signs of chest wall movement, breath sounds, or tracheal deviation. Bilateral decompression for refractory patients is warranted given the potential for masking of these lateralizing signs.

Standard ACLS/pediatric advanced life support (PALS) algorithms apply to dysrhythmias. Epinephrine is likely to be the most useful of the standard drug therapies due to its bronchdilatory effect and should be repeated every 2 to 5 minutes. Correction of acidosis may be necessary to achieve responsiveness to sympathomimetics given the potential for severe respiratory, and later, metabolic acidosis. Empiric use of 50–100 mEq (1–2 ampules) of sodium bicarbonate, or administration guided by arterial pH less than 7.0 is appropriate. The addition of isoproterenol, aminophylline, terbutaline, or magnesium may be considered for improved bronchodilation; however their benefit in asthma-induced cardiac arrest has not been validated.

PREGNANCY

Resuscitation of the pregnant cardiac arrest victim provides added stress to the clinician due to the idea of caring for 2 patients simultaneously. Alleviation of this concern is best dealt with by accepting the conventional wisdom that the best care of the unborn fetus is optimal care for the mother.

Etiologies of cardiac arrest unique to the pregnant patient include maternal hemorrhage, preeclampsia/eclampsia, HELLP syndrome (hemolysis, elevated liver enzymes, low platelet count), amniotic fluid embolus, and adverse effects of maternal care including tocolytic and anesthetic therapies. The likelihood of some nonobstetric etiologies of cardiac arrest also increases in pregnancy including pulmonary embolus, septic shock, cardiovascular diseases such as cardiomyopathy and myocardial infarction, endocrine disorders, and collagen vascular disease. Traumatic causes of arrest should also be considered due to documented increased rates of abuse and homicide in pregnant women.[20,21]

Preparation for emergent cesarean delivery should be made as soon as cardiac arrest is identified in a pregnant patient. Deliveries performed within 5 minutes of arrest of the mother result in the highest survival rates for infants above 24 to 25 weeks gestational age.[17,22] Early delivery may also benefit the successful resuscitation of the mother. Removing the fetus allows for decompression of the inferior vena cava and abdominal aorta, allowing for improved venous return and cardiac output in the mother. Additional staff, including a neonatal intensive care team, should be available to assume care of the fetus after delivery. Obstetric or surgical consultants should be contacted for definitive management after resuscitation if not already present for the perimortem cesarean section.

Initial resuscitation efforts of the pregnant patient should focus on securing a protected airway and removal of blood flow obstruction caused by the gravid uterus. Because of anatomic and physical changes that occur during pregnancy, the likelihood of regurgitation of gastric contents is increased. Bag valve mask ventilation with supplemental oxygen is recommended before intubation attempts due to faster desaturation in pregnant patients.[23] Smaller ventilatory volumes should be used given the diaphragm elevation and increased potential for gastric insufflation due to decreased lower esophageal sphincter tone.[17,22] Endotracheal intubation should occur as soon as possible while maintaining cricoid pressure. Verification of endotracheal placement should be performed by colormetric carbon dioxide detection or waveform capnometry, as decreased lower esophageal sphincter tone may lead to erroneous results or misinterpretation of suction-based esophageal intubation detector devices.

Displacement of the gravid uterus away from the inferior vena cava and aorta likely improves hemodynamics beyond 20 weeks gestation.[22] A one or two-handed technique can be used to move the uterus toward the left upper quadrant of the abdomen. This allows the patient to remain supine for other procedures including chest compressions and intubation. Manual displacement has been shown to be superior to placing the patient in a left lateral tilt position; however, tilting the patient 30° to the left from supine using blanket rolls or a commercially available wedge should be attempted if manual displacement is not successful.[17]

Standard ACLS algorithms require no modification in the care of the pregnant patient. A theoretic need for increased dosing exists due to increased volumes of distribution and higher glomerular filtration; there is no evidence to support this, but some advocate that higher doses of medications should be considered if no response to initial dosing is seen.[24] Whenever possible, venous access and subsequent medication administration should be performed at sites above the diaphragm to avoid failure of the medication to reach central circulation due to decreased venous return.[17] Cardiac arrest occurring during magnesium infusion for treatment of preeclampsia or premature labor requires discontinuing the magnesium infusion and administering 1 g of calcium gluconate intravenously.[25]

POISONING

Cardiac arrest due to poisoning presents a complex challenge to even the most astute clinicians. Information provided from often scant history of present illness may identify toxins suspected in the poisoning, but often multiple drugs are encountered in the case of intentional overdose or an unknown agent is involved in a workplace incident or chemical exposure. In these cases, toxidromes are relied upon to determine the culprit. Masking of clinical toxidromes may be present in the setting of cardiac arrest due to prolonged hypoxia, hypoperfusion, or prehospital management (eg, dilated pupils after atropine administration or cold, wet skin after field decontamination). This may further complicate the choice of specific antidotes or therapies. Once poisoning is suspected in cardiac arrest, immediate consultation with a medical toxicologist or poison control center should occur.

Provider safety should also be a paramount consideration in chemical ingestion or exposures. Gross decontamination including removal of clothing and copious irrigation should occur before entrance to the emergency department. Exposure to ingested or inhaled chemicals may also pose a threat through exhaled air, vomitus, or fecal material.

As with all cardiac arrest patients, immediate resuscitative efforts should begin with assessment and immediate management of the ABCs. Standard ACLS/PALS protocols should be followed. Once these initial interventions have been started, the provider may then address any suspected toxidromes and consider their respective antidotes. Gastrointestinal decontamination therapies including activated charcoal administration, gastric lavage, and whole-bowel irrigation are not recommended in the setting of cardiac arrest. These interventions can, however, be considered if resuscitative efforts are successful, preferably after expert consultation. Immediate consideration for antidote therapy is appropriate in some cases where an agent exposure or ingestion is known or reasonably assumed based on the available history.

Victims in cardiac arrest from smoke inhalation or who are removed from a fire in a confined area should be treated for cyanide toxicity. Hydroxocobalamin (Cyanokit; Meridian Medical Technologies, Inc, St Louis, MO, USA) should be immediately administered (5–10 g over 15–30 min) intravenously if available.[17,26] Additionally, sodium thiosulfate administered intravenously may offer benefit over hydroxocobalamin alone.[17] If hydroxocobalamin is not available, other cyanide antidotes kits may be useful. The effectiveness of classic cyanide antidotes for smoke inhalation is limited, as amyl nitrite administration requires an inhaled route. Additionally, both amyl and sodium nitrite may result not only in hypotension, but also in functional anemia if excessive methemaglobinemia is produced in the setting of concomitant carboxyhemoglobinemia.[27]

Cholinergic agent exposure should be treated primarily with atropine sulfate. Pralidoxime chloride can also be administered for cholinergic poisonings when the offending agent is speculated to be an organophosphorous compound. Both antidotes can be found in the commercially available Mark 1 kit or other similarly packaged nerve agent antidote kit. Adequate patient decontamination and ventilation of the treatment area should be ensured to provide safety for the health care providers during resuscitation.

Opioid overdose that results in respiratory arrest may respond naloxone administration through intravenous, intramuscular, or intranasal routes. While titrated 0.4 mg doses are recommended, higher doses may be necessary if large ingestions are present or if ultrapotent opioids are involved. If a mixed ingestion has occurred or is suspected, the provider may opt for supportive care including intubation to await metabolism of the medication. In situations where cardiac arrest occurs, naloxone is unlikely to provide return of spontaneous circulation.

In contrast to opioid reversal, overdoses involving benzodiazepines should not be treated with a reversal agent such as flumazenil in the emergent setting. This therapy could theoretically precipitate seizures in chronic benzodiazepine use or mixed ingestions. Supportive measures should be the mainstay of therapy.

Antihypertensive agents including beta-blockers and calcium channel blocker overdoses may result in profound hypotension with or without bradycardia. Antidotes such as glucagon, calcium gluconate, or insulin/D50 have had some success in the symptomatic, prearrest patient.[17] There are no data to support their use in cardiac arrest; however, if they are to be successful in aiding in resuscitation, their administration should occur early in arrest rather than waiting to the end of the ACLS algorithm.

In the suspected poisoned patient, wide complex tachycardia may be secondary to conduction delays caused by myocardial sodium channel blocking agents. While unstable wide complex tachycardia should be treated with standard ACLS protocols, 1 to 2 mEq/kg of sodium bicarbonate should be considered improve cardiac function. This is particularly important in suspected poisonings when wide complex tachycardia is refractory to electrical therapy.

ELECTRICAL/LIGHTNING INJURY

As the heart is an electrically driven organ, it is particularly sensitive to electrical injury. Alternating current (AC), standard in household and commercial power supply, is reported to produce VF through a mechanism similar to the R-on-T phenomenon. Lightning is a massive direct current discharge and can produce asystole or VT by depolarizing the myocardium. In addition, secondary arrest can occur in lightning injury, as a patient's spontaneous cardiac activity may return only to suffer a secondary hypoxic arrest due to disruption of central nervous system (CNS) respiratory centers or thoracic muscle paralysis.[28]

No modifications of standard ACLS/PALS algorithms are needed in electrically induced cardiac arrest. The potential for successful resuscitation is higher than other etiologies for arrest given that the patients are typically younger and lack coexisting cardiopulmonary disease, as long as immediate treatment is available and initiated. As opposed to standard care of multiple casualty incidents, patients in respiratory and/or cardiac arrest after a lightning strike should have priority triage and treatment over those victims not in arrest.

Trauma and burn care are often required as they are common sequelae of electric shock and lightning injury. Cervical spine immobilization should be maintained during intubation and resuscitation efforts of these patients.

HYPOTHERMIA

In severe hypothermia, marked depression occurs in all critical organ systems. This may lead to cardiovascular collapse, but may also have a protective effect, allowing for successful resuscitation after prolonged arrest times. For this reason, many feel that a patient cannot be pronounced dead until rewarming has occurred and resuscitative efforts remain futile. However, clinical judgment should still prevail in the decision to attempt resuscitation. Efforts should be withheld in the presence of obvious lethal injuries, lividity, blockage of airways with ice, or if chest compressions are impossible due to advanced freezing.[17] If drowning occurs before hypothermia, chances of resuscitation are reduced. Other etiologies of injury and illness often accompany hypothermia (eg, overdose, hypoglycemia, and trauma) and should be considered and treated appropriately.

If the decision is made to attempt resuscitation, the patient should be immediately intubated and chest compressions begun. Core body temperature should be obtained as soon as possible, which will guide further resuscitation efforts. If available, needle-type electrodes are preferred for cardiac monitoring.

For severe hypothermia (core temperature <30° C), aggressive active internal rewarming should be undertaken, including warmed, humidified oxygen, warmed intravenous fluids, pleural or peritoneal lavage, and partial or complete cardiopulmonary bypass. Hypothermic myocardium may be refractory to defibrillation and ACLS medications. One attempt at defibrillation should be made for VF/VT. Further attempts at defibrillation for VF/VT refractory to the initial shock may be reasonable according to standard basic life support (BLS) algorithm concurrent with rewarming. Similarly, the current recommendation for ACLS drugs suggests it may be reasonable to administer these medications in accordance with standard ALS algorithm concurrent with rewarming.[17]

For moderate hypothermia (30–34° C) or once rewarming has raised the core temperature to 30° C, defibrillation and medication administration should occur per ACLS/PALS guidelines. At this temperature, active internal rewarming should be undertaken or continued. If hypothermia is mild (>34° C) or when rewarming raises core temperature to 34° C, standard ACLS/PALS guidelines may be applied, including decisions regarding termination of resuscitation efforts. During rewarming, intravascular volume expansion will likely be necessary secondary to vasodilation.

SUBMERSION INJURY/DROWNING

Cardiac arrest from submersion is usually due to hypoxia. This may result from suffocation, but it may also be secondary to head or spinal cord injury. For this reason, early intubation is required and should be performed with manual stabilization of the cervical spine. Aspiration of large volumes of fluid with submersion is rare, but increased inspiratory and PEEPs may be required to achieve adequate ventilation and oxygenation due to pulmonary edema or acute lung injury. The beneficial use of pulmonary surfactant has been documented in case reports of fresh water drowning and may be considered.[17]

Standard ACLS/PALS algorithms should be used for cardiac arrhythmias without modification. Electrolyte and acid–base disturbances are unlikely the etiology of cardiac arrest in early presentations of submersion injury and do not warrant empiric correction; however, this should be a consideration in patients who later deteriorate during observation. Hypothermia and trauma are common confounders of submersion injury; treatment of these issues was previously discussed.

Prognosis depends on duration of submersion and the duration and severity hypoxia. In 1 pediatric study, submersion or resuscitative efforts greater than 25 minutes and pulseless arrest on arrival to the emergency department reportedly were associated with universal mortality.[29] A second study correlated the severity of respiratory involvement with mortality, citing 93% mortality for those presenting in arrest.[30]

ELDERLY

The number of people in the United States aged 55 and older continues to rapidly rise. The US Census Bureau reported a 13% increase to 67.1 million between 2000 and 2005, more than 4 times the rate of growth (3%) of the population under 55. In accordance with that trend, the number of senior citizens, aged 65 and older, increased by a factor of 11 in the 20th century, from 3.1 million to 33.2 million. It is estimated that by the year 2030, 20% of Americans will be senior citizens. While most of the aging baby boomers live independently, a growing subset of the population is in nursing home care. Data from the US Centers for Disease Control and Prevention report approximately 1.5 million nursing home residents in over 16,000 nursing homes across the United States.

As age increases, so does the likelihood of having more than 1 disease process. Cardiac disease, cancer, and stroke remain the leading causes of death in the elderly, accounting for 70% of all deaths in this age group.[31] Debilitating conditions like stroke and dementia often leave these patients poor historians and unable to give complete medical information to the health care providers. Therefore, providers often rely on medical records, emergency medical services (EMS), and family for supplemental information. Multiple illnesses, both acute and chronic, often lead to multiple medications, resulting in polypharmacy. Special attention should be paid to the medications of this patient group during resuscitation efforts to look for contributors and possible dysrhythmia-attributing side effects.

ACLS algorithms should be initiated unless the patient has advanced directives stating contrary. Airway management should include attention to any dental apparatus, which may assist in bag valve ventilation, but should be removed before intubation. Early recognition of a potentially difficult airway is crucial in elderly patients with severe kyphosis and degenerative joint disease of the neck and torso. Despite changes in muscle mass and fat composition, along with potentially decreased glomerular filtration rates in this population, there are no current recommended medication adjustments for ACLS therapy.

Advanced directives such as a living will, do not resuscitate order, and durable power of attorney should be ascertained as soon as possible in efforts to honor the wishes of the patient. Early discussion with any available family regarding continuing versus termination of resuscitative efforts and family presence during the resuscitation should occur.

SUMMARY

In certain cardiac arrest situations, modifications to current cardiac resuscitation algorithms may improve patient outcome. These situations are often rare, but when they occur, they house the potential for severe time and resource use, and in some cases specialized skill sets. The decision to apply these modifications to standard care for the cardiac arrest patient may be obvious in some cases or may be applied due to suspicion from the presenting medical history, history of present illness, or physical examination. However, with rare exception, general care of any cardiac arrest patient should include continuous high-quality chest compressions and appropriate airway and ventilatory management.

REFERENCES

1. Lavery GG, McCloskey BV. The difficult airway in adult critical care. Crit Care Med 2008;36:2163–73.
2. Sellick BA. Cricoid pressure to control regurgitation of stomach contents during induction of anesthesia. Lancet 1961;2:404–6.
3. Marco CA, Marco AP. Airway adjuncts. Emerg Med Clin North Am 2008;26: 1015–27.
4. Levitan RM, Kinkle WC, Levin WJ, et al. Laryngeal view during laryngoscopy: a randomized trial comparing cricoid pressure, backward-upward-rightward pressure, and bimanual laryngoscopy. Ann Emerg Med 2006;47:548–55.

5. Serocki G, Bein B, Scholz J, et al. Management of the predicted difficult airway: a comparison of conventional blade laryngoscopy with video-assisted blade laryngoscopy and the GlideScope. Eur J Anaesthesiol 2010;27:24–30.

6. Byhahn C, Iber T, Zacharowski K, et al. Tracheal intubation using the mobile C-MAC video laryngoscope or direct laryngoscopy for patients with a simulated difficult airway. Minerva Anestesiol 2010;76:577–83.

7. Malik MA, Subramaniam R, Maharaj CH, et al. Randomized controlled trial of the Pentax AWS, Glidescope, and Macintosh laryngoscopes in predicted difficult intubation. Br J Anaesth 2009;103:761–8.

8. Cook TM, Hommers C. New airways for resuscitation? Resuscitation 2006;69: 371–87.

9. Littlejohn LF, Devlin JJ, Kircher SS, et al. Comparison of Celox-A, ChitoFlex, WoundStat, and combat gauze hemostatic agents versus standard gauze dressing in control of hemorrhage in a swine model of penetrating trauma. Acad Emerg Med 2011;18:340–50.

10. McManus J, Hurtado T, Pusateri A, et al. A case series describing thermal injury resulting from zeolite use for hemorrhage control in combat operations. Prehosp Emerg Care 2007;11:67–71.

11. 2005 American Heart Association guidelines for cardiopulmonary resuscitation and emergency cardiovascular care. Part 10.7: cardiac arrest associated with trauma. Circulation 2005;112:IV146–9. Available at: http://circ.ahajournals.org/content/112/24_suppl/IV-146.full.pdf+html. Accessed September 2, 2011.

12. Hunt PA, Greaves I, Owens WA. Emergency thoracotomy in thoracic trauma—a review. Injury 2006;37:1–19.

13. Committee on Trauma. Working Group, Ad Hoc Subcommittee on Outcomes, American College of Surgeons. Practice management guidelines for emergency department thoracotomy. J Am Coll Surg 2001;193:303–9.

14. Akinbami LJ, Moorman JE, Liu X. Asthma prevalence, health care use, and mortality: United States, 2005-2009. Natl Health Stat Report 2011;32:1–14.

15. Oddo M, Feihl F, Schaller MD, et al. Management of mechanical ventilation in acute severe asthma: practical aspects. Intensive Care Med 2006;32:501–10.

16. Corbridge TC, Hall JB. The assessment and management of adults with status asthmaticus. Am J Respir Crit Care Med 1995;151:1296.

17. Vanden Hoek TL, Morrison LJ, Shuster M, et al. Part 12. Cardiac arrest in special situations: 2010 American Heart Association guidelines for cardiopulmonary resuscitation and emergency cardiovascular care. Circulation 2010;122: S829–61.

18. National Asthma Education and Prevention Program. Expert Panel Report 3 (EPR-3): guidelines for the diagnosis and management of asthma—summary report 2007. J Allergy Clin Immunol 2007;120:S94–138.

19. Watts JI. Thoracic compression for asthma. Chest 1984;86:505.

20. Gazmararian JA, Lazorick S, Spitz AM, et al. Prevalence of violence against pregnant women. JAMA 1996;275:1915–20.

21. Horon IL, Cheng D. Enhanced surveillance for pregnancy-associated mortality–Maryland, 1993-1998. JAMA 2001;285:1455–9.

22. Atta E, Gardner M. Cardiopulmonary resuscitation in pregnancy. Obstet Gynecol Clin North Am 2007;34:585–97.

23. Cheun JK, Choi KT. Arterial oxygen desaturation rate following obstructive apnea in parturients. J Korean Med Sci 1992;7:6–10.

24. Whitty JE. Maternal cardiac arrest in pregnancy. Clin Obstet Gynecol 2002;45: 377–92.

25. Munro PT. Management of eclampsia in the accident and emergency department. J Accid Emerg Med 2000;17:7–11.
26. Cyanokit [package insert]. Columbia (MD): Meridian Medical Technologies Incorporated; 2011.
27. Kirk MA, Gerace R, Kulig KW. Cyanide and methemoglobin kinetics in smoke inhalation victims treated with the cyanide antidote kit. Ann Emerg Med 1993; 22:1413–8.
28. Fish RM, Geddes LA. Conduction of electrical current to and through the human body: a review. Eplasty 2009;9:e44.
29. Quan L, Kinder D. Pediatric submersions: prehospital predictors of outcome. Pediatrics 1992;90:909–13.
30. Szpilman D. Near-drowning and drowning classification: a proposal to stratify mortality based on the analysis of 1831 cases. Chest 1997;112:660–5.
31. American Geriatric Society Foundation for Health and Aging. Trends in the elderly population. Available at: http://www.healthinaging.org/agingintheknow/chapters_ch_trial.asp?ch=2. Accessed May 11, 2011.

Devices Used in Cardiac Arrest

Steven C. Brooks, MD, MHSc, FRCPC[a,b,c,]*, Alina Toma, MD, FRCPC[d,e],
Jonathan Hsu, BHSc[f]

KEYWORDS

- Cardiac arrest • Cardiopulmonary resuscitation
- Medical devices • Extracorporeal life support

High-quality cardiopulmonary resuscitation (CPR), with an emphasis on adequate compression depth, rate, and consistency, is important in optimizing vital organ perfusion and survival from cardiac arrest.[1] However, even the best-quality conventional CPR is inefficient, resulting in only 25% of normal cardiac output.[2] Over the past several decades, many therapeutic devices have been designed to improve on conventional CPR and increase the probability of survival. This article does not provide a comprehensive review of all devices proposed for this purpose, but reports on a selection of those that have received attention in the medical literature and the most recent 2010 American Heart Association (AHA) guidelines for Emergency Cardiovascular Care and CPR.[3]

This article reviews devices in two main sections. The first section describes devices that are adjuncts to conventional manual chest compressions. These devices include those that provide prompts to the rescuer to guide conventional CPR. This section

This chapter discusses the several devices that may be used in the treatment of cardiac arrest. The ResQPod, Autopulse, Zoll Pocket CPR, Q-CPR, LUCAS, Lifestat, and ECMO devices are approved for use as described in this chapter. At the time of writing, the CPRglove, Lifestick, ResQPump, and CPRmeter devices have not received FDA approval for use on patients in cardiac arrest as described in the chapter.

The authors have nothing to disclose.

[a] Division of Emergency Medicine, Department of Medicine, University of Toronto, 2075 Bayview Avenue, C7-53, Toronto, Ontario, Canada, M4N 3M5

[b] Rescu, Li Ka Shing Knowledge Institute, St Michael's Hospital, 30 Bond Street, Toronto, Ontario, Canada, M5B 1M8

[c] Program for Trauma, Emergency and Critical Care, Sunnybrook Health Sciences Centre, 2075 Bayview Avenue, Toronto, Ontario, M4N 3M5

[d] Department of Internal Medicine, Sunnybrook Health Sciences Centre, University of Toronto, 2075 Bayview Avenue, Toronto, Ontario, Canada, M4N 3M5

[e] Emergency Department, St Michael's Hospital, 30 Bond Street, Toronto, Ontario, Canada, M5B 1M8

[f] Undergraduate Medical Education Program, Faculty of Medicine, University of Toronto, Toronto, Canada

* Corresponding author. Rescu, St. Michael's Hospital, 30 Bond Street, Toronto, Ontario, M5B 1W8

E-mail address: brooksst@smh.ca

also reviews devices used to augment conventional manual chest compressions through improving the physics of the chest wall translation during the compression maneuver or improving the dynamics of the chest cavity pump through other mechanisms. The second section describes devices that have been designed to entirely replace manual chest compressions during CPR as a method of maintaining vital organ perfusion.

DEVICES USED AS ADJUNCTS TO MANUAL CHEST COMPRESSIONS
Devices Used to Prompt CPR Providers

CPR prompting devices are designed to focus the provider's attention on accepted standards of CPR quality. Prompting devices range from basic metronomes to guide the rate of chest compressions to more sophisticated accelerometer or impedance technology that can provide real-time audio and visual feedback in response to other important components of CPR quality. Prompting devices are either stand-alone or incorporated into defibrillator-monitor units. Examples of stand-alone devices are the Zoll PocketCPR (Zoll Medical Corporation Technologies, Chelmsford, MA, USA) and the CPRmeter (Laerdal Medical, Stavanger, Norway), which are puck-like devices that can be placed under the hands of the rescuer during chest compressions. These devices measure aspects of dynamic chest compression and provide audio or video feedback. Prompting devices can be used on mannequins as educational tools during CPR training or as adjuncts during actual resuscitations.

Metronomes

A metronome is a device used to mark time using an auditory or visual stimulus at regular intervals. The use of a metronome during CPR has been studied in the hospital and out-of-hospital settings. Most studies show that metronomes can improve the rate of chest compression delivery closer to recommended rates, and one study reported an associated improvement in survival.[4–6] No studies have shown harm with the use of metronomes.

Force transducers and accelerometers

Force transducers are devices that can measure the force applied to the chest wall during CPR. Accelerometers can detect movement of the chest wall. Data from these devices can be translated into audio or visual feedback on the depth, rate, consistency, and recoil of chest compressions. Supportive evidence for these devices was first reported in a case series of patients using a position-sensing arm that showed encouraging hemodynamic effects when used during in-hospital cardiac arrests. Abella and colleagues[7] showed a reduction in variability of compression rate and ventilation rate in a prospective cohort study of 156 patients using the Q-CPR system (Philips Medical, Andover, MA, USA), which uses an accelerometer for feedback on compression depth and impedance measurements across the chest for feedback on ventilation rate. A prehospital before-and-after study of 284 patients performed with a similar device found that average compression depth increased from 34 ± 9 mm to 38 ± 6 mm ($P<.001$), percent of adequate depth compressions increased from 24% to 53% ($P<.001$), and mean compression rate decreased from 121 ± 18 to 109 ± 12 ($P<.001$).[8] Survival was not significantly different between the groups, with 2.9% surviving to discharge versus 4.3% in the intervention group ($P = .2$).

Edelson and colleagues[9] also used the Q-CPR device in 224 patients and were able to show a decrease in ventilation rate (13 ± 7 vs 18 ± 8; $P<.001$) and an increase in compression depth (50 ± 10 mm vs 44 ± 10 mm; $P<.001$) when the device was used. Niles and colleagues[10] were also able to show that audiovisual feedback in a pediatric arrest population decreases the amount of detrimental leaning performed during chest compressions and therefore promotes better chest recoil. When using an accelerometer, placing a stiff backboard behind the patient experiencing cardiac arrest is important for feedback. One study showed that the feedback can be inaccurate when chest compressions are performed on soft surfaces without a backboard, resulting in delivery of chest compressions with suboptimal compression depth.[11]

Accelerometer and pressure sensing technologies have also been incorporated into novel feedback devices, such as a CPR glove and CPR board. The CPR glove (Altreo Medical, Burlington, Ontario, Canada) is designed to be worn on the hand of the provider giving chest compressions. A small visual display and built-in speaker on the back of the glove provide the user with instructions on the sequence of CPR and feedback about quality of chest compressions. No studies reporting use of the glove have been published at the time of writing. A single Chinese case report described a pressure-sensitive CPR board placed under the patient's body during CPR, which provides feedback about the quality of chest compresssions.[12] No published studies have directly compared feedback devices.

Devices Used to Augment Manual Chest Compressions

Active compression-decompression devices
Active compression-decompression devices have been designed to improve the mechanics of standard chest compressions through facilitating an exaggerated recoil phase of the chest compression cycle. For example, the CardioPump ACD-CPR Device (Advanced Circulatory Systems, Inc., Roseville, MN) uses a suction cup component that attaches to the patient's chest and allows lifting of the chest wall beyond neutral position causing active decompression (**Fig. 1**). This device also includes a force gauge to encourage adequate compression and decompression by the user. Other more simple devices, such as a modified oven mitt with Velcro, have also been developed for this purpose.[13] The intended physiologic mechanism common to all active

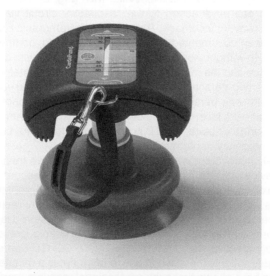

Fig. 1. The CardioPump ACD-CPR Device (Advanced Circulatory Systems, Inc., Roseville, MN, USA) is an active compression-decompression CPR device that uses a suction cup to facilitate active decompression during the recoil phase of manual chest compressions during cardiac arrest. (*Courtesy of* Advanced Circulatory Systems, Inc., Roseville, MN, USA; with permission.)

compression-decompression CPR (ACD-CPR) devices is to create a negative intrathoracic pressure and increased venous return during the active decompression phase. Several studies have shown that improved hemodynamics are possible with this technique compared with standard chest compressions.[14] Evidence for the effectiveness of these devices in humans is mixed, but no data suggest they are harmful.[15–27]

A Cochrane systematic review and meta-analysis (updated in 2010) pooled the data from 12 randomized and pseudo-randomized comparisons involving 4988 patients and found no evidence of mortality benefit with the use of ACD-CPR compared with standard manual chest compressions.[14] The recent American Heart Association (AHA) guidelines for CPR and Emergency Cardiovascular Care concluded that evidence is insufficient to recommend for or against the routine use of these devices in cardiac arrest, but suggest that these may be considered for use when providers are adequately trained and monitored.

Impedance threshold device

During the compression phase of CPR, pressure in the heart chambers and intrathoracic vascular structures increases as external pressure is applied to the chest. The pressure gradient directs blood out of the heart and to the periphery. The recoil of the chest wall during the decompression phase is equally important. The decrease in intrathoracic pressure to subatmospheric levels assists in the venous return of circulation to the heart. This phase is critical for cardiac preload and is thus essential for optimal cardiac output, blood pressure, and vital organ perfusion. However, as the intrathoracic vacuum draws blood back to the heart, it simultaneously draws air into the lungs. This influx of inspiratory gases takes away from the potential hemodynamic benefit of the decompression phase of CPR.

First described in 1995,[28] the impedance threshold device (ITD) is designed to limit this influx of air, increase the negative intrathoracic pressure, and thus enhance circulation during CPR. This device is commercially available as the ResQPOD ITD (Advanced Circulatory Systems, Inc., Roseville, MN) (**Fig. 2**). The ITD is a pressure-sensitive valve that can be attached to the respiratory circuit via an endotracheal tube, supraglottic airway, or facemask. The negative intrathoracic pressure in an intubated patient has been documented to be up to −13 mm Hg, contrasted with a pressure of only −3 mm Hg without the use of an ITD.[29] When used with a facemask, a tight seal between the face and the mask must be continuously maintained during CPR to hold the vacuum. A two-person ventilation technique can be used to maintain this continuous seal, with one person delivering ventilations and another securing the mask against the patient's face. Because of its flexibility in attachment to the respiratory circuit and its portable nature, the ITD is appropriate to use for basic life support in the field and for emergency department resuscitation.

During individual chest compressions, air is allowed to move freely out of the chest and through the device, just as during active ventilation by the rescuer. The lumen within the ITD will remain open, creating no resistance to ventilation. Spontaneous inspiration through the ITD is possible but may be difficult for a recently resuscitated patient. Thus, immediate removal of the ITD once pulse has been restored is recommended.

Besides providing augmentation of negative intrathoracic pressure during CPR decompression to increase venous return, the ResQPOD ITD comes equipped with ventilation timing assist lights that flash at a rate of 10 times a minute to prevent over-ventilation. Studies have shown that even professional rescuers responding to out-of-hospital cardiac arrests may excessively ventilate patients,[30] which can lead to decreased venous return to the heart, decreased coronary perfusion pressure, and increased intracranial pressure.

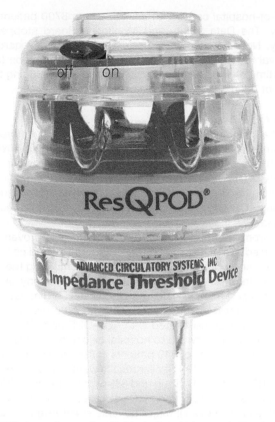

Fig. 2. The ResQPOD impedance threshold device (Advanced Circulatory Systems, Inc., Roseville, MN, USA) is used on the patient's airway to prevent passive influx of respiratory gases during the recoil phase of chest compressions and increase the negative intrathoracic pressure generated. (*Courtesy of* Advanced Circulatory Systems, Inc., Roseville, MN, USA; with permission.)

A systematic review and meta-analysis published in 2008 identified five randomized controlled trials that tested the effectiveness of the ITD in treating out-of-hospital cardiac arrests. The included studies were heterogeneous in that three of them included the use of ACD-CPR in the ITD group and two used conventional CPR. The meta-analysis of these studies found that patients in the ITD group were more likely to experience return of spontaneous circulation (relative risk,1.29; 95% CI, 1.10–1.51) and early survival, defined as survival at 24 hours or intensive care unit admission (relative risk, 1.45; 95% CI, 1.16–1.80). No evidence showed a positive effect on neurologic outcome in survivors or longer-term survival (eg, survival to hospital discharge).

The 2010 AHA guidelines suggested that an ITD may be considered as a circulatory adjunct during CPR by trained personnel in adults in cardiac arrest.[1,3] The moderate strength of recommendation (level IIb) balances the biologic plausibility for benefit with ITD use and the heterogeneous results from clinical studies. Soon after these guidelines were published, preliminary results from the Resuscitation Outcomes Consortium (ROC) PRIMED study were published in abstract form.[31] The PRIMED study was a large multicenter, double-blind, randomized, controlled trial comparing the ITD with a sham device during standard CPR for patients experiencing nontraumatic out-of-hospital cardiac arrest. More than 8700 patients were randomized in this study. The Data Safety and Monitoring Board stopped the trial early because of futility. No difference was seen between groups regarding the primary outcome of survival to discharge with a good neurologic function (modified Rankin score ≤3). At the time of writing, full analysis of the study, including that of important subgroups, had not been published.

Combined use of ACD-CPR and an ITD

Adding the use of an ITD during ACD-CPR may synergistically improve the effectiveness of chest compressions during resuscitation from cardiac arrest. In one small randomized controlled study in humans, airway pressures were not significantly reduced during ACD-CPR alone because inspiratory gases were allowed to flow into the airway during the decompression phase. When an ITD was used on an endotracheal tube during ACD-CPR, significant negative airway pressures were generated (mean, –7.3 mm Hg; SD, 4.5).[29]

Building on data from several smaller studies showing an improvement in short-term survival with combined ACD-CPR and ITD use, Aufderheide and colleagues[32] recently published a multicenter randomized controlled study comparing the use of ACD-CPR with an ITD versus standard CPR without an ITD. In this study of more than 1200 patients who experienced nontraumatic out-of-hospital cardiac arrest, the investigators showed a 53% improvement in survival to hospital discharge with favorable neurologic function in the group treated with ACD-CPR and ITD. The study showed that 47 (6%) of 813 controls survived to hospital discharge with favorable neurologic function compared with 75 (9%) of 840 patients in the intervention group (odds ratio, 1.58; 95% CI, 1.07–2.36; $P = .019$). Similar results were found when assessing 1-year survival rates, with 9% in the ACD group and 6% of the standard CPR group ($P = .03$). Both survival groups had equivalent cognitive skills, disability ratings, and emotional-psychological statuses. The overall major adverse event rate did not differ between groups, but more patients had pulmonary edema in the intervention group (94 [11%] of 840) compared with controls (62 [7%] of 813; $P = .015$).

This study was well-designed but had some limitations. The ACD-CPR device (the ResQPump) also included a pressure gauge feedback device for providers to monitor chest compression quality, and the ITD device included a metronome light to standardize ventilation rate. These two additional sources of feedback should be considered cointerventions. Furthermore, the study was stopped early because of a funding shortage, and early termination of trials can lead to inflated estimates of outcomes.[33] Lastly, the authors declared potential conflicts of interest, which include the fact that one is the coinventor of both tested devices and Chief Medical Officer of the company that sells the devices (Advance Circulatory Systems).

Despite these limitations, in the context of previous studies showing the effective generation of negative intrathoracic pressure and numerous smaller clinical studies showing a short-term survival advantage, this study supports the concept that combining ACD-CPR and ITD to augment negative intrathoracic pressure generation is a viable strategy for resuscitating patients in cardiac arrest and may be associated with improved longer-term survival with good neurologic function. Reproduction of these results in future independent studies will clarify whether this strategy should be broadly implemented.

Interposed abdominal compression devices

The Lifestick resuscitator (Datascope, Fairfield, NJ, USA) is a device that combines ACD-CPR and interposed abdominal compression techniques, which, when used in animal studies, showed an increased coronary perfusion pressure and total cerebral blood flow, higher end-tidal carbon dioxide, and better survival compared with standard CPR.[34,35] One randomized trial and one prospective study investigated outcomes with the Lifestick device in patients experiencing cardiac arrest. The randomized trial included only 50 patients and was not powered to detect differences in survival outcomes, but it did show that the device was not associated with any increase in CPR-related injuries and was well accepted by users.[36] The 2010 AHA guidelines for emergency cardiovascular care and CPR do not include a specific recommendation for the use of this type of device because there is insufficient data supporting or refuting effectiveness.[3]

Devices Used as an Alternative to Manual Chest Compressions

Mechanical chest compression devices
Traditional cardiopulmonary resuscitation for cardiac arrest victims includes the delivery of rhythmic manual chest compressions by a human rescuer. However, several types of mechanical chest compression devices using a variety of mechanisms can provide an alternative to the human chest compressor, including pneumatic vests, load-distributing bands (LDB), and pistons. The feature common to all of them is that a deforming force is applied rhythmically and automatically to the chest wall, simulating the action of manual chest compressions.

Numerous studies have shown that even well-trained, experienced rescuers tend to provide suboptimal compressions with respect to depth, rate, and consistency.[37–40] Human chest compressors are also prone to fatigue and dwindling compression quality over time.[41] In theory, mechanical chest compression devices are not susceptible to these problems. With the understanding that CPR quality and consistency are associated with patient outcomes, mechanical chest compression devices have been proposed as an alternative to imperfect manual CPR. The benefit of these devices may be their ability to provide consistent, high-quality chest compressions with minimal interruptions while liberating rescuers from this duty to tend to other tasks associated with resuscitation and transportation. Mechanical chest compression devices may be particularly useful in scenarios where a prolonged resuscitation may be necessary or where manual chest compressions may be technically difficult (eg, accidental hypothermia, toxicologic causes of cardiac arrest or intra-arrest cardiac catheterization).

Available devices use a variety of mechanisms. Several papers report on the use of a pneumatic vest to facilitate chest compression during cardiac arrest. Similar to an oversized blood pressure cuff, the pneumatic vest is placed circumferentially around the patient's thorax, and chest compression is achieved with the rapid introduction of pressurized air into and out of the vest.[42] The pneumatic vest concept has since evolved into a load-distributing band cardiopulmonary resuscitation device called the AutoPulse (Zoll Medical Corporation, Chelmsford, MA, USA) (**Fig. 3**). The commercially available AutoPulse uses a wide band of material attached to a short backboard. The band is connected to a mechanism that can shorten the band under force in a rhythmic fashion such that the band squeezes the entire chest with each cycle.

Other devices use compressed gas or an electric mechanism to drive a piston placed over the lower sternum of the patient. For example, the Life-Stat (formerly the Thumper) device (Michigan Instruments, Grand Rapids, MI, USA) is a gas-powered piston device with a built-in transport ventilator. Other piston devices, such as the Lund University Cardiac Assist System (LUCAS; Jolife AB, Lund, Sweden), incorporate a suction cup attachment for the piston to facilitate active compression-decompression CPR (**Fig. 4**).

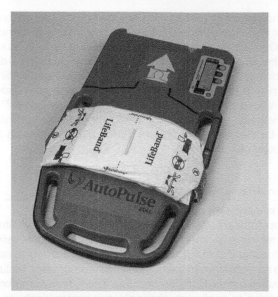

Fig. 3. The AutoPulse Non-Invasive Cardiac Support Pump (Zoll Medical Corporation, Chelmsford, MA, USA) is a mechanical CPR device that uses a load-distributing band that encircles the patient's chest and rhythmically shortens and lengthens to facilitate chest compressions. (*Courtesy of* Zoll Medical Corporation, Chelmsford, MA, USA; with permission.)

The relative effectiveness of mechanical chest compression devices as an alternative to manual chest compressions for improving clinical outcomes after cardiac arrest is not clear. Data suggesting clinical benefit with the use of mechanical chest compression devices are mostly derived from animal and human observational studies. Animal studies have shown that mechanical chest compressions can produce improved cerebral, central, and coronary blood flow[43–45] and improved survival[46,47]

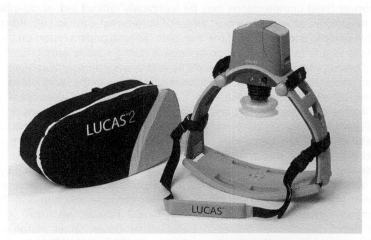

Fig. 4. The LUCAS2 (Jolife AB, Lund, Sweden) is a mechanical chest compression device that incorporates a suction cup attachment for the piston to facilitate active compression-decompression CPR. (*Courtesy of* Jolife AB, Lund, Sweden; with permission.)

compared with manual chest compressions. Several observational studies in humans have shown improved outcomes with the use of mechanical chest compression devices.[48–52] The study by Ong and colleagues[52] was a before-and-after comparison of the AutoPulse device with manual chest compressions in patients with out-of-hospital cardiac arrest treated by paramedics. When comparing 499 patients who received manual chest compressions with 284 patients who received treatment with the AutoPulse device, the authors showed an adjusted odds ratio of 2.27 (95% CI, 1.11–4.77) for survival to hospital discharge favoring the AutoPulse. They report a number-needed-to-treat of 15.

The ASPIRE trial was published in the same issue of the *Journal of the American Heart Association*. In this multicenter, cluster-randomized trial, Hallstrom and colleagues[53] studied 767 patients with out-of-hospital cardiac arrest. They compared the effectiveness of chest compressions delivered by the AutoPulse with that of standard manual chest compressions delivered during advanced life support and basic life support procedures by prehospital personnel. Clusters were based on ambulance station or group of stations, with crossover occurring at intervals ranging from 4 weeks to 2 months. The study recruited patients in five cities, and the protocol for CPR was not uniform across all sites. In fact, the CPR protocol was changed part way through the study at one site. The change involved a 2-minute delay in applying the mechanical device to the patient while paramedics administered manual CPR and a first defibrillation if needed. This change was incorporated in response to quality assurance data from the local emergency medical services system showing "prolonged time" without compressions in the load-distributing band device group. The primary outcome of this study was survival to 4 hours after the 911 call. The Data Safety and Monitoring Board stopped the trial early because of decreased survival to hospital discharge in patients who received mechanical chest compressions (9.9% in the manual CPR group vs 5.8% in the mechanical CPR group). The proportion of patients with a cerebral performance category of 1 or 2 (good neurologic function) at discharge was lower in the mechanical CPR arm of the study (3.1% in the mechanical CPR group vs 7.5% in the manual CPR group).

The results of this study, which is the largest randomized comparison to date, were unexpected. The bulk of previous animal, human physiologic, and observational clinical data had suggested benefit. Many commentators and a more recent reanalysis of the original trial data[54] suggested that the protocol change at one of the sites (resulting in a delay in the application of the device) had been responsible for the negative results. This controversy has highlighted the importance of how devices are incorporated into the sequence of CPR and the need to monitor CPR quality in both arms of the study. The risk is that the use of the devices may introduce interruptions in chest compressions or delay other interventions, such as defibrillations, which may negate any beneficial effects from the mechanical chest compressions that are ultimately provided once the device is in place.

Reflecting on these heterogeneous data, the 2010 AHA guidelines for emergency cardiovascular care and CPR[3] concluded that evidence is insufficient to recommend the routine use of mechanical CPR devices for cardiac arrest, but recommended that properly trained personnel may considered their use in specific settings of cardiac arrest. More clarity is likely to come soon from two ongoing, large, multicenter, randomized studies comparing mechanical chest compression with manual chest compressions.

The PaRAMeDIC study in the United Kingdom (trial registered at http://www.controlled-trials.com/ISRCTN08233942) plans to randomize 4200 patients with out-of-hospital cardiac arrest treated by paramedics to either chest compressions with the LUCAS device or manual chest compressions. They will measure survival to hospital discharge as the primary outcome, and a variety of neurologic and functional outcomes at short- and long-term end points as secondary outcomes. Enrollment is planned to end in 2013.

The Circulation Improving Resuscitation Care (CIRC) study is a multicenter, randomized study enrolling patients with nontraumatic out-of-hospital cardiac arrest from several locations in the United States and Europe. This study will compare the use of the AutoPulse device with manual chest compressions with respect to survival to hospital discharge and several other outcomes, including neurologic outcome. The investigators are planning to recruit 5000 patients in the study, which will be completed sometime in 2012.

The hope is that, with attention to uniform training, early application of the device into the sequence of CPR with minimal interruptions, and careful monitoring of CPR quality in both study arms, these trials will provide a definitive answer regarding the effectiveness of mechanical chest compression devices for cardiac arrest.

Extracorporeal life support

Advances in technology have enabled the rapid deployment of cardiopulmonary bypass since it was first proposed in 1966.[55] The extracorporeal membrane oxygenation (ECMO) device has shown to be effective in the neonatal population for respiratory failure[56] and congenital cardiac defects.[57] More recently, ECMO has been studied in chidren and adults with prolonged arrest after conventional measures have failed.[58–61]

A basic ECMO circuit consists of a gas-exchange device, such as an oxygenator; vascular cannulae to access and return blood; circuit tubing; a pump; and a heater-cooler that regulates blood temperature.[62] ECMO is typically a temporary means of providing oxygenation, carbon dioxide removal, and hemodynamic support to patients with cardiac or pulmonary failure. In instances of cardiac arrest, this device can buy valuable time for resolution of underlying pathophysiologic problems.

When ECMO is used on a patient, blood is removed from the venous system via a catheter, which can be attached to the right atrium. It passes through a membrane oxygenator and is delivered back to the patient's circulatory system through a catheter in the arterial system. Points of attachment can be the aorta or common carotid artery.

Besides the risk of complications, another challenge with ECMO is its deployment during ongoing conventional CPR. Interruptions in chest compressions should be minimized to facilitate favorable outcomes, including best possible coronary perfusion and chance of regaining spontaneous circulation. Thus, a rapid, simple cannulation technique is necessary. Choices for arterial cannulation include the carotid artery or femoral artery, and for venous cannulation include the internal jugular or the common femoral vein. Percutaneous cannulation of the femoral arteries during cardiac arrest has also been shown to be successful in adults.[63]

Although several observational studies and case reports have shown an association between extracorporeal life support for cardiac arrest and increased survival compared with conventional CPR,[64,65] no data are available from randomized controlled trials. The emergent, unexpected nature of cardiac arrest and the complicated nature of deploying this intervention threaten the feasibility of a randomized controlled trial. In the most recent observational report from Seoul, Korea, Shin and colleagues[65] undertook a retrospective analysis of 406 patients with in-hospital cardiac arrest. Using a propensity score–adjusted analysis, which attempted to control for prearrest conditions and CPR variables, the investigators observed that the use of ECMO in 120 adult patients who had greater than 10 minutes of CPR was associated with a reduced risk of mortality and less neurologic impairment (odds ratio, 0.17; 95% CI, 0.04–0.68).

Currently, the practical deployment considerations and high resource use will prohibit the implementation of this therapy in most centers. Data are sparse and from nonrandomized comparisons, but support the feasibility, safety, and effectiveness of extracorporeal life support. The 2010 AHA guidelines found that evidence was insufficient to recommend the routine use of extracorporeal life support but that it may be considered when it is readily available for patients who have a brief period without blood flow and when the condition leading to cardiac arrest is reversible (eg, accidental hypothermia, drug intoxication).[3]

SUMMARY

Good-quality CPR and chest compressions are essential to maximize a patient's chances of survival after cardiac arrest. Even the best manual chest compressions are inefficient at replacing normal cardiac output. This article reviewed several technologies and devices proposed to improve survival after cardiac arrest through optimizing the physics of CPR and vital organ perfusion. Despite promising results from laboratory studies or observational human studies, no single strategy or device has consistently shown improvement in survival over conventional CPR. Recent data supporting the combined use of the ITD and ACD-CPR in cardiac arrest[32] provide rationale for investigating investigating combination strategies that simultaneously use multiple devices with complimentary mechanisms to improve cardiac output during CPR.

The benefit of mechanical chest compression devices remains unclear. Evidence from randomized studies is mixed, with the largest study suggesting harm. Using these devices in cardiac arrest has the potential for delaying or interrupting good-quality manual CPR. For clinicians choosing to use any of these devices, caution and attention to overall CPR quality must be used during the deployment of devices. The answer to the long-debated question of whether human or machine provides the best life-saving chest compressions is likely to be answered shortly as two large randomized trials of mechanical chest compression close enrollment within the next 1 to 2 years. However, regardless of the results, this and other questions around the effectiveness of devices in the treatment of cardiac arrest will likely need to be readdressed continuously as technology and understanding of resuscitation advance.

REFERENCES

1. Berg RA, Hemphill R, Abella BS, et al. Part 5: adult basic life support: 2010 American Heart Association guidelines for cardiopulmonary resuscitation and emergency cardiovascular care. Circulation 2010;122(18 Suppl 3):S685–705.
2. Andreka P, Frenneaux M. Haemodynamics of cardiac arrest and resuscitation. Curr Opin Crit Care 2006;12:198–203.
3. Cave DM, Gazmuri RJ, Otto CW, et al. Part 7: CPR techniques and devices: 2010 American Heart Association guidelines for cardiopulmonary resuscitation and emergency cardiovascular care. Circulation 2010;122(18 Suppl 3):S720–8.
4. Berg RA, Sanders AB, Milander M, et al. Efficacy of audio-prompted rate guidance in improving resuscitator performance of cardiopulmonary resuscitation on children. Acad Emerg Med 1994;1(1):35–40.
5. Chiang WC, Chen WJ, Chen SY, et al. Better adherence to the guidelines during cardiopulmonary resuscitation through the provision of audio-prompts. Resuscitation 2005;64(3):297–301.
6. Fletcher D, Galloway R, Chamberlain D, et al. Basics in advanced life support: a role for download audit and metronomes. Resuscitation 2008;78(2):127–34.

7. Abella BS, Edelson DP, Kim S, et al. CPR quality improvement during in-hospital cardiac arrest using a real-time audiovisual feedback system. Resuscitation 2007;73(1):54–61.
8. Kramer-Johansen J, Myklebust H, Wik L, et al. Quality of out-of-hospital cardiopulmonary resuscitation with real time automated feedback: a prospective interventional study. Resuscitation 2006;71(3):283–92.
9. Edelson DP, Litzinger B, Arora V, et al. Improving in-hospital cardiac arrest process and outcomes with performance debriefing. Arch Intern Med 2008; 168(10):1063–9.
10. Niles D, Nysaether J, Sutton R, et al. Leaning is common during in-hospital pediatric CPR, and decreased with automated corrective feedback. Resuscitation 2009;80(5):553–7.
11. Nishisaki A, Nysaether J, Sutton R, et al. Effect of mattress deflection on CPR quality assessment for older children and adolescents. Resuscitation 2009;80(5):540–5.
12. Wang LX, Zheng JC. Message measurement and feedback cardiopulmonary resuscitation board: a monitor for standard cardiopulmonary resuscitation. Zhongguo Wei Zhong Bing Ji Jiu Yi Xue 2010;22(2):73–5 [in Chinese].
13. Udassi J, Udassi S, Lamb M, et al. Improved chest recoil using an adhesive glove device for active compression-decompression CPR in a pediatric manikin model. Resuscitation 2009;80(10):1158–63.
14. Lafuente-Lafuente C, Melero-Bascones M. Active chest compression-decompression for cardiopulmonary resuscitation. Cochrane Database Syst Rev 2004;4:CD002751.
15. Goralski M, Villéger JL, Cami G, et al. Evaluation of active compression-decompression cardiopulmonary resuscitation in out-of-hospital cardiac arrest. Reanimation Urgences 1998;7(5):543–50.
16. Mauer D, Schneider T, Dick W, et al. Active compression-decompression resuscitation: a prospective, randomized study in a two-tiered EMS system with physicians in the field. Resuscitation 1996;33(2):125–34.
17. Skogvoll E, Wik L. Active compression-decompression cardiopulmonary resuscitation: a population-based, prospective randomised clinical trial in out-of-hospital cardiac arrest. Resuscitation 1999;42(3):163–72.
18. Nolan J, Smith G, Evans R, et al. The United Kingdom pre-hospital study of active compression-decompression resuscitation. Resuscitation 1998;37(2):119–25.
19. Schwab TM, Callaham ML, Madsen CD, et al. A randomized clinical trial of active compression-decompression CPR vs standard CPR in out-of-hospital cardiac arrest in two cities. JAMA 1995;273(16):1261–8.
20. Luiz T, Ellinger K, Denz C. Active compression-decompression cardiopulmonary resuscitation does not improve survival in patients with prehospital cardiac arrest in a physician-manned emergency medical system. J Cardiothorac Vasc Anesth 1996;10(2):178–86.
21. Arai T, Adachi N, Tabo E, et al. Evaluation of efficiency of ACD-CPR and STD-CPR; a multi-institutional study. Masui 2001;50(3):307–15 [in Japanese].
22. Panzer W, Bretthauer M, Klingler H, et al. ACD versus standard CPR in a prehospital setting. Resuscitation 1996;33(2):117–24.
23. Kern KB, Figge G, Hilwig RW, et al. Active compression-decompression versus standard cardiopulmonary resuscitation in a porcine model: no improvement in outcome. Am Heart J 1996;132(6):1156–62.
24. Bertrand C, Hemery F, Carli P, et al. Constant flow insufflation of oxygen as the sole mode of ventilation during out-of-hospital cardiac arrest. Intensive Care Med 2006;32(6):843–51.

25. Plaisance P, Lurie KG, Vicaut E, et al. A comparison of standard cardiopulmonary resuscitation and active compression-decompression resuscitation for out-of-hospital cardiac arrest. French Active Compression-Decompression Cardiopulmonary Resuscitation Study Group. N Engl J Med 1999;341(8):569–75.

26. Plaisance P, Adnet F, Vicaut E, et al. Benefit of active compression-decompression cardiopulmonary resuscitation as a prehospital advanced cardiac life support. A randomized multicenter study. Circulation 1997;95(4): 955–61.

27. Shuster M, Lim SH, Deakin CD, et al. Part 7: CPR techniques and devices: 2010 international consensus on cardiopulmonary resuscitation and emergency cardiovascular care science with treatment recommendations. Circulation 2010; 122(16 Suppl 2):S338–44.

28. Lurie KG, Coffeen P, Shultz J, et al. Improving active compression-decompression cardiopulmonary resuscitation with an inspiratory impedance valve. Circulation 1995;91(6):1629–32.

29. Plaisance P, Soleil C, Lurie KG, et al. Use of an inspiratory impedance threshold device on a facemask and endotracheal tube to reduce intrathoracic pressures during the decompression phase of active compression-decompression cardiopulmonary resuscitation. Crit Care Med 2005;33(5):990–4.

30. Aufderheide TP, Sigurdsson G, Pirrallo RG, et al. Hyperventilation-induced hypotension during cardiopulmonary resuscitation. Circulation 2004;109(16): 1960–5.

31. Aufderheide T, Nichol G, Rea TD, et al. The Resuscitation Outcomes Consortium (ROC) PRIMED Impedance Threshold Device (ITD) cardiac arrest trial: a prospective, randomized, double-blind, controlled clinical trial. Circulation 2010;122(21): S2225.

32. Aufderheide TP, Frascone RJ, Wayne MA, et al. Standard cardiopulmonary resuscitation versus active compression-decompression cardiopulmonary resuscitation with augmentation of negative intrathoracic pressure for out-of-hospital cardiac arrest: a randomised trial. Lancet 2011;377(9762):301–11.

33. Bassler D, Matthias B, Montori V, et al. Stopping randomized trials early for benefit and estimation of treatment effects. JAMA 2010;303(12):1180–7.

34. Tang W, Weil MH, Schock RB, et al. Phased chest and abdominal compression-decompression. A new option for cardiopulmonary resuscitation. Circulation 1997;95(5):1335–40.

35. Wenzel V, Lindner KH, Prengel AW, et al. Effect of phased chest and abdominal compression-decompression cardiopulmonary resuscitation on myocardial and cerebral blood flow in pigs. Crit Care Med 2000;28(4):1107–12.

36. Arntz HR, Agrawal R, Richter H, et al. Phased chest and abdominal compression-decompression versus conventional cardiopulmonary resuscitation in out-of-hospital cardiac arrest. Circulation 2001;104(7):768–72.

37. Abella BS, Alvarado JP, Myklebust H, et al. Quality of cardiopulmonary resuscitation during in-hospital cardiac arrest. JAMA 2005;293(3):305–10.

38. Abella BS, Sandbo N, Vassilatos P, et al. Chest compression rates during cardiopulmonary resuscitation are suboptimal: a prospective study during in-hospital cardiac arrest. Circulation 2005;111(4):428–34.

39. Ko PC, Chen WJ, Lin CH, et al. Evaluating the quality of prehospital cardiopulmonary resuscitation by reviewing automated external defibrillator records and survival for out-of-hospital witnessed arrests. Resuscitation 2005;64(2):163–9.

40. Wik L, Kramer-Johansen J, Myklebust H, et al. Quality of cardiopulmonary resuscitation during out-of-hospital cardiac arrest. JAMA 2005;293(3):299–304.

41. Ashton A, McCluskey A, Gwinnutt C, et al. Effect of rescuer fatigue on performance of continuous external chest compressions over 3 minutes. Resuscitation 2002;55(2):151–5.
42. Halperin H, Tsitlik J, Gelfand M, et al. A preliminary study of cardiopulmonary resuscitation by circumferential compression of the chest with use of a pneumatic vest. N Engl J Med 1993;329:762–8.
43. Halperin H, Paradis N, Ornato JP. Improved hemodynamics with a novel chest compression device during a porcine model of cardiac arrest. Circulation 2002; 106:538.
44. Rubertsson S, Karlsten R. Increased cortical cerebral blood flow with LUCAS; a new device for mechanical chest compressions compared to standard external compressions during experimental cardiopulmonary resuscitation. Resuscitation 2005;65:357–63.
45. Timmerman S, Cardoso L, Ramires J. Improved hemodynamics with a novel chest compression device during treatment of in-hospital cardiac arrest. Prehosp Emerg Care 2003;7:162.
46. Ikeno F, Kaneda H, Hongo Y, et al. Augmentation of tissue perfusion by a novel compression device increases neurologically intact survival in a porcine model of prolonged cardiac arrest. Resuscitation 2006;68(1):109–18.
47. Steen S, Liao Q, Pierre L, et al. Evaluation of LUCAS, a new device for automatic mechanical compression and active decompression resuscitation. Resuscitation 2002;55(3):285–99.
48. Casner M, Andersen D, Isaacs SM. The impact of a new CPR device on rate of spontaneous circulation in out-of-hospital cardiac arrest. Prehosp Emerg Care 2005;9:61–7.
49. Steen S, Sjoberg T, Olsson P, et al. Treatment of out-of-hospital cardiac arrest with LUCAS, a new device for automatic mechanical compression and active decompression resuscitation. Resuscitation 2005;67:25–30.
50. Swanson M, Poniatowski M, O'Keefe M, et al. Effect of a CPR assist device on survival to emergency department arrival in out of hospital cardiac arrest. Circulation 2005;112(17):U1186.
51. Swanson M, Poniatowski M, O'Keefe M, et al. A CPR assist device increased emergency department admission and end tidal carbon dioxide partial pressures during treatment of out of hospital cardiac arrest. Circulation 2006;114(18):554.
52. Ong ME, Ornato JP, Edwards DP, et al. Use of an automated, load-distributing band chest compression device for out-of-hospital cardiac arrest resuscitation. JAMA 2006;295(22):2629–37.
53. Hallstrom A, Rea TD, Sayre MR, et al. Manual chest compression vs use of an automated chest compression device during resuscitation following out-of-hospital cardiac arrest: a randomized trial. JAMA 2006;295(22):2620–8.
54. Paradis N, Young G, Lemeshow S, et al. Inhomogeneity and temporal effects in AutoPulse Assisted Prehospital International Resuscitation—an exception from consent trial terminated early. Am J Emerg Med 2010;28:391–8.
55. Sawa Y. Percutaneous extracorporeal cardiopulmonary support: current practice and its role. J Artif Organs 2005;8(4):217–21.
56. Mugford M, Elbourne D, Field D. Extracorporeal membrane oxygenation for severe respiratory failure in newborn infants. Cochrane Database Syst Rev 2008;3:CD001340.
57. Aharon AS, Drinkwater DC Jr, Churchwell KB, et al. Extracorporeal membrane oxygenation in children after repair of congenital cardiac lesions. Ann Thorac Surg 2001;72(6):2095–102.

58. Chen YS, Chao A, Yu HY, et al. Analysis and results of prolonged resuscitation in cardiac arrest patients rescued by extracorporeal membrane oxygenation. J Am Coll Cardiol 2003;41(2):197–203.
59. del Nido PJ. Extracorporeal membrane oxygenation for cardiac support in children. Ann Thorac Surg 1996;61(1):336–9.
60. Duncan BW, Ibrahim AE, Hraska V, et al. Use of rapid-deployment extracorporeal membrane oxygenation for the resuscitation of pediatric patients with heart disease after cardiac arrest. J Thorac Cardiovasc Surg 1998;116(2):305–9.
61. Ghez O, Feier H, Ughetto F, et al. Postoperative extracorporeal life support in pediatric cardiac surgery: recent results. ASAIO J 2005;51(5):513–6.
62. Royston D. Techniques in extracorporeal circulation. In: Kay PH, Munsch CM, editors. 4th edition. London: Arnold; 2004. p. 354.
63. Schwarz B, Mair P, Margreiter J, et al. Experience with percutaneous venoarterial cardiopulmonary bypass for emergency circulatory support. Crit Care Med 2003; 31(3):758–64.
64. Chen YS, Lin JW, Yu HY, et al. Cardiopulmonary resuscitation with assisted extra-corporeal life-support versus conventional cardiopulmonary resuscitation in adults with in-hospital cardiac arrest: an observational study and propensity analysis. Lancet 2008;372(9638):554–61.
65. Shin TG, Choi JH, Jo IJ, et al. Extracorporeal cardiopulmonary resuscitation in patients with inhospital cardiac arrest: a comparison with conventional cardiopulmonary resuscitation. Crit Care Med 2011;39(1):1–7.

Index

Note: Page numbers of article titles are in **boldface** type.

Emerg Med Clin N Am 30 (2012) 195–201
doi:10.1016/S0733-8627(11)00130-1
0733-8627/12/$ – see front matter © 2012 Elsevier Inc. All rights reserved.

emed.theclinics.com

EmergencyMed **Advance**

All the latest emergency medicine news and research you need, all in one place

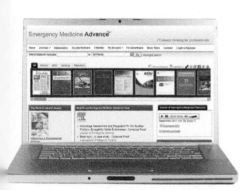

EmergencyMedAdvance.com is a new essential online resource offering valued high-quality content and news for the global community of Emergency Medicine professionals to save time and stay current—from physicians and nurses to EMTs.

Stay current
- Emergency Medicine news
- Upcoming meetings and events

Save time
- Access relevant articles in press from 16 participating journals
- Search across 500+ health sciences journals
- Learn how to submit a manuscript

And more...
- Journals' profiles
- Personalized search results
- Emergency Medicine bookstore
- Sign up for free e-Alerts
- Emergency Medicine jobs

**Bookmark us today at
EmergencyMedAdvance.com**

Printed and bound by CPI Group (UK) Ltd, Croydon, CR0 4YY

03/10/2024

01040457-0004

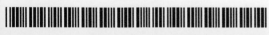